Donald Dutton, PhD
Daniel J. Sonkin, PhD
Editors

D0140287

Intimate Violence: Contemporary Treatment Innovations

Intimate Violence: Contemporary Treatment Innovations has been co-published simultaneously as *Journal of Aggression, Maltreatment & Trauma*, Volume 7, Numbers 1/2 (#13/14) 2003.

Pre-publication REVIEWS, COMMENTARIES, EVALUATIONS . . .

"**E**XCELLENT. . . . Represents 'outside the box' thinking. I HIGHLY RECOMMEND THIS BOOK for everyone working in the field of domestic violence who wants to stay fresh. Readers will be stimulated and in most cases very valuably informed."

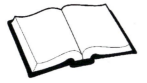

David B. Wexler, PhD
Executive Director
Relationship Training Institute
San Diego, California

More Pre-publication
REVIEWS, COMMENTARIES, EVALUATIONS . . .

" **A** LANDMARK BOOK that presents cutting-edge alternatives to the mainstream for treating men who batter. . . . ANY SERIOUS CLINICIAN OR STUDENT of abuse abatement treatment SHOULD HAVE THIS BOOK IN THEIR LIBRARY. . . . Challenges mainstream views about why men batter and how to get them to stop. . . . Represents the leading edge of the next wave for efforts to end intimate partner violence."

L. Kevin Hamberger, PhD
Professor
Department of Family & Community Medicine
Medical College of Wisconsin

HMTP
Haworth Maltreatment and Trauma Press

Intimate Violence: Contemporary Treatment Innovations

Intimate Violence: Contemporary Treatment Innovations has been co-published simultaneously as *Journal of Aggression, Maltreatment & Trauma*, Volume 7, Numbers 1/2 (#13/14) 2003.

The *Journal of Aggression, Maltreatment & Trauma* Monographic "Separates"

Robert Geffner, PhD, Senior Editor

Below is a list of "separates," which in serials librarianship means a special issue simultaneously published as a special journal issue or double-issue *and* as a "separate" hardbound monograph. (This is a format which we also call a "DocuSerial.")

"Separates" are published because specialized libraries or professionals may wish to purchase a specific thematic issue by itself in a format which can be separately cataloged and shelved, as opposed to purchasing the journal on an on-going basis. Faculty members may also more easily consider a "separate" for classroom adoption.

"Separates" are carefully classified separately with the major book jobbers so that the journal tie-in can be noted on new book order slips to avoid duplicate purchasing.

You may wish to visit Haworth's Website at . . .

http://www.HaworthPress.com

. . . to search our online catalog for complete tables of contents of these separates and related publications.

You may also call 1-800-HAWORTH (outside US/Canada: 607-722-5857), or Fax 1-800-895-0582 (outside US/Canada: 607-771-0012), or e-mail at:

docdelivery@haworthpress.com

Sexual Abuse Litigation: A Practical Resource for Attorneys, Clinicians, and Advocates, edited by Rebecca Rix, MALS (Vol. 3, No. 2 [#6], 2000). *"An interesting and well developed treatment of the complex subject of child sexual abuse trauma. The merger of the legal, psychological, scientific and historical expertise of the authors provides a unique, in-depth analysis of delayed discovery in CSA litigation. This book, including the extremely useful appendices, is a must for the attorney or expert witness who is involved in the representation of survivors of sexual abuse." (Leonard Karp, JD, and Cheryl L. Karp, PhD, co-authors, Domestic Torts: Family Violence, Conflict and Sexual Abuse)*

Children Exposed to Domestic Violence: Current Issues in Research, Intervention, Prevention, and Policy Development, edited by Robert A. Geffner, PhD, Peter G. Jaffe, PhD, and Marlies Sudermann, PhD (Vol. 3, No. 1 [#5], 2000). *"A welcome addition to the resource library of every professional whose career encompasses issues of children's mental health, well-being, and best interest . . . I strongly recommend this helpful and stimulating text." (The Honorable Justice Grant A. Campbell, Justice of the Ontario Superior Court of Justice, Family Court, London, Canada)*

Maltreatment in Early Childhood: Tools for Research-Based Intervention, edited by Kathleen Coulborn Faller, PhD (Vol. 2, No. 2 [#4], 1999). *"This important book takes an international and cross-cultural look at child abuse and maltreatment. Discussing the history of abuse in the United States, exploring psychological trauma, and containing interviews with sexual abuse victims, Maltreatment in Early Childhood provides counselors and mental health practitioners with research that may help prevent child abuse or reveal the mistreatment some children endure."*

Multiple Victimization of Children: Conceptual, Developmental, Research, and Treatment Issues, edited by B. B. Robbie Rossman, PhD, and Mindy S. Rosenberg, PhD (Vol. 2, No. 1 [#3], 1998). *"This book takes on a large challenge and meets it with stunning success. It fills a glaring gap in the literature . . . " (Edward P. Mulvey, PhD, Associate Professor of Child Psychiatry, Western Psychiatric Institute and Clinic, University of Pittsburgh School of Medicine)*

Violence Issues for Health Care Educators and Providers, edited by L. Kevin Hamberger, PhD, Sandra K. Burge, PhD, Antonnette V. Graham, PhD, and Anthony J. Costa, MD (Vol. 1, No. 2 [#2], 1997). *"A superb book that contains invaluable hands-on advice for medical educators and health care professionals alike . . ." (Richard L. Holloways, PhD, Professor and Vice Chair, Department of Family and Community Medicine, and Associate Dean for Student Affairs, Medical College of Wisconsin)*

Violence and Sexual Abuse at Home: Current Issues in Spousal Battering and Child Maltreatment, edited by Robert Geffner, PhD, Susan B. Sorenson, PhD, and Paula K. Lundberg-Love, PhD (Vol. 1, No. 1 [#1], 1997). *"The Editors have distilled the important questions at the cutting edge of the field of violence studies, and have brought rigor, balance and moral fortitude to the search for answers." (Virginia Goldner, PhD, Co-Director, Gender and Violence Project, Senior Faculty, Ackerman Institute for Family Therapy)*

Published by

The Haworth Maltreatment & Trauma Press, 10 Alice Street, Binghamton, NY 13904-1580 USA

The Haworth Maltreatment & Trauma Press is an imprint of The Haworth Press, Inc., 10 Alice Street, Binghamton, NY 13904-1580 USA.

Intimate Violence: Contemporary Treatment Innovations has been co-published simultaneously as *Journal of Aggression, Maltreatment & Trauma*, Volume 7, Numbers 1/2 (#13/14) 2003.

© 2002 by The Haworth Press, Inc. All rights reserved. No part of this work may be reproduced or utilized in any form or by any means, electronic or mechanical, including photocopying, microfilm and recording, or by any information storage and retrieval system, without permission in writing from the publisher. Printed in the United States of America.   Reprint 2006

The development, preparation, and publication of this work has been undertaken with great care. However, the publisher, employees, editors, and agents of The Haworth Press and all imprints of The Haworth Press, Inc., including The Haworth Medical Press® and The Pharmaceutical Products Press®, are not responsible for any errors contained herein or for consequences that may ensue from use of materials or information contained in this work. Opinions expressed by the author(s) are not necessarily those of The Haworth Press, Inc.

Cover design by Lora Wiggins

Library of Congress Cataloging-in-Publication Data

Intimate violence: contemporary treatment innovations /Donald Dutton, Daniel J. Sonkin, editors.
        p. cm.
"Intimate Violence: Contemporary Treatment Innovations has been co-published simultaneously as Journal of Aggression, Maltreatment & Trauma, Volume 7, Numbers 1/2 (#13/14) 2003."
        ISBN 0-7890-2018-1 (hard cover : alk. paper)–ISBN 0-7890-2019-X (soft cover.: alk. paper)
        1. Family violence–Treatment. 2. Victims of family violence–Rehabilitation. I. Dutton, Donald G., 1943- II. Sonkin, Daniel Jay. III. Journal of aggression, maltreatment & trauma.
RC569.5.F3I58 2003
616.85'822–dc21   2003005333

Intimate Violence: Contemporary Treatment Innovations

Donald Dutton, PhD
Daniel J. Sonkin, PhD
Editors

Intimate Violence: Contemporary Treatment Innovations has been co-published simultaneously as *Journal of Aggression, Maltreatment & Trauma*, Volume 7, Numbers 1/2 (#13/14) 2003.

HMTP

The Haworth Maltreatment & Trauma Press
An Imprint of
The Haworth Press, Inc.
New York • London • Oxford

Indexing, Abstracting & Website/Internet Coverage

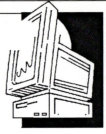

This section provides you with a list of major indexing & abstracting services. That is to say, each service began covering this periodical during the year noted in the right column. Most Websites which are listed below have indicated that they will either post, disseminate, compile, archive, cite or alert their own Website users with research-based content from this work. (This list is as current as the copyright date of this publication.)

Abstracting, Website/Indexing Coverage . . . . Year When Coverage Began

- *Cambridge Scientific Abstracts (Risk Abstracts) <www.csa.com>* 1997

- *caredata CD: the social & community care database*
  <www.scie.org.uk> 1998

- *Child Development Abstracts & Bibliography*
  (in print and online) <www.ukans.edu> 1997

- *CINAHL (Cumulative Index to Nursing & Allied Health Literature),*
  in print, EBSCO, and SilverPlatter, Data-Star, and PaperChase.
  (Support materials include Subject Heading List, Database Search
  Guide, and instructional video) <www.cinahl.com>. 2000

- *CNPIEC Reference Guide: Chinese National Directory*
  of Foreign Periodicals 1997

- *Criminal Justice Abstracts* 1997

- *Educational Administration Abstracts (EAA)* 2001

- *EMBASE/Excerpta Medica Secondary Publishing Division*
  Included in newsletters, review journals, major reference works,
  magazines & abstract journals <URL: http://www.elsevier.nl> . . . 1999

- *e-psyche, LLC <www.e-psyche.net>*. 2001

(continued)

(continued)

Special Bibliographic Notes related to special journal issues (separates) and indexing/abstracting:

- indexing/abstracting services in this list will also cover material in any "separate" that is co-published simultaneously with Haworth's special thematic journal issue or DocuSerial. Indexing/abstracting usually covers material at the article/chapter level.
- monographic co-editions are intended for either non-subscribers or libraries which intend to purchase a second copy for their circulating collections.
- monographic co-editions are reported to all jobbers/wholesalers/approval plans. The source journal is listed as the "series" to assist the prevention of duplicate purchasing in the same manner utilized for books-in-series.
- to facilitate user/access services all indexing/abstracting services are encouraged to utilize the co-indexing entry note indicated at the bottom of the first page of each article/chapter/contribution.
- this is intended to assist a library user of any reference tool (whether print, electronic, online, or CD-ROM) to locate the monographic version if the library has purchased this version but not a subscription to the source journal.
- individual articles/chapters in any Haworth publication are also available through the Haworth Document Delivery Service (HDDS).

Dedicated to the professionals engaged in the daunting and sometimes rewarding task of working with abuse perpetrators.

ALL HAWORTH MALTREATMENT &
TRAUMA PRESS BOOKS
AND JOURNALS ARE PRINTED
ON CERTIFIED ACID-FREE PAPER

Intimate Violence: Contemporary Treatment Innovations

CONTENTS

TREATMENT OF SPECIAL POPULATIONS

SPECIAL ISSUES IN THE TREATMENT OF INTIMATE VIOLENCE PERPETRATORS

ABOUT THE EDITORS

Donald Dutton, PhD, received his PhD in Psychology from the University of Toronto in 1970. In 1974, while on faculty at the University of British Columbia, he began to investigate the criminal justice response to wife assault, preparing a government report that outlined the need for a more aggressive response, and subsequently training police in "domestic disturbance" intervention techniques. After receiving training as a group therapist at Cold Mountain Institute, he co-founded the Assaultive Husbands Project in 1979, a court mandated treatment program for men convicted of wife assault. During the fifteen years he spent providing therapy for these men, he drew on his background in both social and clinical psychology to develop a psychological model for perpetrators of intimate abuse. This model views intimate abusiveness as emanating from a trauma triad and comprised of witnessing abuse, being shamed and experiencing insecure attachment. He has published over 100 papers and three books, including *Domestic Assault of Women* (1995), *The Batterer: A Psychological Profile* (1995) and *The Abusive Personality* (1998). *The Batterer* has been translated into French, Spanish, Dutch and Polish and Dutton has provided numerous workshops to professionals based on this work, including talks at the Sorbonne in Paris, Washington, D.C. and New York City. Dutton frequently serves as an expert witness in civil trials involving domestic abuse and in criminal trials involving family violence, including his work for the prosecution in the O.J. Simpson trial (1995). The latter led to an interest in spousal homicide and to "abandonment killing." He is currently Professor of Psychology at the University of British Columbia, Vancouver, BC, Canada.

Daniel J. Sonkin, PhD, is a Licensed Marriage and Family Therapist in an independent practice in Sausalito, California. His work focuses on the treatment of individuals and couples facing a variety of psychological problems including domestic violence and child abuse. In addition to his clinical experience, he has testified as an expert witness in criminal cases where domestic violence is an issue. He has also evaluated defendants facing the death penalty conducting social histories with a focus on their childhood abuse and its impact on adult criminal behavior. He has also testified as an expert witness in malpractice cases and licensing actions. As one of the early investigators and specialists in the field of family violence, he has developed a widely used protocol for treating male batterers. He is the author of numerous articles and books on domestic violence and child abuse including: *Learning to Live Without Violence: A Handbook for Men*; *The Male Batterer: A Treatment Approach*; *Domestic Violence on Trial: Psychological and Legal Dimensions of Family Violence*; *Wounded Boys/Heroic Men: A Man's Guide to Recovering from Childhood Abuse*; *The JurisMonitor Stabilization Program for Stalkers*; *A Counselors Guide to Learning to Live Without Violence*; and *Domestic Violence: The Court-Mandated Perpetrator Assessment and Treatment Handbook*. He has written software for assessing perpetrators of violence for both Macintosh and IBM compatible computers. He has conducted trainings nationally and internationally for mental health professionals on the treatment of male batterers. He is a former chair of the state ethics committee of the California Association of Marriage and Family Therapists and a former member of the Board of Directors for that organization. In addition to his clinical practice, he is an adjunct faculty in the Department of Counseling at Sonoma State University. Dr. Sonkin provides consultation, training and supervision in his unique model outlined in his books to individuals and agencies providing services to male batterers and their families.

ABOUT THE CONTRIBUTORS

Ibrahim Agabaria, BA, obtained a bachelor's degree in social work from Haifa University, and is a social worker at Beit Noam.

Beni Beili, BA, received a bachelor's degree in social work from Tel-Aviv University and is currently in private practice.

Rosemary Cogan, PhD, ABPP, is Professor of Psychology at Texas Tech University, Lubbock, Texas. She is a Diplomat in Clinical Psychology, American Board of Professional Psychology, a graduate of the Dallas Psychoanalytic Institute, and Certified in Psychoanalysis, American Psychoanalytic Association.

Vallerie E. Coleman, PhD, is a clinical psychologist and psychoanalyst in private practice in Santa Monica, CA. She is on faculty at the Newport Psychoanalytic Institute and Loyola Marymount. In addition to her clinical work, Dr. Coleman has provided expert witness testimony, conducted research, and led numerous workshops on lesbian battering.

Lynn Dowd, PsyD, is a clinical psychologist who provides treatment for adolescents and adults in the Ambulatory Psychiatry Clinic at University of Massachusetts Memorial Health Care. She designed the group treatment format for the Women's Anger Management Program at UMMHC, and has led groups and conducted research on partner aggressive women since 1996. Other treatment and research interests include trauma, mood disorders, substance abuse, and developmental issues related to women's aggression.

Albert J. Grudzinskas, Jr., JD, received his undergraduate degree at Northeastern University and his law degree at Syracuse University. After 12 years of private legal practice Attorney Grudzinskas served as Assistant General Counsel to the Department of Mental Health of the Commonwealth of Massachusetts for eight years. Currently Attorney Grudzinskas is Assistant Professor of Psychiatry in Law at the University of Massachusetts Medical School and Coordinator of Legal Studies in the Law and Psychiatry Program. Attorney Grudzinskas is active in the National Association of Counsel for Children and the American Academy of Psychiatry and the Law having contributed to the APPL Journal, served as a member of the Journal's Editorial Board and presented at national conferences. Attorney Grudzinskas consults widely to state governments and court systems. He lectures frequently on such topics as police training for encounters with persons in crisis, involuntary outpatient commitment, diminished capacity, substance abuse, the presentation of expert testimony, and trial tactics.

Richard E. Heyman, PhD, is Research Associate Professor in the Department of Psychology at the State University of New York at Stony Brook. Dr. Heyman's research on assessing and treating families and on the risk factors and causes of family maltreatment is internationally known. He is the author of over 50 publications in scientific journals and scientific books. His research has been funded by the National Institute of Mental Health, the Centers for Disease Control, the U.S. Army and the U.S. Air Force. Dr. Heyman is a licensed clinical psychologist and maintains a private practice in Stony Brook, NY.

Ophra Keynan, BA, received a bachelor's degree in social work from Tel-Aviv University, and is the Chairperson of the Noam association.

Robert Kiyoshk, MA, is of Anishinabe (Ojibway) ancestry, and lives in Vancouver, British Columbia. His family is involved in the ceremonial life and culture of the Eagle Sundance Society, where he is member of the Red Blanket Society. He served two terms as a director of the BC Association of Counsellors of Abusive Men, and founded the Change of Seasons Society, a program that provides free counselling to First Nations men who abuse their partners/spouses. He is President of the Warriors Against Violence Society, an agency that also provides free counselling to Aboriginal men, women and children. He holds a Bachelor's degree in Law and Justice, and a Master's degree in Management and Leadership. He has published numerous articles, and recently completed a review of Aboriginal Family Violence for the Aboriginal Nurses Association of Canada and the Royal Canadian Mounted Police.

Penny A. Leisring, PhD, is currently Assistant Professor of Psychology at Quinnipiac University in Hamden, CT. She received her PhD in Clinical Psychology from the State University of New York at Stony Brook in 1999. Her clinical interests focus on the prevention and reduction of aggressive behavior in adults and children. She conducts research examining male- and female-perpetrated relationship aggression, parental discipline styles, and child behavior problems.

Shlomit Levin, BA, received a bachelor's degree in social work from Tel-Aviv University, and is currently in private practice.

Ariel Mor, BA, received a bachelor's degree in education from Beit-Berl College.

Michal Nir, MSW, received a master's degree in social work from Tel-Aviv University, and is currently a family and sexual therapist in private practice.

John H. Porcerelli, PhD, ABPP, is Associate Professor, Department of Family Medicine, Wayne State University School of Medicine, Detroit, Michigan. He is a Diplomat in Clinical Psychology, American Board of Professional Psychology, and a graduate of the Michigan Psychoanalytic Institute.

Alan Rosenbaum, PhD, is Professor in the Department of Psychology at Northern Illinois University and the Center for the Study of Family Violence and Sexual Assault. He founded the Marital Research and Treatment Program at the University of Massachusetts Medical School and served as its director for sixteen years. This program included the Men's Educational Workshop, one of the largest university based batterers' treatment programs in the U.S., as well as anger management programs for men, women, and adolescents. Research interests include outcome evaluation of batterers' treatment, the etiology of intimate partner aggression, female aggression, and the contributions of biological factors to domestic violence.

Hannah Rosenberg, MSW, received her degree from Bar-Ilan University. She is Executive director of the Noam association.

Mindy S. Rosenberg, PhD, is a clinical and community psychologist in private practice in Sausalito, California. She is a consultant to a domestic violence unit of a probation department in Northern California and has been on the faculty of several psychology departments. Her research and clinical interests are in child and adolescent maltreatment, children of battered women, forensic issues, neuropsychological evaluation, and post-intervention outcome for men and women arrested for domestic violence. Dr. Rosenberg has published numerous articles and chapters on these subjects, including three books: *Prevention of Child Maltreatment: Developmental and Ecological Perspectives* (with D. J. Willis and E. E. Holden), *Multiple Victimization of Children: Conceptual, Developmental, Research and Treatment Issues* (with B. B. R. Rossman), and *Children and Interparental Violence: The Impact of Exposure* (with B. B. R. Rossman and H. M. Hughes).

Karin Schlee, PhD, was trained in the research and treatment of domestic violence and intimate partner violence at the State University of New York at Stony Brook. She received experience working with various traumatized populations working at the National Crime Victims Research and Treatment Center, the Medical University of South Carolina, and the Ralph H. Johnson Veterans Administration Medical Center in Charleston. She is now a licensed psychologist in New York who shares a private practice and serves as a consultant psychologist.

Avi Tefelin, BA, received a bachelor's degree in social work from Tel-Aviv University, and is currently in private practice.

Robert Wallace, MA, MSW, CSW, and **Anna Nosko, MSW,** both social workers, co-led abuser groups at The Family Service Association of Toronto for over ten years. Their treatment model, which borrowed from Social Group Work Theory, Affect Theory and Attachment Theory, provided the basis for several articles and conference presentations throughout North America. They also participated in research evaluating the efficacy of this approach. Most recently, they have continued to work together in training and consulting with clinicians involved in the delivery of group services to those experiencing HIV and depression.

Jennifer Waltz, PhD, is Associate Professor of Psychology at the University of Montana. She has ten years of experience providing training in Dialectical Behavior Therapy. In addition, she conducts research on the impact of psychological trauma.

William J. Warnken, PsyD, is Assistant Professor of Psychiatry at the University of Massachusetts Medical School, where he is also on the faculty of the Law and Psychiatry Program. Dr. Warnken is the Director of

Psychology Training at the University of Massachusetts Medical School and is the Coordinator of Forensic Service at Worcester State Hospital. He is a diplomate with the American Board of Forensic Psychology. He has presented nationally on such topics as risk assessment and training of forensic psychologists. He has authored and coauthored articles and book chapters on issues related to domestic violence.

Preface

It is with pleasure that we publish this innovative volume, edited by Donald Dutton and Daniel J. Sonkin. For too long, there has been an emphasis on treating domestic violence offenders with a unilateral psychoeducational approach. Even though many researchers and practitioners have been stating for a decade that we need alternative approaches for treatment that are based upon the specific characteristics of the offenders, policies and standards in many states of the United States, in the provinces of Canada, and in other countries have not followed this. In addition, many of those working with victims or offenders have not wanted to consider that alternative treatment modalities might be more effective with certain clients, or to acknowledge that special populations might also need different approaches. This volume not only addresses these issues, it presents innovative approaches by those who have worked in the field of family violence for many years.

This volume provides current information on various techniques for working with both males and females who commit intimate partner abuse. Recent research and approaches have begun to focus on a few key issues as important for long-term success in the treatment of offenders. Two major ones are shame and attachment. It is important to be open to approaches in which these key issues are explored in treatment since they had not been emphasized in many more traditional approaches. It is time that we focus more on alternative approaches that may be effective with certain populations, that we not assume that all offenders are the same, that we move away from a "one size fits all" mentality, and that we begin to emphasize the importance of treatment

[Haworth co-indexing entry note]: "Preface." Geffner, Robert. Co-published simultaneously in *Journal of Agression Maltreatment & Trauma* (The Haworth Maltreatment & Trauma Press, an imprint of The Haworth Press, Inc.) Vol. 7, No. 1/2 (#13/14), 2003, pp. xxvii-xxviii; and: *Intimate Violence: Multidimensional Psychotherapeutic Perspectives in Treatment* (ed: Donald Dutton, and Daniel J. Sonkin) The Haworth Maltreatment & Trauma Press, an imprint of The Haworth Press, Inc., 2003, pp. xxiii-xxiv. Single or multiple copies of this article are available for a fee from The Haworth Document Delivery Service [1-800-HAWORTH, 9:00 a.m. - 5:00 p.m. (EST). E-mail address: docdelivery@haworthpress.com].

http://www.haworthpress.com/store/product.asp?sku=J146
© 2003 by The Haworth Press, Inc. All rights reserved. *xxiii*

being based upon an assessment and tailored to the individual needs so that long term changes in attitudes, beliefs, and behaviors can be achieved. Outcome research to verify the effectiveness of the various approaches is needed as well. This volume is an important step in the right direction to meet these needs, and it adds to the prior volumes published in this series to help all of us think and operate "out of the box" when we work with offenders and/or their partners to eliminate such family violence. I am proud that we are able to offer this volume in the effort to move the field forward.

Robert Geffner, PhD
Senior Editor
Journal of Aggression, Maltreatment & Trauma

Acknowledgments

We would like to thank Dr. Robert Geffner for his dedication to the field of domestic violence and child abuse. His vigorous energy for quality publications has helped to create a highly respected series of journals and books that have been a valuable asset to researchers and clinicians alike. We would especially like to thank Ms. Jennifer Zellner, our editor at the Family Violence and Sexual Assualt Institute Journals Department. Through her expertise on the written language, and sensitivity to the sometimes tempermental writer's nature, she has helped to bring this project from rough manuscript to coherent book so that each author can be proud to have been a contributor. Lastly, we would acknowledge all the authors for their innovative contributions to the field of domestic violence. It takes a lot of courage to stand apart from the crowd, especially when the subject matter itself is likely to generate intense controversy. We thank you for your creativity and willingness to express your ideas no matter how much they diverge from the party line. Because you thought outside the box, we are hoping that it will inspire our readers to do the same.

Introduction:
Perspectives on the Treatment
of Intimate Violence

Donald Dutton
Daniel J. Sonkin

SUMMARY. The authors describe the rationale for a publication that explores new and innovative approaches to treating domestic violence perpetrators. A brief history is also presented on perpetrator treatment, the feminist perspectives on treatment and how recent research findings suggest that perpetrators of domestic violence need more than education and attitude adjustment. *[Article copies available for a fee from The Haworth Document Delivery Service: 1-800-HAWORTH. E-mail address: <docdelivery@haworthpress.com> Website: <http://www.HaworthPress.com> © 2003 by The Haworth Press, Inc. All rights reserved.]*

KEYWORDS. Domestic violence, perpetrators, treatment

Treatment for men who assault their wives began in the late 1970s, pioneered by Anne Ganley at the Veteran's Administration Center in Tacoma, Washington. Dr. Ganley developed a cognitive-behavioral

[Haworth co-indexing entry note]: "Introduction: Perspectives on the Treatment of Intimate Violence." Dutton, Donald, and Daniel J. Sonkin. Co-published simultaneously in *Journal of Aggression, Maltreatment & Trauma* (The Haworth Maltreatment & Trauma Press, an imprint of The Haworth Press, Inc.) Vol. 7, No. 1/2 (#13/14), 2003, pp. 1-6; and: *Intimate Violence: Contemporary Treatment Innovations* (ed: Donald Dutton, and Daniel J. Sonkin) The Haworth Maltreatment & Trauma Press, an imprint of The Haworth Press, Inc., 2003, pp. 1-6. Single or multiple copies of this article are available for a fee from The Haworth Document Delivery Service [1-800-HAWORTH, 9:00 a.m. - 5:00 p.m. (EST). E-mail address: docdelivery@haworthpress.com].

modification model, based on principles derived from social learning theory, to enable men to modify and regulate their anger and abusive behavior. Her model was especially applicable to court-mandated treatment as it strongly affirmed a sense of personal responsibility for one's actions and taught men applications through which anger could be modified. Nevertheless, the model came under intense criticism, especially from feminist-activists who claimed it did not produce results and that abuse was not related to anger or psychological phenomena but was an outgrowth of patriarchal social systems and the suppression of women. Many treatment groups came under attack for everything from diverting funds to shelters to promising false hope to battered women. In some areas, therapists treating batterers were told they must be accountable to shelter activists who in most cases knew nothing of therapeutic practice or the psychology of perpetrator populations. Indeed, if patriarchal social systems cause wife assault, most men should be assaultive and there would be no therapeutic objective in treating individuals (see also Dutton, 1994).

Two results of this political assault on treatment were the development of feminist models of treatment and intense scrutiny of the outcome success of treatment groups. Of the feminist models, the most widely known was the "Duluth Model." Developed in Minnesota, this model utilized community resources and "attitude readjustment" for clients toward a more feminist view of their relationship. There are several problems with the Duluth approach. It assumes that attitudes control abusive behavior when research data suggest that both attitudes and behavior are symptoms of deeper personality factors (Dutton 1995a, 1995b, 1998a) and have a bidirectional form of influence. Also, attitude "readjustment" may generate reactance in men who do not share feminist values, and may inadvertently create shame reactions in clients that recapitulate their early victimization experience. My [D.D.] own research on the developmental precursors of abusiveness found that exposure to shaming experiences was a major contributor to adult tendencies to externalize blame, reject feedback and experience chronic levels of high anger (Dutton, 1995b; Dutton, Starzomski, & van Ginkel, 1995). In this volume, Robert Wallace and Anna Nosko write eloquently of "vicarious detoxification" of shame in group therapy with batterers. A therapeutic implication of the salience of shame (shame-proneness) in batterers is to structure therapy so as not to recreate early shaming experiences. One example is to have clients write their own "violence policy" in response to the statement "I feel it is acceptable to be violent when . . . ." Most clients will answer "in defense of my self and my family." Other answers can become material for group discussion. The point is that all ensuing therapeutic interventions can be presented as helping the client to remain consistent with their own policy, not an externally imposed policy that can generate shame and resentment.

The failure of the Duluth model to deal with deeper psychological issues lends superficiality to the method that produces, according to one report, a 40% recidivism rate (Shepard, 1992). This rate approaches the 50% recidivism rate we obtained for treatment dropouts in a long-term follow up study (Dutton, Bodnarchuk, Kropp, Hart, & Ogloff, 1997b). By comparison, the eleven-year recidivism rate for "anger management" treatment completers was 23%.

Treatment groups for batterers have been scrutinized more closely than any other treatment form. Meta analyses (Smith & Glass, 1977) yield effect sizes that tell us the mean difference between treated and untreated clients of subsequent manifestation of problem behaviors. The most successful treatment is that given to motivated neurotics with a specific problem that they want to change. The least effective is that given to criminal justice populations, especially sex offenders. Batterer treatment falls somewhere in the middle.

An unstated motive for the attack on treatment efficacy by feminists is the desire to see "within the system" approaches to domestic violence fail, necessitating the argument for radical social change. Shelter house activists who see the same women return even after their husbands receive treatment generalize that observation to the incorrect conclusion that the treatment failure must occur for all men. In fact, the worst candidates for treatment are psychopaths, but the failure of treatment for them should not be generalized to all clients (Dutton, Bodnarchuk, Kropp, Hart, & Ogloff, 1997a). Radical social change is beyond the control of national governments, let alone activist groups. What can we do to diminish family violence in the current context that is within our control?

It is, of course, possible to criticize some elements of current group practice: In many jurisdictions, the practice has not developed beyond the original anger management or attitude readjustment models. The Duluth model is particularly widespread and even legislated in some states, including California. Yet our knowledge of the psychology of batterers has developed extensively in the past decade. My [D.D.] own work on cyclical batterers has implicated shaming, insecure attachment and witnessing of parental violence as interactive contributors to an abusive personality that sees, feels and acts differently than most men during intimate conflict. It stands to reason that acknowledgment of attachment, shaming and trauma precursors to battering should become an integral part of treatment.

In this volume, we contributed a chapter on the treatment of attachment insecurity which, in our opinion, will only grow in therapeutic importance as its adult ramifications become more fully realized. Robert Wallace and Anna Nosko contribute a chapter on shaming. The interested reader is referred to excellent source material on the former topic by Robert Karen (1994) and the latter topic by Helen Block Lewis (1971). The adult personality resulting from childhood exposure to shaming, violence and insecure attachment is a form of borderline personality organization (Dutton, 1994, 1995a, 1995b, 1998c). Working with borderlines, even the less extreme form, is notoriously difficult for a therapist. In this collection, Jennifer Waltz describes the application of a treatment model for borderlines developed by Marsha Linehan to working with batterers.

At present, there is no one "treatment of choice" in working with physically abusive clients. No research demonstrates clear and consistent superior effectiveness for one treatment strategy. In the present publication, Rosemary Cogan and John H. Porcerelli outline psychoanalytic strategies for working with people in abusive relationships, and Richard E. Heyman and Karin Schlee describe a couples treatment approach. Each represents an alternative to current practice.

We make no claim of exhausting the therapeutic possibilities for new approaches to working with intimately violent men. Most batterers suffer from some form of extreme tension held in the body. Both "body work" and Reichian breathing are useful in teaching them to control and reduce their tension through nonviolent means. We had originally attempted to obtain an article on body work for this volume but the treatment form is notoriously difficult to describe verbally. Its practice is probably better learned in a form of oral tradition or through direct experience with a qualified practitioner. We learned of its benefits from a marvelous clinician, Bob Berger, who practices in Crescent Beach, south of Vancouver. Reichian breathing, which comes from the same tradition as bodywork, again teaches alternative tension reduction techniques by combining stretching and breathing. Clients learn to vocalize on exhales, opening the throat and dissipating more stored tension. Exercises can be practiced in group, as part of an opening routine, or to demonstrate anger reduction in an individual client.

In addition to new treatment techniques, the present volume also presents articles for treating special populations. Robert Kiyoshk describes integrating native spiritual healing with conventional anger management for use in native treatment groups. Although this article is specific to working with indigenous populations in Canada, the issue of spirituality is an important element to the treatment process, and his ideas described in this article can be applied to other ethnic groups as well. Vallerie E. Coleman describes the psychoanalytic treatment of lesbian batterers. Her article thoroughly discusses the etiology of violence in lesbian relationships and how clinicians can address this problem from a psychodynamic perspective. Ophra Keynan and colleagues describe Beit Noam, an innovative residential program in Israel, and their unique approach to treating Israeli perpetrators of woman battering. Lastly, Penny A. Leisring, Lynn Dowd and Alan Rosenbaum discuss the treatment of female batterers. With the advent of mandatory arrest laws for domestic violence, more and more women are being mandated into treatment programs. These clients present a unique challenge to clinicians in that a significant percentage of them are not only perpetrators of violence, but current victims of domestic violence. They discuss how clinicians treating women must learn how to incorporate the treatment of trauma with acting-out/violence containment strategies in order to effectively treat these clients.

In the final section of the publication, we have two articles that all clinicians working with perpetrators will find extremely useful. First, Alan Rosenbaum, William J. Warnken, and Albert J. Grudzinskas, Jr. provide an excellent discussion of the legal and ethical issues confronting individuals treating the court-mandated perpetrators of domestic violence. Although theory and techniques are important, clinicians must be aware of and prepared to address the numerous legal and ethical issues they are likely to encounter in treating the court-mandated clients. Issues of confidentiality, dangerousness, child abuse and boundaries are frequently encountered with this clinical population, and addressing these issues effectively not only increases the likelihood of successful treatment outcome, but also reduces the therapist's exposure to civil and legal liability. Historically, outcome studies have focused on the reoccurrence of violence (Dutton, Bodnarchuk, Kropp & Ogloff, 1997b) rather than asking treatment participants about their experience of the intervention. In the final article, Mindy S. Rosenberg presents findings from a post treatment interview with treatment clients asking them what the experience was like, and which skills worked best for them. Clinicians can learn from their clients as well as the empirical data.

Research has also indicated that batterers have histories of being abuse victims. I [D.D.] have written about the high levels of trauma symptoms found in batterers (Dutton, 1995a, 1995b) and have attempted to show how a trauma model better accounts for their psychological features than other models, including social learning theory (Dutton, 1998a, 1998b). In this collection, we have attempted to reconcile this work with treatment practices and to point to new opportunities for treatment. It is sometimes difficult, in working with an abusive client, to remember that the person was once an abuse victim. Nevertheless, integrating these two parts of that client's overall personality ensures a more complete therapeutic stance. We need never accept bad behaviors in order to acknowledge the human essence of the client.

REFERENCES

Dutton, D. G. (1994). Patriarchy and wife assault: The ecological fallacy. *Violence & Victims*, 9(2), 125-140.

Dutton, D. G. (1995a). Male abusiveness in intimate relationships. *Clinical Psychology Review*, 15(6), 567-581.

Dutton, D. G. (1995b). *The batterer: A psychological profile*. New York: Harper Collins.

Dutton, D. G. (1998a). Traumatic origins of intimate rage. *Aggression and Violent Behavior*, 4(4), 431-448.

Dutton, D. G. (1998b). *The limitations of social learning analyses applied to intimate abusiveness*. Claremont Graduate School Symposium: Sage Publications.

Dutton, D. G. (1998c). *The abusive personality: A trauma model*. New York: Guilford.

Dutton, D. G., Bodnarchuk, M., Kropp, R., Hart, S., & Ogloff, J. (1997a). Client personality disorders affecting wife assault post treatment recidivism. *Violence & Victims*, 12(1), 37-50.

Dutton, D. G., Bodnarchuk, M., Kropp, R., Hart, S., & Ogloff, J. (1997b). Wife assault treatment and criminal recidivism: An eleven year follow-up. *International Journal of Offender Therapy and Comparative Criminology*, 41(1), 9-23.

Dutton, D. G., Starzomski, A., & van Ginkel, C. (1995). The role of shame and guilt in the intergenerational transmission of abusiveness. *Violence & Victims*, 10(2), 121-131.

Karen, R. (1994). *Becoming attached*. New York: Warner Books.

Lewis, H. B. (1971). *Shame and guilt in neurosis*. New York: International Universities Press.

Smith, M. L., & Glass, G. V. (1977). Meta-analysis of psychotherapy outcome studies. *American Psychologist*, September, 752-760.

THEORETICAL APPROACHES TO THE TREATMENT OF INTIMATE VIOLENCE PERPETRATORS

Treatment of Assaultiveness

Donald Dutton

SUMMARY. Assaultiveness and abusiveness have a psychology that must be addressed in therapy; they are not merely the product of "bad attitudes" or social roles, nor can they be narrowly defined as the robotic imitation of action. Perceptions and feelings about the world of intimate relationships both sustain and are sustained by abusive actions. These provide points of intervention for cognitive behavioral therapy (CBT). Given the tendency to shame easily, abusive men must not be confronted too quickly or too strongly. On the other hand, given their well-established denial system and tendency to minimize the consequences of their abusiveness, some confrontation must occur. Hence a "Zen" line of least resistance must be found between the opposites of acceptance and con-

[Haworth co-indexing entry note]: "Treatment of Assaultiveness." Dutton, Donald. Co-published simultaneously in *Journal of Aggression, Maltreatment & Trauma* (The Haworth Maltreatment & Trauma Press, an imprint of The Haworth Press, Inc.) Vol. 7, No. 1/2 (#13/14), 2003, pp. 7-28; and: *Intimate Violence: Contemporary Treatment Innovations* (ed: Donald Dutton, and Daniel J. Sonkin) The Haworth Maltreatment & Trauma Press, an imprint of The Haworth Press, Inc., 2003, pp. 7-28. Single or multiple copies of this article are available for a fee from The Haworth Document Delivery Service [1-800-HAWORTH, 9:00 a.m. - 5:00 p.m. (EST). E-mail address: docdelivery@haworthpress.com].

http://www.haworthpress.com/store/product.asp?sku=J146
© 2003 by The Haworth Press, Inc. All rights reserved.
10.1300J146v07n01_02

frontation. Treatment outcome studies indicate moderate success for cognitive behavioral treatment (CBT) for batterers. Treatment is less successful with men who have personality disorders, especially psychopathy. *[Article copies available for a fee from The Haworth Document Delivery Service: 1-800-HAWORTH. E-mail address: <docdelivery@haworthpress.com> Website: <http://www.HaworthPress.com> © 2003 by The Haworth Press, Inc. All rights reserved.]*

KEYWORDS. Treatment, batterer, shame, attachment, trauma, CBT, personality disorder, anger

As cited in an article on pharmacological treatment for assaultive males, Maiuro and Avery (1996) developed a three-stage program termed 'biopsychosocial intervention.' The biological aspect involves administering pharmacological treatment for depression, irritable temperament, hyper-reactivity, emotional lability, pathological anxiety, obsessiveness, compulsiveness, and post-concussive or other related syndromes. The biological treatment intervention was based on the assumption that pharmacological agents such as antidepressants, anxiolytics, and serotonin re-uptake moderators might aid in treating certain aspects of the abusive personality. However, as the researchers point out, this form of intervention cannot be substituted for social change or psychological (group) treatment. Instead it must be viewed as an adjunct to the broader forms of intervention: psychological and sociocultural. The following were listed as potential *psychological* treatment targets: defenses against acknowledgment of responsibility (e.g., denial, minimizing, blame projection), anger management (detection and control of anger responses), assertiveness, bargaining and communication skills, attitudes toward women, family of origin modeling influences, relationship enhancement skills, and relapse prevention skills. I agree that these appear to be reasonable targets for psychological intervention. Yet both the narrower biological and psychological interventions must be set within a social context of activism concerning general cultural acceptance of violence, violence toward women, women's safety, and male sex-role conditioning.

Dr. Anne Ganley (1981), then a psychologist at the Veterans' Administration Hospital in Tacoma, Washington, developed a treatment group approach for assaultive males in the late 1970s. Following from a social learning perspective, Dr. Ganley's treatment model was based on the notion of abusiveness as a learned behavior. We adopted her treatment model and, in line with our own experience, revised it somewhat. This model is outlined here, including extended applications relating to borderline personality disorder, psychopathy, attachment issues, and trauma. I then examine the outcome research on treatment effectiveness. The clinical goals of treatment are relatively simple: to get the man to recognize and accept responsibility for his abusiveness, and to develop control over and reduce the frequency of such behavior. The treatment program described below is simply one means of achieving these objectives. Notice that each week has both a 'didactic' (skills acquisition) and a process (group dynamic) component (see Appendix A). The interested reader is referred to Yalom's (1975) classic text on this subject.

SIXTEEN WEEKS IN A TREATMENT GROUP

Court mandated treatment models arose in a number of locations in the early 1980s and range in length from eight to fifty-two weeks. The criminal justice system needed an effective way for judges to settle wife assault cases before them, and treatments were developed to meet that need. Many men who are sent by the courts for wife assault treatment have had no experience with psychotherapy. They imagine their worst fears and weaknesses being exposed; consequently, the experience is initially terrifying.

Bob Wallace and Anna Nosko (1993) have described the opening night ritual in such groups as a "vicarious detoxification" of shame (also see Wallace & Nosko, 2002). Men who come to group, assuming they are 'normally' socialized, experience high levels of shame as a result of their violent behavior. Hearing other men in the group discuss their own violence allows the man to 'vicariously detoxify'; that is, to face his own sense of shame. This sense of shame, were it not detoxified, would maintain the man's anger at a high level and preclude his opening to treatment. The anger is maintained to keep the shame at bay. Anger allows blame to be directed outwardly, preventing shame-induced internalized blame.

For this reason, we start very slowly in our groups, simply asking men on opening night to describe "the event that led to your being here" (e.g., the assault). Their stories provide them with a sense of mutual affliction and of shame detoxification that furthers the bonding process.

Moreover, these stories provide us with an initial assessment of the man's level of denial and willingness to accept responsibility for his violence. The only other treatment objective on opening night is to review the group rules with the clients. These rules are reproduced in Appendix B.

Apart from common sense rules such as attending consistently in a sober condition, these rules also outline the confidential nature of the group and the exceptions to this rule (such as disclosures of child abuse or of direct threats towards another person). As straightforward as these rules may be, they still trigger resentment concerning the criminal justice system's handling of the man's case. Many men feel poorly treated by the system, view their wives as also needing anger management, and see therapists as extensions of the system that unfairly depicted them as the perpetrator and their wives as the victim. These feelings frequently surface during discussion of the participation agreement. It is important to acknowledge and empathize with these feelings while still maintaining a focus on stopping abusive behavior (see Waltz, 2002). Differentiation of the feelings from the behavior and exploring how the feelings may interfere with change are important tools to be used in this regard.

At the end of group one, we ask men how they feel at this juncture. Generally, they express relief about "surviving" the first group, and about being in a group composed of men with similar problems. Their relief generally has to do with not feeling judged; this aspect proves to be particularly important given the shame feelings often experienced by abusive males, as described by Wallace and Nosko (1993). For this reason, I would not recommend confrontation on opening night.

Immediately following the beginning of group, therapists should interview female partners to assess her safety plans, her perception of personal risk, the man's current level of abuse, and any feedback he may have brought home from his first group experience. One danger sign, for example, is the use of the group to minimize one's abuse: "You think I'm bad, you should hear these other guys in my group." The therapist should also ascertain what information can safely be fed back to the man. If the woman is not comfortable with direct feedback (attributed or traceable to her), present the issue during group in general terms. Ask the men if they have any lingering reactions to what they heard the preceding week and discuss "defensive social comparison," where one uses the group to deny or to minimize one's abuse. The point should be that each man, regardless of his level of abuse, has to take responsibility for that abuse. In other words, it is irrelevant that someone else may be more violent than he.

The second meeting should begin with addressing residual feelings from week one. It is useful to get the clients to focus on and describe such feelings; this begins a weekly 'check-in' exercise that will initiate the group process for each week to come. It can also lead into a simple exercise for week two: differentiating feelings from "issues" and actions. We present this as an exercise: Men are asked, "What do you argue about? How do you feel after these arguments?" and "How do you act when you are arguing?" This exercise is again deceptively simple; it outlines some apparent distinctions between feelings and actions. At the same time, it again shows the client that other men share many of the same issues. This revelation furthers the bonding process in the group (i.e., group cohesiveness) and facilitates shame detoxification. We tend not to confront men much during these initial few weeks. We describe what confrontation is and distinguish it from attack or put down. We explain that confrontation is a device to help someone change, whereas attack is simply done to make the attacker feel powerful. We warn men that we will later use confrontation as a part of treatment. However, if a group is particularly woman-blaming it is important to initiate the confrontation process earlier, before a negative form of group cohesiveness develops that is built on shared commiseration about how difficult women can be. Reorienting the men from an other-blaming orientation to a self-control orientation typically has to be repeated during early sessions. A self-control orientation, as the guiding philosophy, emphasizes personal responsibility and control of self (along with negotiation with, rather than control over, others).

Week three also begins by checking-in on the feelings generated from the previous meeting, and then examines what is meant by "abuse." The various forms of abuse (physical, sexual, and emotional) are discussed, and the "power wheel," developed during the program in Duluth, Minnesota (Pence & Paymar, 1986), is explained. A working definition of abuse also includes the motive of harming the partner's self-esteem or restricting her autonomy. Men are informed that, for the duration of the group, they will be asked to report any abuse committed that fits the aforementioned definitions.

At this point, there is one practical issue regarding the 'check-in' exercise that deserves mention: It can run for an hour and a half in a ten-man group, reducing group time for other exercises. If this begins to happen, get the men to respond succinctly to three questions: Was there any abuse this week (if so describe), did you handle your anger well on any occasion, and do you need any group time for special problems?

Week four examines the gains and losses each man experiences through the use of violence. This leads to asking the men to develop a personal "violence policy" for the following week. This violence policy must answer the question "I believe it all right to be violent under the following circumstances." Each man has to develop his personal policy as a homework exercise. Again, from a process perspective, this is a test of the man's commitment to the groupwork. Most men will cite self-defense or protection of family as justification for violence, while others may cite reactions to situations such as home invasion. Few men will cite that violence is acceptable during arguments with their wife. It is important that this policy come from the client. This undercuts his erroneous conviction that actions and beliefs are being imposed upon him by the "system" (including the therapist). If it is his own policy, a policy that the therapist will hold him to, there exists a greater feeling of co-authorship between the client and therapist. The therapeutic bond is strengthened and the resistance to perceived threats to the clients' autonomy is removed.

Note that men who have a policy that is at odds with the group philosophy will need to have their attitude directly identified and confronted. The role of the 'pro-violence' attitude in sustaining destructive behavioral patterns must also be addressed. If the man refuses to change his attitude, the therapist must decide whether this is a 'protest gesture' (i.e., against the therapist who is seen as an extension of the criminal justice response) or a bona fide attitude that impedes the client's progress. This is a situation where confrontation by another group member or by a 'catalyst' (e.g., a man returning from a prior group to co-facilitate and act as a catalyst) is especially helpful. However, in the face of prolonged failure, men who refuse to change their pro-violence attitude may be asked to leave the group; their refusal to adopt a more constructive perspective is contradictory to a commitment to change.

Week five introduces the anger diary or anger log. This anger diary is the basic tool to improve the men's ability to detect and to manage their anger. It requires them to specifically state what triggered their anger as objectively as possible (under the trigger column), to list how they knew they were angry (what physical cues told them so?), to rate their anger severity on a scale where ten is their own personal extreme, and to describe their "talk up" (their thoughts as their anger escalates) and their "talk down" thoughts (their thoughts as their anger diminishes). Most clients have some initial difficulty with the latter. A list of talk down statements is provided to help them with this (see Table 1). Men are in-

TABLE 1. Self-Talk

Both research and experience show that when people with anger problems change their self-talk, their anger de-escalates and they regain control. When you notice your cues escalating or start to feel angry, take a TIME-OUT and read these statements to yourself.

- I don't need to prove myself in this situation.
- As long as I keep my cool, I'm in control of myself.
- No need to doubt myself, what other people say doesn't matter. I'm the only person who can make me mad or keep me calm.
- Time to relax and slow things down. Take a time out if I get uptight or start to notice my cues.
- My anger is a signal. Time to talk to myself and to relax.
- I don't need to feel threatened here. I can relax and stay cool.
- Nothing says I have to be competent and strong all the time. It's okay to feel unsure or confused.
- It's impossible to control other people and situations. The ONLY thing I can control is myself and how I express my feelings.
- It's okay to be uncertain or insecure sometimes. I don't need to be in control of everything and everybody.
- If people criticize me, I can survive that. Nothing says that I have to be perfect.
- If this person wants to go off the wall, that's their thing. I don't need to respond to their anger or feel threatened.
- When I get into an argument, I can use my control plan and know what to do. I can take a time-out.
- Most things we argue about are stupid and insignificant. I can recognize that my anger comes from having my old primary feelings restimulated. It's okay to walk away from this fight.
- It's nice to have other people's love and approval, but even without it, I can still accept and like MYSELF.
- People put erasers on the ends of pencils for a reason; it's okay to make mistakes.
- People are going to act the way they want to, not the way I want.
- I feel angry, that must mean I have been hurt, scared or have some other primary feeling.

structed to select a statement that feels soothing to them personally, and to use it during their anger arousal.

Comparison of the 'trigger' and the talk-up columns of the anger diary will assist the therapist in making explicit the interpretations and assumptions that color the client's perception of the trigger. Assumptions of malevolent intent (that the action of the other person was done intentionally, to hurt them) are frequent with angry clients. Group discussion should clarify that other interpretations are possible and more likely. This exercise can also be used to evaluate the client's ability to empathize with the other person. Assuming the client's perception of the event that precipitated their action is accurate (this needs checking), the therapist must assess the extent to which they can imagine and accept another interpretation for the other persons' emotional response.

Week six should focus on the feelings that can be converted to anger, such as guilt, shame, or humiliation. Some teaching of theory (for example, how shame or fear can be converted to anger because anger is more consistent with the 'male sex role') helps here, but it is also important to return to the anger diary and to ensure that each client can and is completing it weekly. We also institute a "gut-check" on honest participation around this time by asking the men to describe (on a written note) who they think has been the most and least honest in the group (see Appendix C). They are also asked whom it is that they feel they know the least in the group. When these notes are collected from each man, the therapist asks whether or not they would like feedback. At this point, a summary of the notes can be delivered either individually or collectively. The former involves telling an individual how the group rates him, while the latter involves tallying all of the ratings on a grid.

DESC scripts are the men's introduction to assertive communication and function to replace previously used coping mechanisms, including abuse and repression of feelings. DESC is an acronym that stands for Describe, Express, Specify, and Consequences. This term was borrowed from an excellent book on assertive communication by Gordon Bower and Sharon Bower called *Asserting Yourself* (1976). These DESC scripts take the internal work of the anger diary and transform it into an interpersonal tool for improving communication (see Appendix D). The key is to get the men to improve at recognizing irritations sooner, and to express them. The concept here is that relationships are "yoked-outcome" situations, where what is good for one party improves the other's lot in life as well. The DESC script initiates this process. Men should be cautioned not to expect to "get their way" by using these scripts. The rules for using a DESC script are outlined in Appendix E.

Week eight focuses on teaching breathing and stretching exercises to improve stress management. Wilhelm Reich (1945/1972) describes character armor as the result of storing tension in the fascia or connective tissue of the body. Since many assaultive men react to a buildup of internal tension, it is important to teach them how to maintain tension within acceptable levels through daily routines of breathing and stretching. A variety of useful stretching programs exist that can be combined with breathing and breath-control exercises to develop useful tension self-management techniques (see, for example, Kabat-Zinn, 1990). The therapist can demonstrate these in the group session and encourage participation. Some therapists like to teach these techniques much sooner in the schedule and to start each group with breathing and stretching exercises. The didactic goal here is to teach effective tension management so that the reliance on abusive outbursts to diminish tension is lessened. Borderline clients can benefit from this aspect of the group, as cyclical tension build-ups are a major part of their abusiveness. In working with cyclical or borderline clients, it is also important to ensure that the therapist is consistent from week to week. Any alterations in the therapist's relationship with the client can then be pointed out as part of the clients' changeability and cues can be elicited to help the client track their changes (see also Dutton & Winters, 1999).

Weeks nine and ten involve confronting the men's family of origin issues. We ask each of them the following questions: How did your father/mother express his/her anger? What did he/she do? How did this make you feel? How did others react? Did you ever talk to brothers/sisters about it? How did they feel? What message do you take from this for raising your own children? These questions typically produce strong emotion because many of these men will have experienced an abusive childhood. This also marks the completion of the group bonding process that began during week one. Because of the intensity of feelings produced by these topics, is it suggested that the group be broken into smaller subgroups for more intimate discussion.

Weeks eleven to fourteen involve consolidation of the techniques developed during the group. These sessions function to improve communication, which in turn sets the men up for effective couples counseling. We focus on using "I" statements, on improving empathy, and on distinguishing between argument versus acknowledgment.

During week fifteen, we prepare the men for the end of treatment by asking them to spend the week considering what they learned, what they changed, what they still have to work on, and how they will replace the honest male-to-male communication developed in the group once they leave. We sensitize them to relapse prevention, asking them what plan they could develop for a "worst case scenario," that is, if they were to relapse and to abuse again. There is no fixed need to run these treatment groups in sixteen weeks. Longer treatment periods (e.g., in California, the courts mandate one year) allow more in-depth work on early issues, attachment issues, and anxieties related to loss that often underlie abuse of power in relationships. I strongly recommend reading the Rosenberg article (2002) for an insightful retrospective view of the group experience from the clients' perspective.

SPECIAL POPULATIONS

Borderlines

Jennifer Waltz's article (2002) focuses on one treatment approach to working with borderline men called Dialectical Behavioral Therapy (DBT; Linehan, 1987). Dutton (2002) has written an integrative chapter that focuses on commonalities in DBT and cognitive behavioral therapy. Waltz carefully outlines the pros and cons of applying this technique to a batterer group. If you have men who exhibit borderline traits in your group (extreme swings in positivity-negativity towards their spouse, yourself, and/or the groupwork), some special treatment needs should be addressed. First, you must keep in mind that your group has a limited therapeutic goal: to stop abusiveness. It is not designed for deeper work on personality disorders. Nevertheless, there are some therapeutic imperatives that may benefit borderline men in their ability to self-soothe and self-control. Notice the thinking errors common to borderlines, listed in Table 2.

These are issues that need to be addressed in most groups anyway, especially the issues surrounding lack of integration of the other and of personalization (see Table 3). The latter will come up through the interpretation of anger diaries. Again, interviews with partners are an invaluable source of information about the man's mood and temper swings. These are the men who go through the 'abuse cycles' of tension build-up, abuse outburst, and contrition (Dutton, 1998). In a tracking study of cyclical males, Dutton and Winters (1999) found that the men's wives were better at tracking their swings than were the men. It is important to help these men become more aware of how they are storing tension, what cues they can use to anticipate an outburst, and what alternative tension-reduction methods are available. Borderlines vary in the extent to which their cycles are demonstrated publicly. A strong channel of communication with the man's partner can be used effectively with men whose tension build-ups are solely expressed in their intimate bond. Be sure to check with the partner as to how safe it is to confront the man based upon her report. We include a didactic session on the 'Cycle of Violence' in Week eight. Refreshers can be used when risk of recurrence is reported. Start with the general lesson and then ask the men if any of them are currently experiencing 'cyclical symptoms' (e.g., increasing anger, irritability, withdrawal, or increasing frequency of negative thoughts about their partner). Be prepared for partner blaming, and counter this by using historical material (waxing and waning of

TABLE 2. Borderline Thinking Errors

- **Dichotomous (black and white) thinking:**
  - – e.g., splitting of intimate other; splitting of self-concept
- **Personalization:**
  - – tendency to excessively relate external occurrences to the self
  - – includes self-blame
- **Catastrophizing:**
  - – inability to differentiate others' wishes from demands

Source: Arntz (1994). Klein & Swales. Psychiatry online. Available: <www.cityscape.couk/users/ad88/html>.

TABLE 3. Borderline Treatment

- **Consistency of therapist**
- **Direct attention to clients' fluctuations in:**
  - (1) affect
  - (2) perception of self
  - (3) perception of partner
  - (4) perception of others
  - (5) general optimism-pessimism
- **Challenge fundamental assumptions:**
  - (1) others are dangerous and malignant
  - (2) client is powerless and vulnerable
  - (3) client is inherently bad/unacceptable
- **Differentiate problem behavior (abuse) from client's self**

negative thoughts about the partner in the past). Eventually, focus on the client in question. Ask him if this has been a problem in the past. Does he consider it to be something he would like to change? How could he improve at spotting the cues? The trick here is to move him from attributing changes to external factors to attributing changes to internal states and to encourage him to focus on changing such states. A cognitive-behavioral borderline treatment was developed by Arntz (1994) that is quite compatible with the Ganley (1981) model and much less labor-intensive than the Linehan (1987) approach. Arntz emphasizes the importance of the therapist remaining consistent from week to week. Any changes in the borderline's reaction to the therapist can then be more clearly attributed to the client. Some men may be so deeply personality disordered that individual therapy (such as DBT) is required in conjunction with treatment for wife assault.

Psychopaths

There is some question, of course, of whether or not psychopaths are treatable at all (Hare, 1995). Psychopaths lack the ability to develop emotional relationships with significant others and with therapists, do not see themselves as having psychological problems, and, in some studies, are the worst recidivists. However, the research suggesting that psychopaths are completely untreatable is far from conclusive. Losel (1998) reviews this literature and concludes "structured behavioral, cognitive-behavioral, skill-oriented, and multimodal measures, based on social learning theories have better effects on antisocial behavior (characteristic of most but not all Psychopaths) than other modes of treatment" (p. 101). Also of note is Losel's suggestion regarding a Therapeutic Community (TC). He describes a permanent TC in an incarcerated setting, lasting for at least one year. A three-hour per week group is a poor substitute, and there is a risk that the Psychopath will con the therapist, take advantage of another client, and recidivate anyway. All I can do is warn you. I would recommend reading Hare (1993, 1995) so that you will know what you are dealing with.

DO TREATMENT GROUPS WORK?

The assessment of psychotherapeutic treatment efficacy is typically done as follows: Groups of treated and untreated men and their partners report on the man's abusiveness both before and after treatment (for the treated group) or for a comparable time period (for the untreated group). The "outcome study" assumes that the two groups are either randomized or matched for their level of pre-violence before any meaningful comparison can be made. The difference in reduction or cessation of violence between the two groups is called the "effect size." Effect size is the standardized difference between the mean recidivism rate of the treatment group and the mean of the untreated group, divided by the pooled standard deviation for the two groups' scores. The analysis is strengthened by combining these differences across a number of independent studies in what Gene Glass (1976) calls "meta-analysis."

Meta-analyses yield summaries of several studies and are believed to be superior to data offered by any single study. This method cancels out the interpretative problems, due to the methodological variation that exists between independent studies, associated with any single design. Eligible studies are viewed as a population to be systematically sampled and surveyed. Individual study results are then quantified, coded, and assembled into a database.

The strongest finding to emerge from meta-analytic studies is that psychological treatment is generally effective. In a broad ranging review of 302 meta-analytic studies, Mark Lipsey and David Wilson (1993) found only six that produced negative results (the control group showing greater improvements than the treated group), with 85% of the studies obtaining effect sizes of .2 or greater. By comparison, the effect size for coronary bypass surgery is .15, while for breast cancer chemotherapy, it is .09.

To make effect size more intuitively understandable, psychologist Robert Rosenthal (1983) suggests a "binomial effect size display" (BESD), which is a depiction of the proportion of treated versus untreated clients who reach or exceed a common success criterion. In practical terms for the treatment success criterion, a "binomial" effect size of .4 translates into about a 24% spread between treated and untreated groups. A .2 binomial effect size translates into about a 10% spread. The importance of the spread size depends largely on the behavior in question. For example, in regard to lives saved through some intervention, a 5% spread size would be considered pretty important to clients or patients. Lipsey and Wilson (1993) report an effect size of .67 for cognitive-behavioral therapies; for offender treatment programs, it is said to be .20. How would wife assault treatment compare?

Barry Rosenfeld (1992) assessed the outcome of treatment programs for spouse abusers. He examined twenty-five treatment outcome studies, five of which focused on court-ordered clients. Although Rosenfeld did not do a formal meta-analysis, he reported aggregate outcome results that allow for the general assessment of effect sizes. For example, he found that according to police recidivism data, 8.4% of treated men and 23.4% of untreated men with comparable prior spouse abuse rates re-offended. This translates roughly into a 15% difference or about a .30 effect size. This midrange result is somewhat higher than offender treatment program results, while it is somewhat lower than treatment outcomes in general. These findings, in turn, probably reflect differences in individual clients' motivation to change.

THE PROCESS OF CHANGE

Psychologist James Prochaska and his colleagues (Prochaska, DiClemente, & Norcross, 1992) have examined the role of destructive addictions and motivational factors in the process of change. Essentially, by examining studies of change for a variety of addictions, Prochaska et al. were able to derive some general principles of change, stemming from various stages in a change process.

Abusiveness can be thought of as a destructive addiction; the perpetrator knows only one way to reduce tension and to regain feelings of control. In this sense, the Prochaska, DiClemente, and Norcross model of change applies to abusive men as it does to cigarette addicts or to alcoholics. Prochaska et al. describe a "pre-contemplation" stage in which the person is not yet convinced that he/she has a problem. Friends and family may believe that he/she has a problem, but the person him/herself is not convinced. With addicts, a familiar phrase is "I know I can quit, I've done it a dozen times." Others include statements that classify the problem as minor. With abusive men, denial and minimization of the problem is commonplace. Men attending court-ordered therapy for wife assault are often catapulted from the pre-contemplation phase into the "action" phase; thus, they often enter treatment with a mixed motivational set. Experienced therapists know that some men will accept treatment as necessary and overdue, while others will still believe that the problem is with their wife, the courts, or the criminal justice system. According to the Prochaska et al. study, however, all of these men will undergo a spiral process on the way to "termination" (permanent cessation of their abusiveness). This means that the expectation that one sixteen-week treatment group will automatically end abusiveness is somewhat naive or optimistic. Therapists should build in "relapse prevention" mechanisms, such as allowing men to drop in on new groups when they feel stressed, or emphasizing the importance of re-entering treatment if relapse occurs. From the outcome research perspective, the implication offered by Prochaska's model is that some recidivism will occur in the treated group. As such, the emphasis should probably be on hastening the man's path towards cessation, rather than on expecting an "instant" improvement following treatment. In this light, my colleagues and I (Dutton, Bodnarchuk, Kropp, Hart, & Ogloff, 1997b) tracked men who had come to our treatment program for up to eleven years. We used national police data to ascertain whether these men, after initial contact, had any repeat assault charges against them. These data are displayed in Table 4.

One hundred fifty-six men had completed treatment ("completers"; attended at least twelve sessions), 167 had dropped out ("non-completers"; attended 0-11 sessions), 32 were rejected for treatment ("rejects"; typically because of lack of motivation), and 91 men never even pre-

TABLE 4. Post-Contact Crime Variables for TOTAL Sample (*N* = 446)

	Total	Completers	Non-Completers	Rejects	No Shows
N	446	156	167	32	91
Average Years At Risk	5.19	5.20	4.85	5.91	5.59
Post-contact crimes					
Mean # crimes*	1.67	1.26	2.08	2.16	1.45
Mean # violent-crimes*	0.61	0.47	0.74	0.88	0.49
Mean # assaults*	0.46	0.32	0.55	0.81	0.40
% age with at least 1 assault	25.3	23.2	28.0	37.5	21.0
Mean # wife assaults*	0.26	0.23	0.50	0.29	0.23
% with at least 1 wife assault		17.9%	22.2%	31.3%	16.5%
Total # wife assaults	116	36**	84***	9	21

* Denotes statistically significant difference between Completers and Non-Completers
** 6 wife assaults by one man
*** 11 wife assaults by one man

Source: Dutton, D. G., Bodnarchuk, M., Kropp, R., Hart, S. D., & Ogloff, J. P. (1997). Wife assault treatment and criminal recidivism: An eleven year follow-up. *International Journal of Offender Therapy and Criminal Recidivism,* *41*(1), 9-23.

sented for assessment ("no shows"). These groups were followed for 5-6 years on average. Almost a third of the rejects re-offended compared to 22.2% of the treatment group drop-outs and 17.9 % of the completers. Since this was not a randomized design, we could not say whether these differences were due to treatment per se, or to motivational or psychological differences in the men. All groups demonstrated the following result pattern: The majority was non-violent, a small minority was violent once, and an even smaller minority was serial batterers. One man in the drop-out group had eleven repeat wife assault convictions, and one man in the treated group had six.

These data seem to suggest that treatment works for most but not all abusive men. Who are the treatment risks? The man who completed treatment and re-offended six times had neurological problems as a result of head trauma. He was beyond the scope of our treatment model. Other psychological profiles that do not lend themselves well to treatment include those suggesting an antisocial or a borderline personality disorder. Extreme personality disorders simply require deeper, long-term, or adjunct treatment (Dutton et al., 1997a).

One final point: Various attempts have been made to evaluate treatment groups for assaultive men. It is important to keep two things in mind with regard to outcome evaluation. The first is that appropriate controls are almost always lacking. The second is the result described above: Treatment outcomes are extremely skewed. Most group completers have no recidivist offenses, a smaller group has one re-offense, and a tiny group continues to be chronic offenders. They are not normal distributions; hence, 'significant' differences, based on statistical tests that assume normality, are hard to find.

Court mandated treatment groups for batterers will persist because the criminal justice system needs them as a viable sentencing option. They can improve by beginning to incorporate treatments for special groups of batterers (such as borderlines) or special features of battering (attachment disorders). This book presents some ideas behind the new generation of batterer treatment; I expect many more to follow soon.

REFERENCES

Arntz, A. (1994). Treatment of borderline personality disorder: A challenge for cognitive-behavioral therapy. *Behavior, Research and Therapy 32*(4), 419-430.

Bower, S. A., & Bower G. H. (1976). *Asserting yourself: A practical guide for positive change*. Reading, MA: Addison-Westley.

Dutton, D. G. (1998). *The abusive personality: Violence and control in intimate relationships*. Guilford Press: New York.

Dutton, D. G. (2002). *The abusive personality: Violence and control in intimate relationships* (2nd ed.). Guilford Press: New York.

Dutton, D. G., Bodnarchuk, M., Kropp, R., Hart, S., & Ogloff, J. (1997a). Client personality disorders affecting wife assault post treatment recidivism. *Violence & Victims, 12*(1), 37-50.

Dutton, D. G., Bodnarchuk, M., Kropp, R., Hart, S., & Ogloff, J. (1997b). Wife assault treatment and criminal recidivism: An eleven year follow-up. *International Journal of Offender Therapy and Comparative Criminology, 41*(1), 9-23.

Dutton, D. G., & Winters, J. (1999). *Tracking cyclical abuse*. Unpublished manuscript. Department of Psychology, University of British Columbia.

Ganley, A. (1981). *Participant's manual: Court-mandated therapy for men who batter–A three day workshop for professionals*. Washington, DC: Center for Women Policy Studies.

Glass, G. (1976). Primary, secondary, and meta-analysis of research. *Educational Researcher, 5*, 3-8.

Hare, R. D. (1993). *Without conscience: The disturbing world of psychopaths among us*. New York: Simon and Schuster.

Hare, R. D. (1995). Psychopathy: A clinical construct whose time has come. *Criminal Justice and Behavior, 23*, 25-54.

Kabat-Zinn, J. (1990). *Full catastrophe living: Using the wisdom of your body and mind to face stress, pain and illness.* New York: Delta.

Linehan, M. (1987). Dialectical behavior therapy for borderline personality disorder. *Bulletin of the Menninger Clinic, 51*(3), 261-276.

Lipsey, M., & Wilson, D. B. (1993). The efficacy of psychological, educational and behavioral treatment. *American Psychologist, 48*(12) 1181-1209.

Losel, F. (1998). Treatment and management of psychopaths. In D. C. Cooke, A. E. Forth, & R. D. Hare (Eds.), *Psychopathy: Theory, research and implications for society* (pp. 89-113). Dordrecht: The Netherlands.

Maiuro, R. D, & Avery, D. H. (1996). Psychopharmacological treatment of aggression. *Violence & Victims, 11*(3), 239-262.

Pence, E., & Paymar, M. (1986). *Power and control: Tactics of men who batter.* Duluth, MN: Minnesota Program Development, Inc.

Prochaska, J. O., DiClemente, C. C., & Norcross, C. C. (1992). In search of how people change: Applications to addictive behaviors. *American Psychologist, 47,* 1102-1127.

Reich, W. (1945/1972). *Character analysis.* New York: Touchstone/Simon & Schuster.

Rosenberg, M. S. (2002). Voices from the group: Domestic violence offenders' experiences of intervention. *Journal of Aggression, Maltreatment, & Trauma, 7*(1/2), 305-317.

Rosenfeld, B. D. (1992). Court-ordered treatment of spouse abuse. *Clinical Psychology Review, 12,* 205-226.

Rosenthal, R. (1983). Assessing the statistical and social importance of the effects of psychotherapy. *Journal of Consulting and Clinical Psychology, 51*(1), 4-13.

Wallace, R., & Nosko, A. (1993). Working with shame in the group treatment of male batterers. *International Journal of Group Psychotherapy, 43*(1), 45-61.

Wallace, R., & Nosko, A. (2002). Shame in male spouse abusers and its treatment in group therapy. *Journal of Aggression, Maltreatment, & Trauma, 7*(1/2), 47-74.

Waltz, J. (2002). Dialectical behavior therapy in the treatment of abusive behavior. *Journal of Aggression, Maltreatment, & Trauma, 7*(1/2), 75-103.

Yalom, I. (1975). *The theory and practice of group psychotherapy.* New York: Basic Books.

APPENDIX A. Treatment Outline

	Didactic Exercise	Group Process Goals
Week 1	Describe the assault that led to your being here	Shame detoxification
	Participation Agreement	Group Cohesiveness
		Assessment of denial levels
Week 2	Conflict issues: Emotions, actions	Group cohesiveness; shame detoxification
Week 3	What is "abuse"? Definitions, power wheel	Hierarchy in group; Authority issues
Week 4	Explanation of confrontation; first group check-in	Attitude confrontation
Week 5	Violence policy	Authority issues
Week 6	Anger diaries	Emotion detection
Week 7	Stress Management: Reichian Breathing	Repeat of above
Week 8	Abuse cycle	
Week 9	DESC scripts	
Week 10	Family of origin: How did your mom/dad show their anger?	
Week 11	Continuation: How did you/your siblings feel?	
Week 12	DESC scripts role play	
Week 13	Detection of other prevalent emotion: shame, resentment, guilt, etc.	
Week 14	Consolidation of communication skills	
Week 15	Preparation for the end: Relapse prevention	
Week 16	What did you learn? What continues to be a problem? What other therapies are available?	

APPENDIX B

ALTERNATIVES TO VIOLENCE PROGRAM

Participation Agreement

I_____ , agree to join the Alternatives to Violence Program. I understand that the group will give me an opportunity to,
1. Take responsibility for my behaviour.
2. Learn to manage anger and express feelings in appropriate ways.
3. Learn new and constructive ways of coping with stresses and difficulties in my life.

I agree to cooperate with the following group rules.

1. I will attend every week and will be on time for all group sessions. If I miss more than two sessions, I may be expelled from the group. My probation officer will be notified of this and I may be charged with a breach of the terms of my probation.

2. I will attend all sessions in a sober condition and not under the influence of any mood altering drugs. If I come to a group under the influence of alcohol or drugs I will not be allowed into the group for that evening. This will count as one missed session and my probation officer will be notified about this.

3. I will participate to the best of my ability by sharing honestly my thoughts and feelings and by completing all written assignments.

4. I am in the group to learn skills for respectful and healthy relationships. If I am violent or abusive I will report this at the next group session. Failure to do so may result in my being expelled from the group.

5. I have been given a copy of the "time-out" procedure and will use this to increase my ability to create healthy relationships in all areas of my life.

6. I understand that what is said or done in the group sessions is confidential and I should not discuss information about other group members outside the group. I am free to share my own thoughts, feelings and experiences about being in the group with those who are close to me in my own life.

7. If I am seeing a counselor, psychologist, psychiatrist or other professional for either individual or group counseling I understand I may be asked to sign a release to share information so that the Alternatives to Violence staff may consult with these professionals in order to coordinate the help I am receiving. Withholding my consent for this will not be grounds to expel me from the program.

8. I understand that my wife (partner) will be interviewed as part of the assessment process. The purpose will be to better understand my life situation, give her information about the program, obtain my wife's point of view and provide information for her regarding counseling or support for herself. The program staff will not repeat information given by my partner to me, nor will they share information, given by me, with her. Her participation with this interview is voluntary and will in no way reflect upon my status.

9. I understand that if the therapists have reason to believe that I could be a physical risk to anyone they will contact the appropriate authorities and the person(s) who may be at risk.

10. I understand that I will be asked to complete brief weekly written assignments to help me understand my anger. I will not be admitted to the group without a completed assignment. This will count as one missed session.

11. If I am attending on a probation order a one page summary of my attendance and progress will be given to my probation officer upon my completion or expulsion from the group. I can receive a copy of this report if I wish.

My signature below indicates that I have read this agreement and understand it; having had a chance to ask questions and have them answered.

Date _____

Signature _____

Name _____

Witness _____

APPENDIX C

"Gut Check"

1. How honest am I being in the group?

    1 10

    not at all   completely

2. How much effort am I putting into the group?

    1 10

    not much   a lot

3. How much feedback am I giving to others in the group?

    1 10

    not much   a lot

4. Who do I know the most/least about in the group?

5. Who is denying his violence most/least in the group?

6. How much am I getting out of the group?

    1 10

    not much   a lot

APPENDIX D

Writing Your Own DESC Script

⇒**Your DESCRIBE Lines**
- Does your description clarify the situation, or does it just complicate it?
- Replace all terms that do not objectively describe the behaviour or problem that bothers you. Be specific.
- Have you described a single specific behaviour or problem, or a long list of grievances? Focus on one well-defined behaviour or problem you want to deal with now. One grievance per script is generally the best approach.
- Have you made the mistake of describing the other person's attitudes, motives, intentions? Avoid mind-reading and psychoanalyzing.
- Revise your DESCRIBE lines now, if necessary.

⇒**Your EXPRESS Lines**
- Have you acknowledged your feelings and opinions as your own, without blaming the other person? Avoid words that ridicule or shame the other person. Swear words and insulting labels (dumb, cruel, selfish, racist, idiotic, boring) very likely will provoke defensiveness and arguments.
- Have you expressed your feelings and thoughts in a positive, new way? Avoid your "old phonograph record" lines that your partner is tired of hearing and automatically turns off.
- Have you kept the wording low-key? Aim for emotional restraint, not dramatic impact.
- Revise your EXPRESS lines now, if necessary.

⇒**Your SPECIFY Lines**
- Have you proposed only one small change in behaviour at this time?
- Can you reasonably expect the other person to agree to your request?
- Are you prepared to alter your own behaviour if your partner asks you to change? What are you prepared to change about your behaviour?
- What counterproposals do you anticipate and how will you answer them?
- Revise your SPECIFY lines now, if necessary.

⇒**Your CONSEQUENCES Lines**
- Have you stressed positive, rewarding consequences?
- Is the reward you selected really appropriate for the other person? Perhaps you should ask what you might do for the other person?
- Can you realistically carry through with these consequences?
- Revise your CONSEQUENCES lines now, if necessary.

APPENDIX E

Rules for Writing Asserive DESC Scripts

	No.	Do	Don't
D			
E	D1	Describe the other person's behaviour objectively.	Describe your emotional reaction to it.
S			
C	D2	Use concrete terms.	Use abstract, vague terms.
R	D3	Describe a specified time, place, and frequency of the action.	Generalize for "all time."
I			
B	D4	Describe the action, not the "motive."	Guess at your partner's motives or goals.
E			
E	E1	Express your feelings.	Deny your feelings.
X	E2	Express them calmly.	Unleash emotional outbursts.
P	E3	State feelings in a positive manner, as relating to a goal to be achieved.	State feelings negatively, making put-down or attack.
R			
E	E4	Direct yourself to the specific offending behaviour, not to the whole person.	Attack the entire character of the person.
S			
S			
	S1	Ask explicitly for change in your partner's behaviour.	Merely imply that you'd like a change.
S	S2	Request a small change.	Ask for too large a change.
P	S3	Request only one or two changes at one time.	Ask for too many changes.
E	S4	Specify the concrete actions you want to see stopped, and those you want to see performed.	Ask for changes in nebulous traits or qualities.
C			
I			
F	S5	Take account of whether your partner can meet your request without suffering large losses.	Ignore your partner's needs or ask only for your satisfaction.
Y			
	S6	Specify (if appropriate) what behaviour you are willing to change to make the agreement.	Consider that only your partner has to change.
C			
O	C1	Make the consequences explicit.	Be ashamed to talk about rewards and penalties.
N			
S	C2	Give a positive reward for change in the desired direction.	Give only punishments for lack of change.
E			
Q	C3	Select something that is desirable and reinforcing to your partner.	Select something that only you might find rewarding.
U			
E			
N	C4	Select a reward that is big enough to maintain the behaviour change.	Offer a reward you can't or won't deliver.
C			
E	C5	Select a punishment of a magnitude that "fits the crime" of refusing to change behaviour.	Make exaggerated threats.
S			

Psychoanalytic Psychotherapy with People in Abusive Relationships: Treatment Outcome

Rosemary Cogan
John H. Porcerelli

SUMMARY. Psychoanalytic perspectives on violence between partners is described and forms a foundation for an approach to group and individual psychotherapy of men and women in relationships in which there is physical violence between partners. The empirical results of a study of the outcome of psychoanalytically oriented psychotherapy are described. Nineteen men and 16 women completed research measures before beginning psychotherapy and after completing 16 sessions of group psychotherapy. Twelve people who completed group psychotherapy continued in individual psychotherapy and completed measures again after 16 sessions of individual psychotherapy, and nine people completed measures again after the 16 sessions of group and 32 sessions of individual psychotherapy. Statistical analyses addressed outcomes in terms of verbal and physical aggression and dysphoric affects and anger. Both research and clinical outcomes are discussed. *[Article copies available for a fee from The Haworth Document Delivery Service: 1-800-HAWORTH. E-mail address: <docdelivery@haworthpress.com> Website: <http://www.HaworthPress.com> © 2003 by The Haworth Press, Inc. All rights reserved.]*

Address correspondence to: Rosemary Cogan, PhD, ABPP, Department of Psychology, Texas Tech University, Lubbock, TX 79409-2051.

[Haworth co-indexing entry note]: "Psychoanalytic Psychotherapy with People in Abusive Relationships: Treatment Outcome." Cogan, Rosemary, and John H. Porcerelli. Co-published simultaneously in *Journal of Aggression, Maltreatment & Trauma* (The Haworth Maltreatment & Trauma Press, an imprint of The Haworth Press, Inc.) Vol. 7, No. 1/2 (#13/14), 2003, pp. 29-46; and: *Intimate Violence: Contemporary Treatment Innovations* (ed: Donald Dutton, and Daniel J. Sonkin) The Haworth Maltreatment & Trauma Press, an imprint of The Haworth Press, Inc., 2003, pp. 29-46. Single or multiple copies of this article are available for a fee from The Haworth Document Delivery Service [1-800-HAWORTH, 9:00 a.m. - 5:00 p.m. (EST). E-mail address: docdelivery@haworthpress.com].

http://www.haworthpress.com/store/product.asp?sku=J146
© 2003 by The Haworth Press, Inc. All rights reserved.
10.1300J146v07n01_03

KEYWORDS. Psychoanalytic, psychotherapy, partner violence

How one thinks about a clinical population or problem necessarily leads to a view of how to intervene in a helpful way. Our intent in what follows is to describe a way of looking at men and women in abusive relationships from a psychoanalytic perspective. From this vantage point, we will first discuss some cases. We will then consider somewhat more abstractly what general statements we might make about these cases and others like them and link these more general statements to empirical literature and to a therapeutic perspective. Finally, we will summarize the results of a study of the outcome of group treatment based upon our theoretical perspective and reflect on the implications of the treatment outcome data for understanding the dynamics of abusive relationships. We begin with the work of a noted psychotherapy researcher, Lester Luborsky.

Luborsky (1984) recognized that the stories people tell about themselves and others reflect a relationship template, also called internalized object relations. As he listened to people in psychotherapy, Luborsky realized that the stories about relationship episodes could be organized around three elements: a wish, need, or intention; a response of others; and a response of the narrator. He realized, further, that the core themes of the stories about present relationships, past relationships, and ideas about the relationship with the therapist often have the same dominant theme. Luborsky concluded that he had found a way of empirically studying Freud's concept of transference (Luborsky & Crits-Christoph, 1990; Luborsky, Crits-Christoph, & Mellon, 1986).

Luborsky had found a way of getting acquainted with people in either a clinical or a research setting by way of people's Core Conflictual Relationship Themes (CCRT; Luborsky, 1984). In a research setting, the CCRT can be identified from an interview. The person is asked simply to describe ten episodes important to them that have happened between them and another person, telling something about what happened and how the episode ended. The relationship episodes are recorded and transcribed. From the transcriptions, the CCRT of the person can be formulated and other interpretive coding can be done as well. The narratives are not understood as necessarily reflecting historical reality but are considered as having to do with representations of reality in the person's mind. This focus on narrative truth may help the reader in considering what is to come.

Our illustrative cast of characters includes four people met in the context of a research project. The first two people we will describe are a man and a woman who began psychotherapy with their partners in a psychotherapy research project for people in physically abusive relationships. The next two people are a man and a woman who completed the research protocol as non-clinical volunteers. Each of these people is representative of their respective groups in ways that matter to our thinking about abusive relationships. One sample relationship episode of each of the four people, each chosen as representative of a set of ten relationship episodes that the person described, is shown in Table 1.

CORE CONFLICTUAL RELATIONSHIP THEME

Consider without knowing any more about these people what we might learn about each from these episodes. We will begin with Luborsky's CCRT and then make inferences about underlying processes.

In the sample episode, Mr. A., a man in a physically abusive relationship, wants to be with both the other woman and his wife, and is concerned that other people–his wife in particular–will find out about his badness. He got mad at his son and wanted to hurt him by sending him away. Overall, his CCRT was this: He wants to have things his own way; others get mad at him and threaten to leave him; and he gets mad and hits them. At a more abstract level, this is a man who worries about a part of himself that he considers bad and greedy. The underlying danger is that his wife will find out what a bad person he is and leave him, which is quite frightening for him. Someone tells on him and Mr. A. becomes frightened and angry. He has few resources for dealing with his fears and is more comfortable being angry than being frightened. He turns the tables on his son and threatens him with what worries Mr. A. the most–abandonment. Mr. A.'s story is in real contrast to the representative episode of the man in a non-abusive relationship. Mr. N. says he wants to be treated fairly. He tells a story in which he experiences another man as being dishonest, and in response Mr. N. gets angry and decides not to do business with that person. His anger does not generalize to all people (nor to his family!) and is modulated.

In her sample episode, Mrs. A., a woman in an abusive relationship, presents herself as a young woman who wants to understand what her uncle is doing. He ignores her anxious confusion and intrudes by taking off his clothes, and she feels bewildered. Altogether, her CCRT was

TABLE 1. Representative Relationship Episodes of Men and Women in Abusive and Non-Abusive Relationships

---

Abusive Relationships

Mr. A.: I got up in the morning and started screaming at my son–he squealed on me about seeing that other lady. I'm screaming at him that I'm going to send him away. I just wanted to hurt him. Cause he, cause he hurt me.

Mrs. A.: I just go in my uncle's house. He comes out of the bathroom and he's naked and he sits down and watches TV and we talk as normal. I don't know. Before my aunt comes home, he puts his clothes on. I don't understand that.

Non-Abusive Relationships

Mr. N.: When the job was completed, I paid him for the work. He didn't pay the person he got the materials from and they sued me. To me there is a right and wrong. I'm very resentful toward that person and I don't do any business with him.

Mrs. N.: I picked up a word here and there that my son's girlfriend might be pregnant. I asked him: "Is she pregnant?" He just said, "No." And I knew if I pushed him he would fly off the handle. So I haven't said any more about it.

---

this: She wants to be left alone by confusing men; they bother her sexually; and she does not understand. Five of her episodes involved invasive sexual behavior by an adult toward a child. At a more abstract level, Mrs. A. is a woman who is worried about blatantly unacceptable behavior by grownups important to her and is concerned, in particular, about sexual matters. When her uncle exposes himself to her, she becomes confused, worries, and says with distress that she does not understand. "Not understanding" is one way Mrs. A. deals with anxiety and the fact that she goes to the house of this strange uncle (that is, this is something that has happened many times before) tells us something about her being drawn to the situation with her uncle, perhaps in the hope of being able to master her anxieties. In real contrast is the sample episode of a woman in a non-abusive relationship. Mrs. N. also wants to understand something about what happens between a man (her son) and a woman. She wants to understand her son in a non-intrusive way, without getting him too worried. He will not talk about what is going on, and she lets it go for the time being. She can manage her own concerns and respect her son's need not to talk quite yet.

Cogan, Porcerelli, Sharp, and Ballinger (2001) have explored the CCRTs of men and women in abusive relationships who were entering psychotherapy. For men in abusive relationships, the most frequent CCRT was this: He wants to dominate, others become either angry and resentful or unhelpful and uncooperative, and he becomes angry and resentful. For women in abusive relationships, the primary CCRT was this: She wants to overcome domination by avoiding conflicts or by dominating others, others become angry and resentful, and she becomes either angry and resentful or passive and submissive.

OBJECT RELATIONS

Relationship episode narratives can also be used to assess other enduring characteristics of the respondent, including object relations, which are another aspect of the templates that mediate interpersonal relations (Cogan & Porcerelli, 1996; Cogan, Porcerelli, & Dromgoole, 2001; Westen, 1991). In terms of object relations, Mr. A. has a marked lack of empathy. He makes no effort to understand why his son would tell on him, and his threatened punishment is extreme: "I'll send you away!" He expects relationships to be malevolent and punishments to be severe and traumatizing. His feelings involve rage and fear of abandonment. He might also be understood as saying in the interview, "Don't hold me responsible, or I will leave." One might expect that in psychotherapy, being found out and finding out about himself will be quite difficult for Mr. A.

In terms of object relations, Mr. N. experiences *some* individuals as being dishonest but this does not color his expectations of business people in general. It is *some* and not *all* contractors with whom he will not do business again as *some* people can be unjust. Mr. N. has internal standards of right and wrong. The episode may suggest that Mr. N. has concerns about aspects of himself having to do with dishonesty, and if he were to present for psychotherapy Mr. N. might be especially concerned about the right and wrong behavior of both himself and his therapist.

Mrs. A. experiences others as blatantly sexually inappropriate, over stimulating, confusing, and unempathic. The degree of her confusion suggests that she does not expect others to come to her aid in understanding this chaos and, in fact, there are no helpers in the sample story. Her relationship episodes were bleak and involved stories of sexual boundary violations by her stepfather and her mother, whom she describe as having run away with Mrs. A.'s first boyfriend, and wistful stories of herself as the helper of the down-and-out including physically, mentally, and emotionally disabled children. In her ten relationship episodes, only one helper appears, an aunt who rescues her from authorities searching for her when she ran away from home as a child. Her aloneness is evidently quite frightening to her and not wanting to be alone provides another unconscious reason for visiting the uncle. Given the lack of helpers or positive relationships in her thoughts, and given that the only helper who presented at all in her episodes was the rescuer of Mrs. A. when she was a runaway, one could anticipate that forming a therapeutic relationship will be difficult for her. In contrast is Mrs. N., who experiences others as doing things for reasons and experiences people as being invested in and concerned about each other. She experiences concern for her son and an emotional investment in protecting his feelings and their relationship.

HISTORIES OF MR. A. AND MRS. A.

To this point, we have made inferences about Mr. A. and Mrs. A. based on the stories they told about their relationships in an interview. Let us consider next something of their histories.

Mr. A. was a Hispanic man in his mid-thirties who presented himself as a kind of tough guy with bravado in the face of danger. He had a high school education and worked as a mechanic. He and his wife of six years had three children and were separated. They saw an announcement of the psychotherapy program in the local newspaper. They were interested in participating in the research as a full payment of fees for psychotherapy and came in the hope of getting back together again. Mr. A. had fights with a variety of people including men he worked with, men in his family, friends, and his wife. On the Conflict Tactics Scale (CTS; Straus, 1979) he said that once in the past year he had hit or tried to hit his wife with something. (Mrs. A., on the other hand, said he had threatened her with a knife or gun several times.) On the CTS, he reported that his wife had stomped out of the house once during a conflict. (She said that she had hit or tried to hit him with something twice.) Although Mr. A. was within normal limits on the Millon Multiphasic Clinical Inventory-II (MCMI-II; Millon, 1985), in his relationship interview he talked more than most other people about times when he had been drinking. On the MCMI-II, his wife showed a borderline profile with avoidant features.

Mrs. A. was a Caucasian woman in her early twenties who had completed two years of junior college. She and her husband had been married for a year and had no children when they were referred for psychotherapy by their employer because their fighting with each other was interfering with their work, which had to do with residential care of a special population. She seemed sad and somewhat preoccupied. On the CTS, she reported that within the past year her husband had beaten her up several times and she had slapped him half a dozen times. (Her husband reported that he had kicked, bit, or hit her with a fist once and that she had slapped him once in the past year.) On the MCMI-II, Mrs. A. showed a dependent, histrionic, and depressed profile and her husband showed elevations characteristic of someone with a borderline personality with manic-depressive features and drug dependence.

MEN AND WOMEN IN ABUSIVE RELATIONSHIPS

Mr. A. and Mrs. A. are like many of the people in abusive relationships who present for psychotherapy. We know that family violence is pervasive (e.g., Maguire & Pastore, 2001). In his work on couples, Kernberg (1995) writes of cycles of violence (see also Dutton, 2002), considering partner violence in the context of superego pathology. From Kernberg's psychoanalytic stance, there are both conscious and unconscious aspects of victimization, and people with long-standing personality problems distort their experiences of reality and involve others as part of an effort to reduce uncomfortable inner feelings, such as guilt.

Both the victim and the victimizer aspects of the person have to do with parts of the personality coming from feelings of vulnerability and helplessness from childhood. The internal experience of the man may be that the woman, through real or symbolic abandonment threats, is the victimizer. In his own mind, the man may experience himself as the threatened victim and he attacks to protect himself from his feelings of vulnerability and helplessness (e.g., Cogan, Porcerelli, & Dromgoole, 2001). This dynamic has to do with his internal experience and cannot be captured by an external view. The woman may respond to the development of the aggressor or victimizer part of herself by projecting it onto the man and the same defensive dynamic can develop as she experiences herself as the victim. For the man, the passivity of the victim experience is generally more threatening than the victimizer experience. For the woman, aggression is likely to be more threatening than the passive position and it is likely to be more bearable for the woman to experience the man as the aggressor. When aggression is expressed by the woman, it may be less severe, taken less seriously by both partners, and is often more symbolic.

Accepting the projections from the partner can confirm one's own bad feelings about himself or herself. If this same person can get the other to argue and fight, they can feel justified in allowing the victimizer part of him or herself to emerge. This can be rationalized as "fighting back to protect oneself." This is an example of Kernberg's (1995) descriptions of abusive couples engaging in sadomasochistic exchanges in sometimes interchangeable roles.

About 30% of the men and about 15% of the women who came to the psychotherapy research project for people in physically abusive relationships were referred by a legal or social service agency. When people come to see us for psychotherapy because they are unhappy and are concerned about what is happening for them, we are likely to be able to work together in psychotherapy. When someone comes to see us for psychotherapy but seems to have no wish to change, we take as our first task confronting the referred client in an effort to create an area in which shared work in psychotherapy may become possible.

PSYCHOANALYTIC GROUP AND INDIVIDUAL PSYCHOTHERAPY

Both the group and the individual psychotherapy were adapted from the psychoanalytic psychotherapy treatment manual of Luborsky (1984).

Group work. Group psychotherapy has been advocated in the family violence literature for both ideological and pragmatic reasons (c.f., Dutton, 1995; Edleson & Syers, 1990; Geffner & Rosenbaum, 1990).

In group psychoanalytic psychotherapy in this project, men's and women's groups are each led by a man and a woman who are advanced doctoral students in psychology, working as co-therapists. The groups are closed and meet for two hours twice a week with a fixed 16-session time limit, after which members choose to continue in individual psychotherapy, completing the research protocol after each 16 sessions of psychotherapy.

The groups are unstructured and the therapists work to understand and articulate what is happening in the group. The emphasis is on using the relationship of the group with the co-therapists as a vehicle through which thoughts and feelings could emerge and be talked about, understood, and integrated (i.e., process therapy). In our experience with both men's and women's groups, group members generally begin by allying with the same-sexed co-therapist and looking to the co-therapist of the same sex as the person who will supply answers. The group begins by almost completely excluding the co-therapist of the other sex. As the group settles itself and the avoidance of dealing with the co-therapist of the other sex becomes very clear, the co-therapist of the same sex brings to the attention of the group the fact that they seem to be avoiding the co-therapist. With that, it becomes possible for the group to talk with each other and the co-therapist of the same sex about the thoughts and feelings they have about the other sex and about how they imagine the relationship between the co-therapists to be (cf. shame detoxification in Wallace & Nosko, 2002). In men's groups, women are often experienced as powerful and withholding and the female co-therapist may find the resultant hostility of the men in group palpable and somewhat frightening. It becomes, then, the task of the male co-therapist to comment on the men's anxious denigration of his therapist-partner. In women's groups, the male co-therapist is often the object of considerable group hostility and denigration and the female co-therapist is able to bring this to the attention of the group. As affects of the group are experienced and articulated, it becomes possible to talk about the ideas associated with the feelings. As uncomfortable feelings and distressing thoughts are more understood, group members are more able to recognize and deal adaptively with what is happening (in group and in their lives). With improved adaptation, rage and other dysphoric affects should decrease and group members should be more able to experience positive affects.

In both men's and women's groups, it becomes increasingly possible to talk about partner violence in the context of feelings of helplessness, reality based dangers, and fears that are not quite in awareness (i.e., loss of the other, loss of love, concern about bodily integrity, and feelings of guilt; cf. Freud, 1926/1962). Partner violence can also be discussed in terms of the person's repeating actively what they have experienced as having been done passively to them at other times. For the reader interested in learning more about this kind of group work, important works include Bion (1961/1992), who provides a lively "experience near" description; Bennis and Shepard (1956), offering a more theoretical treatment; and Jennings (1987), who has discussed unstructured group psychotherapy for battering men (see also Dutton, 2002).

Individual work. In individual psychoanalytic psychotherapy, it becomes possible to work with the more specific conflictual themes of the individual. The regular schedule of 50-minute individual therapy sessions is arranged by agreement between the person and the therapist.

The therapist maintains a position of listening and entering the conversation to help the person to explore their thoughts and feelings. As themes become clear, the therapist puts the operative theme into words. Because what happens in the relationship with the therapist is especially vivid and fruitful in helping people understand themselves, the work emphasizes what is happening in the therapeutic relationship. The dynamics of the relationship with the therapist can then be seen also in the relationships of the person with their partner and others in the wider world and the links to early past relationships can be recognized and talked about.

People in psychoanalytic psychotherapy are usually surprised to realize that they have themes in their relationships with others and surprised also to begin to recognize some of the ways they defend themselves from what worries them. Mr. A., who experienced other people as getting mad at him and threatening to leave, knew he did not want his wife to leave him; however, before psychotherapy he had not realized that his fear of being abandoned was originally a childhood fear. For quite a while, Mr. A. really believed his therapist would leave him for one reason or another. He was not at all aware that his terrible anxiety about being left contributed, paradoxically, to his behaving quite badly to the people he cared most about. He was in a perpetual rage toward his wife ("She's cheating on me," and "She's going to leave–I just know she is") and behaved so badly toward her that, indeed, she *did* leave him! He also behaved badly toward his therapist, but in the therapeutic relationship it was possible to point this out to Mr. A. ("You keep expecting me to leave and then you miss an appointment or come late when you have the idea that missing or being late will make me get mad and leave. You're trying to set things up so you'll make me leave. If you run me off, you won't have to worry about my leaving you because you'll have made it happen all by yourself and that's not as scary for you as waiting around to be left by me").

By becoming aware, talking about, and tolerating uncomfortable feelings associated with unfamiliar or unwanted aspects of the self, the person can develop a more integrated, cohesive picture of himself or herself. The person can begin to accept, partly by identifying with the tolerance of the therapist, their own wishes, fears, and ways of managing anxiety and depression, and can develop a greater sense of self-acceptance. For some people in treatment, past and present can be linked. Eventually a person may be able to experience the long-standing conflicts and fears associated with infantile conflicts and can begin to deal with past hurts and fears with an adult mind (e.g.,

"When I need my wife and she's busy taking care of our little boy, that doesn't mean she's left me. I can go and be with my family instead of getting mad").

To make it possible for core conflictual relationship themes to come into the therapeutic relationship where they can be most directly experienced and talked about, the therapist is rather neutral. It may seem at first somewhat paradoxical that the person coming in for psychotherapy in a program for people in abusive partner relationships is, working this way, not directed to talk about any particular subject. In one instance, 16 sessions of psychotherapy focused (superficially) almost entirely on the man's softball games: Was his wife mad at him because he was on a softball team? Would she and the children come and watch the big game and cheer when he did well? Would she be there when he got home? If she was at home, would there be dinner? Would he be too tired to do chores? It was a productive psychotherapy and the conversations about softball were really all about his relationship with his wife and family.

The very lack of direction of this kind of therapeutic conversation creates considerable anxiety for the person because the non-directive presence of the therapist makes it inevitable that the person will construct the situation to reflect what they expect and fear in all significant relationships. For example, if the person expects to "con" the therapist, once this becomes evident, the therapist is able to comment on the "con" and can put pressure on the person's ways of trying to avoid anxiety until the person does experience anxiety. An example of such a confrontation might be: "You're telling me it's everybody else's fault but you didn't show up last week and you were ten minutes late tonight. Seems like you're trying to con me like you've tried to con everybody else. Evidently you'd rather go back to jail than get serious." Although limits can be and are set as necessary to prevent potentially harmful acting out by the person, in working with people in abusive relationships, our experience has been that about two-thirds of the people who come to see us are already quite anxious and able to work without any remarkable limit-setting or confrontations.

For the reader interested in knowing more about this approach to individual psychotherapy, Luborsky (1984) and Book (1997) provide clear descriptions, and Auld and Hyman (1991) provide a more detailed discussion of theoretical and pragmatic aspects of psychoanalytic psychotherapy. Young and Gerson (1991) are among those who have written about some of the defensive mechanisms involved in partner violent relationships and Lundberg (1990) has described a two track treatment approach in which an insight-oriented treatment is available for people with greater ego-strength.

OUTCOME OF PSYCHODYNAMIC GROUP PSYCHOTHERAPY

As part of a psychotherapy outcome study, we present here some of the outcome results of psychoanalytic psychotherapy. These men and women came to see one of us (R.C.) in the context of a university-based research program studying the dynamics of spouse abuse and change in psychotherapy. The program required that the person have experienced at least one incident of physical abuse in a relationship with a partner in the previous twelve months, that substance abuse not be a major interfering problem, and that the person could read and write in English to complete a research-oriented intake of several hours. Of 59 people who began group therapy, 24 dropped out and 19 men and 16 women completed 16 sessions of group.[1] Eleven people, including five men and six women, continued in psychotherapy and completed 16 sessions of group and then 16 sessions of individual psychotherapy. Of these eleven, nine people, including five men and four women, continued in individual psychotherapy and completed a third set of 16 sessions, then stopping psychotherapy.[2]

To have enough people to form a group, there was sometimes a delay of as long as six weeks before people could begin psychotherapy. When this happened, people were asked to complete the research measures a second time a day or two before they began group. Although the intake itself may have had implicit properties of an intervention, this test-retest control condition is a useful backdrop for considering the effects of group psychotherapy. Statistical comparisons were made of the first and second pre-treatment control reports of 17 people, and there were no differences between the two reports. Here we will compare changes over time among men and women after 16, 32, and 48 sessions of psychoanalytic psychotherapy.

Participants

Data from 19 men and 16 women who completed 16 or more sessions of group psychotherapy are included here. The men averaged 33.6 years of age and 13.4 years of education. The women averaged 34.4 years of age and 13.0 years of education. Fourteen men and 13 women were

White (non-Hispanic), and four men and two women were Hispanic. Most were employed, including 16 of the men and 10 of the women. Among those who completed 16 sessions of group psychotherapy, 45% of the men and 19% of the women had been referred by a legal or social service agency.

Measures

The measures to be considered here were chosen for a variety of reasons. Partner violence was a presenting problem and for a treatment to be considered effective certainly partner violence would have to be reduced. The theory of psychotherapy makes affects of special importance and the literature of family violence shows that depression and anger are marked among men (Beasley & Stoltenberg, 1992; Bland & Orn, 1986; Dutton, 1988; Hamberger & Hastings, 1988; Tolman & Bennett, 1991) and women (Bland & Orn, 1986; Dutton & Painter, 1981). In response to psychotherapy, unpleasurable affects should ultimately be reduced and positive affect increased.

Partner violence. Partner violence was measured with the Conflict Tactics Scale (CTS; Straus, 1979). The CTS is an 18-item self-report measure that assesses reasoning (3 items), verbal aggression (6 items), and physical violence (8 items). Of the eight physical violence items, five describe severe violence or battering by the respondent, and their report of the occurrence of each by their partner. Respondents indicate the frequency of occurrence of each item in a given time period on a 7-point scale ranging from "never" to "more than 20 times."

Affect. Affect was measured with the Multiple Affect Adjective Checklist (MAACL; Zuckerman & Lubin, 1965) and the State Anger Scale (SAS; Spielberger, Jacobs, Russell, & Crane, 1983). The MAACL is a 132-item self-report measure on which respondents check the adjectives that apply to them. Dysphoria (Hunsley, 1990; Zuckerman, Lubin, & Rinck, 1983) is the factor that we will consider here. The SAS includes 15 self-report items. Respondents rate each item on a scale ranging from "almost never" to "almost always"; scores range from 10 to 40, with higher scores indicating more anger. State anger concerns feelings of anger at the time of response.

Data Analyses

Data were analyzed using a series of multivariate factorial repeated measures analysis of variance tests comparing the responses of men and women before and after treatment blocks and with follow-up analysis of variance tests.

RESULTS

Violence. As can be seen in Figure 1, violence of the men and the women decreased[3] with treatment. Among the women, violence decreased in relation to amount of psychotherapy. Among the men, however, with 16 sessions of group psychotherapy, physical violence had not completely dropped out even with the scrutiny and support of on-going psychotherapy. Although physical violence was absent for most men, two men reported episodes of severe violence during psychotherapy. After 32 sessions of psychotherapy (16 sessions of group followed by 16 sessions of individual psychotherapy), verbal and physical aggression had both decreased. After 48 sessions of psychotherapy (16 sessions of group followed by 32 sessions of individual psychotherapy), physical aggression reported by the men remained at low levels while verbal aggression increased. We know that character change requires several years of intense psychoanalytic treatment, generally lasting for about five years (Doidge, 1997; Doidge, Simon, Gillies, & Ruskin, 1994). In the present study, anger became less problematic; after 48 sessions of psychotherapy, these men were able to experience and express anger verbally without escalating to physical violence (see also reference to Prochaska et al. in Dutton, 2002).

Affect. Among both men and women, dysthymia decreased early in psychotherapy (i.e., after 16 sessions of group psychotherapy) and remained at reduced levels as psychotherapy continued. State anger decreased slightly among the men and remained stable over the course of psychotherapy among the women (see Figure 2).

CONCLUSIONS

We have discussed how psychoanalytic psychotherapy can be an effective treatment modality for men and women in abusive relationships. Violence can be limited, depression and anxiety reduced, and positive feelings can increase. With 16 sessions of group psychotherapy, people can begin to recognize that factors outside of their awareness operate to lead them into unhappy situations. As they become aware of repetitive

FIGURE 1. Verbal and Physical Aggression by Men and Women Before Psychotherapy and After 16, 32, or 48 Sessions of Psychotherapy

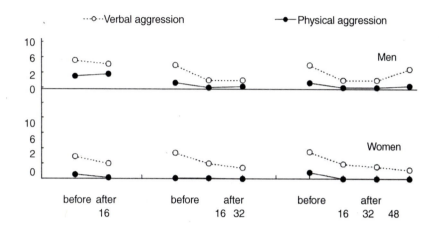

FIGURE 2. Dysthymia and Anger in Men and Women Before Psychotherapy and After 16, 32, or 48 Sessions of Psychotherapy

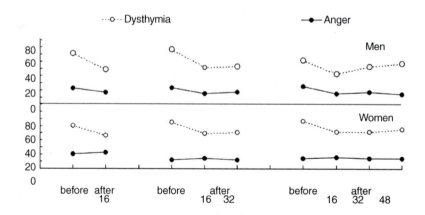

maladaptive patterns they can become less driven to unhappy outcomes. We recall, for example, one man (representative of several who were court referred and unlikely to continue beyond 16 sessions of psychotherapy) for whom we organized his theme quite simply: "When you feel bad about yourself, it seems like you shoot yourself in the foot." In 16 sessions of psychotherapy, this man began to recognize when he was about to "shoot himself in the foot," and he was better able to recognize that he must be feeling bad about himself for some reason and then to stop the self-defeating behavior. The therapeutic results were of value to him even though the work was quite limited. In contrast is the outcome of a woman in the abusive families treatment program who completed a planned termination after about two years of psychotherapy with a considerable understanding of her own dynamics. Not only was her marriage free from further violence, but she and her partner were also able to enjoy themselves together!

It is not easy for people to continue in psychotherapy. Our experience has been that people are more likely to complete group than individual psychotherapy (and least likely of all to complete couples therapy). People are more likely to continue in the intensive individual psychotherapy, which we believe is most effective, after an experience with group psychotherapy. Clinically, it seems likely that in group therapy, the felt safety provided by other group members makes it possible for people in abusive relationships to get acquainted with therapists and therapy without the intensity of the individual therapeutic relationship. While group therapy can be practical, it is not and cannot always be available because arranging for groups also presents practical problems and individual psychotherapy can be a viable option in working with men and women in abusive relationships.

In psychoanalytic psychotherapy, as conflicts outside of awareness are understood and re-worked, there is less distortion of the other people. When experiences of others are not so distorted, others can also be treated with more empathy and more understanding because they are experienced as individuals with their own particular qualities. As changes occur and the partner can be seen as a person with his or her own thoughts and feelings, and his or her own strengths and weaknesses, the partner can be appreciated and, finally, loved.

NOTES

1. Of 101 people who completed intakes before group psychotherapy, 35% completed 16 sessions. In contrast, of 69 people who completed intakes before individual psychotherapy, 19% completed 16 sessions. This difference in the likelihood of completing psychotherapy is congruent with the findings of Harris, Savage, Jones, and Brooke (1988).

2. Several people continued in individual psychotherapy for several years.

3. In 9 instances, both partners completed the first treatment block and completed both pre- and post-treatment measures. The reports of these people about violence by their partners confirmed the self-reports of both men and women.

REFERENCES

Auld, F., & Hyman, M. (1991). *Resolution of inner conflict: An introduction to psychoanalytic therapy*. Washington, D.C.: American Psychological Association.

Beasley, R., & Stoltenberg, C. D. (1992). Personality characteristics of male spouse abusers. Professional Psychology: *Research and Practice, 23,* 310-317.

Bennis, W. G., & Shepard, H. A. (1956). A theory of group development. *Human Relations, 9,* 415-437.

Bion, W. R. (1961/1992). *Experiences in groups and other papers.* New York: Routledge.

Bland, R. C., & Orn, H. (1986). Family violence and psychiatric disorder. *Canadian Journal of Personality, 31,* 129-137.

Book, H. E. (1998). *How to practice brief psychodynamic psychotherapy: The core Conflictual Relationship Theme method.* Washington, D.C.: American Psychological Association.

Cogan, R., & Porcerelli, J. H. (1996). Object relations in abusive partner relationships: An empirical investigation. *Journal of Personality Assessment, 66,* 106-115.

Cogan, R., Porcerelli, J. H., & Dromgoole, K. (2001). Psychodynamics of partner, stranger, and generally violent male college students. *Psychoanalytic Psychology, 18,* 515-533.

Cogan, R., Porcerelli, J. H., Sharp, D., & Ballinger, B. (2001). Core Conflictual Relationship Themes of men and women who are violent toward their partners. *Psychological Reports, 89,* 672-674.

Doidge, N. (1997). Empirical evidence for the efficacy of psychoanalytic psychotherapies and psychoanalysis: An overview. *Psychoanalytic Inquiry, 17* (Suppl.), 102-150.

Doidge, N., Simon, B., Gillies, L. A., & Ruskin, R. (1994). Characteristics of psychoanalytic patients under a nationalized health plan: DSM-II-R diagnoses, previous treatment and childhood traumata. *American Journal of Psychiatry, 151,* 586-590.

Dutton, D. G. (1988). Profiling of wife assaulters: Preliminary evidence for a trimodal analysis. *Violence and Victims, 3,* 5-29.

Dutton, D. G. (1995). *The domestic assault of women: Psychological and criminal justice perspectives* (Rev. ed.). Vancouver, BC: UBC Press.

Dutton, D. G. (2002). Treatment of assaultiveness. *Journal of Aggression, Maltreatment, & Trauma, 7*(1/2), 7-128.

Dutton, D., & Painter, S. L. (1981). Traumatic bonding: The development of emotional attachments in battered women and other relationships of intermittent abuse. *Victimology: An International Journal, 6,* 139-155.

Edleson, J. L., & Syers, M. (1990). Relative effectiveness of group treatments for men who batter. *Social Work Research & Abstracts, 26,* 10-17.

Freud, S. (1962). Inhibitions, symptoms and anxiety. In J. Strachey (Ed. & Trans.), *The standard edition of the complete psychological works of Sigmund Freud* (Vol. 20, pp. 75-156). London: Hogarth Press. (Original work published 1926).

Geffner, R., & Rosenbaum, A. (1990). Characteristics and treatment of batterers. *Behavioral Sciences and the Law, 8*, 131-140.

Hamberger, L. K., & Hastings, J. E. (1988). Skills training for treatment of spouse abusers: An outcome study. *Journal of Family Violence, 3*, 121-130.

Harris, R., Savage, S., Jones, T., & Brooke, W. (1988). A comparison of treatments for abusive men and their partners within a family-service agency. *Canadian Journal of Community Mental Health, 7*, 147-155.

Hunsley, J. (1990). Dimensionality of the Multiple Affect Adjective Check List–Revised: A comparison of factor analytic procedures. *Journal of Psychopathology and Behavioral Assessment, 12*, 81-91.

Jennings, J. L. (1987). History and issues in the treatment of battering men: A case for unstructured group therapy. *Journal of Family Violence, 2*, 193-213.

Kernberg, O. F. (1995). *Love relations: Normality and pathology*. New Haven: Yale University Press.

Luborsky, L. (1984). *Principles of psychoanalytic psychotherapy: A manual for supportive-expressive treatment*. New York: Basic Books.

Luborsky, L., & Crits-Christoph, P. (1990). *Understanding transference: The Core Conflictual Relationship Theme Method*. New York: Basic Books.

Luborsky, L., Crits-Christoph, P., & Mellon, J. (1986). The advent of objective measures of the transference concept. *Journal of Consulting and Clinical Psychology, 54*, 39-47.

Lundberg, S. G. (1990). Domestic violence: A psychodynamic approach and implications for treatment. *Psychotherapy, 27*, 243-248.

Maguire, K., & Pastore, A. L. (Eds.). (2001). *Sourcebook of criminal justice statistics*. Retrieved August 26, 2002, from <http://www.albany.edu/sourcebook/>.

Millon, T. (1985). *Millon Clinical Multiaxial Inventory-II*. Minneapolis, MN: National Computer Systems.

Spielberger, C. D., Jacobs, G., Russell, S., & Crane, R. S. (1983). Assessing anger: The State-Trait Anger Scale. In J. N. Butcher & C. D. Spielberger (Eds.), *Advances in personality assessment* (Vol. 2, pp. 159-187). Hillsdale, NJ: Erlbaum.

Straus, M. A. (1979). Measuring intra-family conflict and violence: The Conflict Tactics (CT) Scale. *Journal of Marriage and the Family, 41*, 75-88.

Tolman, R. M., & Bennett, L. W. (1991). A review of quantitative research on men who batter. *Journal of Interpersonal Violence, 5*, 87-118.

Wallace, R., & Nosko, A. (2002). Shame in male spouse abusers and its treatment in group therapy. *Journal of Aggression, Maltreatment, & Trauma, 7*(1/2), 47-74.

Westen, D. (1991). Social cognition and object relations. *Psychological Bulletin, 109*, 429-455.

Young, G. H., & Gerson, S. (1991). New psychoanalytic perspectives on masochism and spouse abuse. *Psychotherapy, 28*, 30-38.

Zuckerman, M., & Lubin, B. (1965). *Manual for the Multiple Affect Adjective Check List*. San Diego: Educational and Industrial Testing Service.

Zuckerman, M., Lubin, B., & Rinck, C. M. (1983). Construction of new scales of the multiple affect adjective check list. *Journal of Behavioral Assessment, 5*, 119-120.

Shame in Male Spouse Abusers and Its Treatment in Group Therapy

Robert Wallace
Anna Nosko

SUMMARY. The authors offer a social group work model for working with abusive men. They integrate affect and attachment theory in their exploration of the theoretical linkages between shame and anger. Through exploring the ways in which group structure and processes evolve, they demonstrate that group provides a framework through which men's shame and anger can be unlinked. They also demonstrate that the social relatedness group generates can help repair earlier attachment anxieties. This permits men to acquire non-violent means of dealing with the shame-based responses that are at the core of violent and abusive behavior. The authors also provide a description of the interventions used to detoxify shame in a group context. *[Article copies available for a fee from The Haworth Document Delivery Service: 1-800-HAWORTH. E-mail address: <docdelivery@haworthpress.com> Website: <http://www.HaworthPress.com> © 2003 by The Haworth Press, Inc. All rights reserved.]*

KEYWORDS. Partner abuse, abusiveness, social group work, shame, anger, affect theory, attachment theory

Address correspondence to: Robert Wallace and Anna Nosko, Family Service Association of Toronto, 355 Church Street, Toronto, Ontario, M5B 1Z8, Canada.

[Haworth co-indexing entry note]: "Shame in Male Spouse Abusers and Its Treatment in Group Therapy." Wallace, Robert, and Anna Nosko. Co-published simultaneously in *Journal of Aggression, Maltreatment & Trauma* (The Haworth Maltreatment & Trauma Press, an imprint of The Haworth Press, Inc.) Vol. 7, No. 1/2 (#13/14), 2003, pp. 47-74; and: *Intimate Violence: Contemporary Treatment Innovations* (ed: Donald Dutton, and Daniel J. Sonkin) The Haworth Maltreatment & Trauma Press, an imprint of The Haworth Press, Inc., 2003, pp. 47-74. Single or multiple copies of this article are available for a fee from The Haworth Document Delivery Service [1-800-HAWORTH, 9:00 a.m. - 5:00 p.m. (EST). E-mail address: docdelivery@haworthpress.com].

http://www.haworthpress.com/store/product.asp?sku=J146
© 2003 by The Haworth Press, Inc. All rights reserved.
10.1300J146v07n01_04

Recent years have seen growing attention paid to the issue of shame and psychotherapy. Of interest is the fact that the anger literature often intersects with that on shame (Lewis, 1971, 1987; Morrison, 1989; Nathanson, 1987a, 1989, 1992; Kaufman, 1989, 1992; Kohut, 1978; Miller, 1981), leading to a consideration of the relationship between shame and the genesis and treatment of violent behaviour. The treatment model developed over ten years of clinical work with abusive men by Wallace and Nosko (Nosko & Wallace, 1988; Wallace & Nosko, 1993) is based on the understanding of this linkage as provided by affect theory. The model is designed to select, through an assessment process, men whose anger is paired with shame. This therefore excludes men whose pathology is unrelated to the experience of shame (e.g., anti-social personality disorders). Shame and its relationship to anger and violence are kept foreground in the entire treatment framework informing all aspects of group structure. The groups we have delivered have been 20 to 24 weeks in duration, but we believe that an ideal group would extend for at least 36 weeks. This chapter will operationalize the treatment of shame in group work with male spouse abusers. It is important to state, however, that the work reflected in this material has been applied primarily to a screened voluntary population. As many authors have pointed out (Dutton, 1995; Saunders, 1992), the population of abusers is not homogenous; different categories of men may require different therapeutic approaches.

THE LITERATURE OF SHAME

In their seminal psychoanalytic study of shame and guilt, Piers and Singer (1953) argued that shame was an outgrowth of the failure to achieve the goals of the ego ideal, positing it as separate from the super-ego. They suggested that "behind the feeling of shame stands not the fear of hatred, but the fear of contempt which, on an even deeper level of the unconscious, spells the fear of abandonment, the death by emotional starvation" (p. 29). This theme was reiterated by Erich Fromm (1956), who suggested that "The awareness of human separation, without the reunion by love–is the source of shame" (p. 8). In later years, Helen Block Lewis (1971, 1987) elaborated on the relational aspect of shame, arguing that it was an inherently social affect. She also related shame to the experience of narcissism, suggesting that grandiosity represented a defense against the hatred of the self-experienced in shame. Experientially, shame, to her, "is a negative experience of the self; it is an 'implosion' or a momentary 'destruction' of the self in acute self denigration" (1987, p. 95). The idea that shame was related to the very quality of the self also appeared in Wurmser (1987), while the relationship between shame and narcissism was carried forward by Morrison (1986, 1987, 1989). Writing from the perspective of Self Psychology, he argued that there is a tension-generating dialectic between "narcissistic grandiosity and desire for perfection, and the archaic sense of self as flawed, inadequate, and inferior following the realization of separateness from, and dependence on, objects" (1989, p. 66).

Shame receives a different treatment in affect theory. Tomkins (1987) maintains that it is one of nine innate affects that are physiological in origin. Tomkins defines affect as the physiological basis of emotion: It is a predetermined biological response to stimuli, which manifests on various sites on the body. Feeling is the conscious awareness of the physiological arousal of affect; this is differentiated from emotion, which is the memory of associated affective experiences (Nathanson, 1987a, 1992). The majority of the effects of shame are evident on the face, or "the display board of the affect system" (Nathanson, 1994). Each of the nine affects has a range of experienced intensity and can be amplified or moderated by a change in stimulus or by co-assembly with other affects (Tomkins, 1987). Nathanson (1992) and Kaufman (1989) also suggest that affects can be co-assembled or linked with one another, with drives or with cognitions, so that the experience of one affect may produce the experience of others. Finally, affect broadcasts from individual to individual; thus, it has a contagious quality (Nathanson, 1992).

As Nathanson (1992) points out, Tomkins (1987) argued that groups of affective responses are linked over time to produce scenes which themselves link together to form scripts. Scripts embody generalized rules and assumptions about the nature of life and can themselves generate further affect in a feedback process.

Among the nine basic affects, shame is seen as auxiliary, existing only in relation to other affects and specifically serving to inhibit, but not eliminate, the affective arousal of the interest-excitement and/or enjoyment-joy continuums. The purpose of inhibition is to ensure the protection of the individual by decreasing interest when interest is not reciprocated or is mismatched. On a social level, however, this means that when experiencing shame, individuals pursue the resumption of relationship with the other as it was before relations became problematic (Tomkins, 1987).

SHAME AND ANGER

The association between shame and anger has a lengthy history. Helen Block Lewis (1987) argues that shame produces humiliated fury "that is inevitably directed against the offending other, and retaliating impulses are evoked to 'turn the tables' on the other" (p. 102). Anger then becomes a method of by-passing shame, which she describes as an excruciating experience of the self as imploded. The relationship of shame to anger is also evident in studies of narcissism. Kohut (1978), Miller (1981) and Morrison (1989), for example, see anger and rage as a manifestation of narcissistic vulnerability. Retzinger (1991) proposes that in the context of lost or endangered emotional bonds, rage is "a protective measure utilized as an insulation against shame" (p. 39).

In affect theory, anger and rage are affects embedded in the defensive scripts designed to contain shame (Kaufman, 1989; Nathanson, 1987a, 1992). To Kaufman (1989, 1992), anger changes the interpersonal field in a way that attributes power to the self rather than to the shame-inducing other. Anger wards off the terror of abandonment and, in establishing dominance interpersonally, allows the individual to induce shame in the other (see Dutton, this issue).

Nathanson (1992) also sees anger as a defensive script that is activated as the last stage in the process of negotiating shame. The first stage consists of the triggering event, which impedes positive affect. The second involves physiological arousal. Stage three, the cognitive phase, provides access to the repertoire of scripts that organize all the experiences of shame. In stage four, defensive patterns are activated. An understanding of the individual's reactions to shame is produced by exploring the cognitive phase of shame where memories from previous life experiences are identifiable (see Sonkin & Dutton, 2002).

Nathanson (1992) describes four major defensive patterns, each of which embodies a library of scripts that help the individual manage his/her experience of shame. The first two patterns represent a polarity between withdrawal and avoidance. Withdrawal into self and so away from others is accompanied by the affects of distress and fear; avoidance involves the use of strategies that create smoke screens and so distract from and disavow shame. It is accompanied by excitement, fear, and enjoyment. The second set of patterns include "attack self" and "attack other." In "attack other," the goal is to attribute the state of inferiority, powerlessness, or estrangement to the other in a process of projective identification. The associated affect is anger. "Attack self" scripts accept "a reduced sense of self" to protect from the sense of isolation that shame confers and are associated with self-disgust and self-dismissal. In the treatment of abusers, the attack other strategy is most commonly encountered and forms the focus of treatment because it is central to the use of violence as a controlling behaviour. This is not to say, however, that the other strategies do not present themselves in relation to different stimuli, such as those found in a work environment, and that they therefore do not need to be addressed.

It is also important to note Nathanson's (1992) argument that shame can become central in the organization of the self. Following Stern (1985), he suggests that the self is an 'experiential integration' rather than a cognitive construct. It is a summation of experience born in an interpersonal context. Shame can produce, then, "a sense of an incompetent self" (p. 210) that adopts a defensive style falling within the 'compass of shame.' Shame and its defensive strategies always have significance for the interpersonal relationships that the individual forms. This idea suggests a natural linkage with attachment theory that, Nathanson (1992) argues, lacks an analysis of the emotional dimensions of attachment. As we will later suggest, this is important in the context of understanding the role of anxious attachment and shame in the abusive relationship.

RESEARCH ON ABUSERS

Descriptions of characteristics of male abusers are varied in the literature profiling abusers. They can be summarized as follows. Abusive men are highly social but lack the internal dynamics or balance to achieve positive social interaction (Bersani, Chen, Pendleton, & Denton, 1992); they are less assertive (Dutton & Strachan, 1987); they exhibit low self esteem (Goldstein & Rosenbaum, 1986); they have high power needs (Dutton & Strachan, 1987); they experience more depression (Hastings & Hamberger, 1988); they may exhibit characteristics of personality disorders including borderline, narcissistic, passive dependent, and passive aggressive (Caesar, 1988; Hamberger & Hastings, 1986; Hastings & Hamberger, 1988); they are likely to experience chronic alcohol abuse (Tolman & Bennett, 1990); they are more likely to feel angry in situations of conflict or relationship anxiety (Tolman & Bennett, 1990); and they exhibit difficulty with developing intimate relationships based on mutuality, show rapid decompensation in their problem-solving abilities, and tend to be moody, impulsive, self-centered, demanding, and aloof (Barnett & Hamberger, 1992).

Dutton and his colleagues have also done considerable work exploring the dynamics of the abuser. Following Hastings and Hamberger (1988), Dutton and Starzomski (1993) argue that there is an increasing body of evidence correlating abuse with psychopathology, and in particular with a Borderline Personality Organization (BPO), which is defined as a tendency to (1) form intense, unstable interpersonal relationships characterized by the "intermittent undermining of the significant other, manipulation, and masked dependency; (2) an unstable sense of self, with intolerance of being alone and abandonment anxiety; and (3) intense anger, demandingness and impulsivity, usually tied to substance abuse or promiscuity" (p. 327). The results of their study of 120 abusers showed that the BPO and anger scores of the men correlated significantly with wives' reports of both physical and psychological abuse.

Two other studies by Dutton and his associates are important to note. In the first, BPO scores significantly correlated with self-reported verbal and physical abuse leading to the conclusion that "high BPO men are more angered and more assaultive in response to intimacy issues and may be angered by the very experience of intimacy" (Dutton, 1994a, p. 274). In another study, they found that a high correlation exists between BPO scores and fearful attachment with a lesser but still significant correlation between BPO scores and preoccupied attachment. The authors therefore concluded that anxious attachment patterns could be a risk factor for abuse (Dutton, Saunders, Starzomski, & Bartholomew, 1994).

Finally, in a study of 140 abusers, Dutton, van Ginkel and Starzomski (1995) shifted their attention to the issue of shame, exploring the relationship between shame-proneness (measured by childhood recollection of parental shaming behaviors), features of abusiveness (anger, BPO, and chronic trauma symptoms) and abusiveness itself. Their findings demonstrated a significant correlation between shame scores, BPO scores, and anger scores. Also of interest, they found that childhood shaming experiences were of greater importance than a history of physical abuse in the "abusive personality" (Dutton, van Ginkel & Starzomski, 1995, p. 10), although the presence of violence in childhood was found to have a modeling influence. In other words, the experience of violence was a necessary but not a sufficient condition for the perpetration of violence in adulthood. In *The Batterer: A Psychological Profile*, Dutton (1995) also added insecure attachment to the mother to the other two preconditions. Dutton, van Ginkel and Starzomski (1995) further hypothesized that attacks on the global self, which were at the heart of shaming experiences, directly related to the formation of Borderline Personality Organization.

In summarizing his research findings, Dutton (1995) noted the strong correlation between borderline scores and the following features of cyclical abusiveness: anger, jealousy, and a tendency to blame women for relationship difficulties. In synthesizing his findings, Dutton argued that jealousy was consistent with abandonment fears and that high borderline scores correlated with angry or ambivalent attachment, leading him to suggest that ambivalent attachment and the borderline personality are almost synonymous. He wrote that "These findings reinforced a common early origin of borderline personality . . . : childhood abuse, shaming, and weak attachments" (p. 154).

The treatment model that we have developed over the last eleven years draws upon the theoretical and research findings summarized above. As we have seen, abusive men tend to conform to the profile of the Borderline Personality Organization, which involves an unstable sense of self, masked dependency, intense and unstable personal relationships, and intense anger, demandingness, and impulsivity. Dutton and colleagues linking of Borderline Personality Organization with anxious attachment, early life recollections of shaming, and abusive behaviors is consistent with the notion that for many abusers, violence is a manifestation of a shame-based personality, in which shame, or an experience of self as inherently defective, is masked in a defensive script. In this scenario, shame and the anger-rage continuum are co-assembled and linked to scripts governing assumptions about the insecure nature of relationships. The result is an investment in "Attack Other" defensive strategies, which protect the individual from the painful experience of seeing self as defective and, therefore, unlovable. In this respect, anger, and violence become a means of ensuring that the other does not leave the orbit of the self through real or feared separation (Wallace & Nosko, 1993). This argument provides a bridge to attachment theory, which posits that the function of anger "is to dissuade the attachment figure from carrying out the threat (of abandonment)" (Bowlby, 1988, p. 30). For the insecurely attached individual, anger thus becomes the means of repairing the interpersonal bridge that is always put in jeopardy by the experience of shame. On this basis, we believe that there is a strong link between shame, which is at the heart of the fear of abandonment, and the anger accompanying it.

In summary, we suggest that in a substantial subsection of abusers, anger and rage, controlling behaviors, and violence mask shame. As

Kaufman (1989) suggests, they represent an attempt to alter the interpersonal field by shifting the focus of perceived dominance. In experiencing himself as angry and powerful, the abuser uses violence to defend against the fear of abandonment central to shame and to project the shame onto the other in a process of projective identification (Dutton, 1995; Wallace & Nosko, 1993). This is consistent with the suggestions of Alonso and Rutan (1988), Morrison (1987, 1989), and Hahn (1994) that projective identification provides an important defense against the experience of shame and helps us understand the purpose of the abuser's controlling behaviors. It also reinforces the importance of group as the preferred method of treatment.

SOCIAL FACTORS IN THE ETIOLOGY OF VIOLENCE

Before applying this analysis to our intervention model, however, it is useful to consider the impact of male socialization as a factor in abuse. We do not argue that abuse is purely psychological in origin; it has a social dimension as well. As Nathanson (1992) points out, the defensive strategy used in dealing with shame is impacted by circumstance and notions of what is socially acceptable. Thus, an individual may use "attack self" strategies in an employment situation, and "attack other" strategies in an intimate relationship. It must then be asked what influences the individual's choice of defensive strategies in a given context.

Although we do not believe that the individual's adoption of violence is usefully explained by sociological theory (it is a different order of explanation unsuited to understanding a particular individual's life choices), abusers do live in a social context that establishes the boundaries of acceptable action. For this reason, feminist theories are useful in understanding the broader context of abuse but are very limited in their ability to predict or explain individual behavior. Characteristics develop and exist within certain contexts; therefore it is important to understand the interplay between personality traits and environment and situation factors (Bersani et al., 1992). We agree with Dutton's (1994b) argument that wife assault must be understood in an ecological context factoring in the effects of the broader culture, the subculture, the family, and individually learned characteristics. He also argues that microsystems and ontogenetic factors have the greatest explanatory power. For this reason, a psychological understanding of the dynamics of violence is critical to engineering effective treatment. Educative approaches primarily addressing women's oppression will not effectively impact on the emotional capacities of the abuser and, in our analysis, could in fact have the opposite effect by enhancing shame and proneness to violence.

MALE SOCIALIZATION

Having said this, it is still important to note that male socialization as a macro phenomenon does impact how men manage shame and relationships. Osherson and Krugman (1990), O'Leary and Wright (1986), Wright (1987), and Kaufman (1989, 1992) note that men are socialized to experience dependency as shameful. Bergman (1991) suggests that men are socialized to reject relationality itself and to see connecting with women as an impediment to achieving a masculine identity. The consequence is an inability to be intimate coupled with a repressed yearning for connection. This is consistent with Wright's belief that men are socialized to present themselves as powerful (Wright, 1987, 1994) and Osherson and Krugman's (1990) argument that self-reliance is a central cannon of male socialization. Others have pointed out that men's entitlement to experience emotional vulnerability is constricted by social norms (Goldberg, 1976, 1979; Kaufman, 1989, 1992; Osherson & Krugman, 1990; Wright, 1987, 1994). Nathanson (1992) specifically suggests that men in our culture are taught to "experience shame as an excuse or a stimulus for anger and describe shame in the language of insult and threat" (p. 158).

For the individual man, then, situations that confront traditional socialization by evoking dependency needs, powerlessness, or vulnerable emotions such as shame will potentially trigger an experience of failed masculinity. In other words, such situations will have the potential to trigger shame and its co-assembled affects and beliefs. Where this is the case, there is an intersection between the effects of socialization and the micro and ontogenetic factors that come into play in explaining how an individual man mediates both attachment insecurities and shameful experiences. How the individual male reacts to attachment and vulnerability is a product of biology in relation to life history, but is also influenced by broader social values. Socialization alone is unable to account for the individual's particular strategies for dealing with shame and the associated threatened loss of attachment.

THE GROUP MODEL

The Therapeutic Objective

Before discussing the details of our model, it is important to identify the critical elements of therapeutic intervention within the framework of affect theory. Obviously, the primary goal of intervention is to detoxify dysfunctional affective experience. In the context of shame-based clients, this means that the therapeutic process must serve to increase the individual's ability to tolerate shame without activating other co-assembled affects (e.g., anger and rage) or defensive scripts. In our framework, this involves structuring group process in such a way that the abusers are induced to experience shame. The role of the leaders is to enhance the safety of the group environment in such a way that the activated defenses of "attack other" are subject to exploration and change.

As Nathanson (1992) points out, however, defensive scripting involves cognitive processes that follow physiological arousal and precede the experience of shame. These cognitive processes reflect the life scripts of individuals and the meaning ascribed to the experience of affective states over time. This means that effective therapy also involves helping abusers identify the cues of physiological arousal, the cognitive processes attached to that arousal, and the life history that contributes to overall scripting.

In the context of our model, we assume that shame is the core affective experience in violent incidents and that work with the abuser must address the fusion of anger and shame by helping differentiate the two states and by increasing tolerance for shame. In order to do this, it is necessary to begin by helping men recognize and change their anger in order to give access to co-assembled affects. This means that interventions are first designed to structure affective responses through a variety of techniques, including requiring each group member to confront his shame through confessing to the others his worst incident of violence (Wallace & Nosko, 1993). The structured induction of emotion also occurs through the use of visualization, through mirroring, and through working with the interpersonal exchanges of men in group process. By learning to tolerate shame, each man is then better able to tolerate the abandonment fantasies inherent in shame.

Cognitive/Behavioral Interventions

At the same time, the physiological dimension of the anger that masks shame is addressed through having the men complete exercises (e.g., anger charts, anger logs) that inform them about their own physiological experience of anger and other affects. This is coupled with skill building around anger management (e.g., relaxation, self talk) in order to help the men to minimize their anger sufficiently to allow the shame to emerge and be contained.

Cognitive restructuring is partly accomplished through teaching on topics such as the nature of emotion in relation to behavior and physiology, self-talk in the context of angry exchanges, the definitions of violence, effective communications, and transactional analysis concepts of ego states. The latter's concept of Parent (critical and nurturing), Child (emotionality), and Adult (reasoning and logic) provides a simple and practical model that can help men understand, identify, and change their way of managing their affects (Harris, 1973). The goal of teaching is to provide new information that the men can use to generate a different framework through which life experiences and affect can be filtered. Group process is the medium for actualizing these concepts in here and now exchanges. Cognitive restructuring is also the main tool for helping the men redesign their defensive scripts. For example, the exploration of early life shaming experiences and their relationship to anger allow the men an opportunity to identify, challenge, and modify their scripts in relation to their sense of their own value and their sense of relationships with others. Dealing with abandonment fears is an important part of this discussion.

As we intimated earlier, skill building emerges out of the teaching interventions coupled with practice both within and outside the group. Skill building occurs in the areas of anger management (e.g., time outs, shifting the physiology of anger through techniques such as deep breathing, progressive relaxation and self talk) and effective interpersonal communications (e.g., role playing conflictual situations, addressing and resolving actual conflicts and tensions within the group itself). Another important function of skill building is to allow the men to shift their perception of the source of their own power. Rather than resort to violence to enhance their sense of self and project inadequacy onto their partner, they develop the capacity to experience internally generated power as a consequence of effective and appropriate communications.

The Group as a Resocialization Experience

Finally, socialized responses to the expression of affect, particularly anger and shame, can be shifted within the group context. Given that the group is a micro society (Klein, 1972), it affords an opportunity for the men to encounter one another in the context of norms that differ from those of society at large. These norms encourage and legitimize a broader range of affective expression and interpersonal encounters in a non-judgmental context. For example, the group demands that the men view one another as equals, that they accept a woman co-leader in a role of power, that they acknowledge emotion as it is experienced, that they tolerate differences and vulnerability, and that they provide mutual support. These norms lie in opposition to traditional Western male values that dictate that men should be competitive, invulnerable, and powerful and should hold more status than women. Apart from the effect of group itself, re-socialization is effected by the use of male-female co-leadership, and through discussions of men's expectations of themselves.

The Rationale for Group as the Medium for Resolving Shame

What remains to be discussed is the question of why group treatment is the preferred medium for these interventions. Like many others (Bersani et al., 1992; Dutton, 1995; Edelson & Syers, 1991; Gondolf, 1985; Wright, 1987, 1994), we believe that group therapy and group dynamics provide the framework through which the men's shame can be addressed. As Wright (1994) suggests, there are features of group therapy that contribute to uncovering men's feelings, allowing them to learn about themselves. Group provides an interpersonal atmosphere of safety where emotions can be experienced and expressed. Shame, therefore, becomes accessible. In providing support, the group counters men's fears of isolation and abandonment, thus functioning as an "antidote to shame."

This is consistent with Klein's (1972) view that the introduction of social group work norms and values create the outer boundary of what he calls a new micro society. Within this micro society, support and safety can be generated, which allow men to access emotions normally inaccessible to them. The creation of the structure through the introduction of norms permits various group dynamics and processes to unfold. The norms and values include the concept of equal status for all group members, acceptance of interpersonal need, tolerance for interpersonal difference, mutual aid, support for affective expression, and taking responsibility for one's emotions. These norms address Nathanson's (1987b) definition of healthy pride that is counter to social values that put a developing child in a comparative and competitive situation through seeking status. In supporting these norms, the group assists men in developing healthy pride; members are permitted to access and begin to tolerate shame as apart from the identity of self. This further allows them to experience themselves as worthwhile as opposed to inherently flawed.

The structure of the group provides the foundation for moving a collection of individuals into a therapeutic entity called group, characterized by a sense of cohesion and an experience of belonging. The implied movement to group cohesion is essential for therapeutic processes to occur, including those fundamental to the reparation of shame. These processes include *projective identification*, which allows members to see and name in others what they can't fully see and experience in themselves (Alonso & Rutan, 1988; Hahn, 1994; Wright, 1994). For example, in the confessional process, members may project disgust onto the person disclosing his violence towards his partner. This can then lead to the labeling and the exploration of self-disgust that has been projected onto the other member. As defensive strategies are thus exposed, shame is accessed within the group and becomes available for *vicarious detoxification*, which makes shame more bearable through identification with its safe experience by another individual(s) in the group (Alonso & Rutan, 1988). For example, when the group leaders explore underlying shame in the above illustration, it is possible for members to experience their own shame without resorting to strong defensive scripts. In witnessing this, others members have an opportunity to begin vicariously experiencing their own shame within a context of safety, therefore making shame less toxic to themselves. *Group contagion* contributes to the process of resolving shame in groups. It is the process by which emotions experienced by a group member stimulate feelings that are present but not consciously experienced in others. In relation to shame, this gives permission for the experience and expression of the feeling (Alonso & Rutan, 1988; Wright, 1994). This is necessary if group members are to confront their attachment styles and shift from a position of anxious attachment. Again, the goal of accessing shame through these processes is to reduce dependence on "attack other" strategies.

For example, one of our main interventions to access shame is "the confession" (Wallace & Nosko, 1993). Through the first several sessions of the group, time is allotted for each member to describe in detail the worst incident of violence perpetrated against his partner. The female leader takes the lead in this process, taking each man in a detailed retelling of the incident in question. As the questioning unfolds, particularly in the early sessions, the men in the group often react with anger and denial as more details are elicited and as rationalizations are challenged. This anger represents the attempt to intimidate the female co-leader and generate in her his split-off sense of vulnerability and shame. As the projective identification breaks down through the interchange with the group leaders, the shame begins to emerge, permitting vicarious detoxification. As each member listens to the confessor, his own shame is encountered. The distribution of this experience through the group represents contagion.

The emergence of these processes provides a groundwork for the experience of some of Yalom's (1985) therapeutic factors. For example, universality involves the recognition that members are not alone and provides an attachment experience that relieves shame. Altruism, which emerges out of the experience of helping one another, counters the isolation that is at the heart of the shame experience (Wright, 1994). Out of the successful negotiation of shame experiences in the group, imitative behavior (Yalom, 1985) or modeling (Wright, 1994) emerges as group members use one another and the group leaders as models for the appropriate expression and resolution of various affects, in particular anger and shame. As we have said, group provides a re-socializing experience which addresses Yalom's (1985) factor, the development of socializing techniques. The confession, described above is an example of how these therapeutic factors are operationalized. Indeed, all the interventions summarized above are designed to support the processes emerging out of and informing the structure of the group as well as the therapeutic factors associated with them.

Co-Leadership

The co-leadership system is the most powerful subsystem within the group as a whole, and needs to be so in order to establish and maintain the structure that provides safety to group members. Essential to our model is a male-female co-leadership team that models equal power for each gender and provides men with an opportunity to address the male-female issues that are projected onto their partners and reenacted in group (Nosko & Wallace, 1997). Co-leadership offers the opportunity to model non-stereotypic behaviors. For example, the leaders can alternate cognitive and affective functions, ensuring that the female is in an equal power position when addressing cognitive material. This challenges the stereotype that women are primarily affective in orientation. Conversely, having the male co-leader assume a strong emotional role challenges their experience of male socialization. Challenging the members' expectations of male-female behavior and interaction is a recurrent issue in abusers' groups, and effective intervention depends on the application of two core strategies.

First, it is essential that the male co-leader not enter into collusion with the other men in the group by avoiding active support for his female partner. Second, the leadership subsystem needs to be vigilant about the projections transferred onto the female co-leader by group members. It is important that such projections be addressed and supported without evoking an entrenched defensive response. For example, if a group member gets angry at the female co-leader for a challenging statement the male co-leader has made, it is essential for the female to not react in a personal, emotional way, but instead for the co-leadership to label the displacement of anger from the male to the female and to explore the relevance of this dynamic to their daily lives.

It is critical for the co-leaders to actively negotiate how such confrontations from group members will be handled in order to ensure that the leadership remains cohesive and intact. The male leader can support the female leader, for example, by taking the lead in labeling the displacement and by trusting the female leader's competence to negotiate a resolution within the group itself. In group terms, the leaders model group norms supporting an atmosphere of safety by demonstrating tolerance for the emotions underlying the "attack other" script. This provides an opportunity for the group to explore the cognitions associated with anger and begin to access the underlying shame. By reacting in unexpected but supportive ways, the co-leaders permit the men to tolerate shame-evoking interpersonal exchanges without depending on anger. In other words, the way in which the leadership presents new models of male-female interaction will influence members' readiness to internalize and operationalize the values of the group as a whole. It will also significantly impact on the group's movement from one stage to another since there is an automatic dissonance between the values men bring into the group and the values of the co-leadership subsystem.

Stages of Group Development

The foundation of intervention strategy for this model is found in social group work theory, which supposes that groups undergo a maturational process involving movement through various stages. We will explore each stage as it relates to the therapeutic process used to address shame and its defensive scripts. We will also review the interventions that typically apply at each of the stages of group development.

Preparation for Group

The pre-group phase (Garvin, 1981), or the planning process stage (Toseland & Rivas, 1984), focuses primarily on ensuring appropriate group composition in relation to the preset group purpose. Included is "role induction" which involves using the intake interview to orient group members to the group's purpose and norms. This phase includes not only assessment, but also the preliminary work of ensuring that the community is aware of the nature and goals of the program. In the context of this particular model, it is important that potential referral sources are aware of exclusion criteria and the nature of the target population (i.e., voluntary self-referrals). Exclusion criteria include on-going drug and alcohol abuse; sociopathic, paranoid, and/or psychotic disorders; organic brain disorders; and those with developmental handicaps. A critical admission criterion is the capacity to experience shame in relation to abuse through the course of the assessment interview.

Assessment is done by either group leader in a structured interview designed to collect data relevant to the exclusion criteria, provide information about the group, and to determine the client's ability to tolerate a challenge to the defensive scripting associated with his violence. It also functions to establish the basic blueprint that will govern the process and structures of the group itself. In order to meet these goals, the assessment interview has a sequential structure. Clients are first asked to describe the history of their violent behavior, starting with the most recent event. In the course of questioning about the client's violence history, questions are also asked that assess the safety of his partner and any children. The assessor obtains factual information relevant to some of the exclusion criteria. For example, the client is asked questions about alcohol and drug consumption and about any history of brain injury. Finally, the group leader provides information about the nature of group process.

A very important purpose of the assessment interview is to determine whether or not referrals meet the core admission requirement of the program (i.e., the ability to tolerate some shame). In a non-judgmental way, the group co-leader supportively challenges the denial and projections that are part of the defensive scripts associated with abusive behavior.

For example, if the man states that his wife is responsible for the violence because of an action she took, the assessor challenges the denial by suggesting that it is difficult to take responsibility for his actions and his fear of abandonment.

Challenging the defensive scripts often engenders anger towards the assessor as the "attack other" response is triggered. It is critical that the co-leader tolerates the anger and supports the underlying shame. This is often done by acknowledging unspoken emotions and reframing the men's experience in traditional male metaphors. For example, the anger expressed toward the assessor may be reframed as fear of being seen as vulnerable and out of control. Similarly, the experience of vulnerability in the here and now can be reframed as an act of courage given social prohibitions on men's experience of vulnerable emotions. This process creates a bridge between the defensive scripts and shame. If a man is able to acknowledge what is beneath the anger and does not fall within the exclusion criteria, he is accepted into group. It is also important to note that the assessment interview mirrors the structure and process that will emerge and be harnessed in group.

Another function of the assessment process is role induction, in which men are introduced to the structure and norms of the group. In assessing, the co-leaders convey their belief that all group members are entitled to respect, that each member is equal to the others by virtue of experiencing a shared problem, that value is placed on acknowledging and accepting responsibility for emotions and behaviors, and that men and women are equal to one another. Group expectations are defined regarding attendance. Once a candidate is deemed as appropriate for group, the co-leader outlines the contracts the man will be expected to sign and adhere to as a member of the group. The questions directed to the men, the leader's response to what the men present throughout the interview, and the information given about group expectations enact the process of role induction.

Pre-Affiliation

Pre-affiliation (Garland, Jones, & Kolodny, 1973) represents the first stage of group process and is focused on the creation of safety through establishing the outer boundary of the group or microsociety (Klein, 1972). Safety will begin to emerge through the reinforcement of the norms introduced in the assessment process.

The first group session of the program involves the members accepted into group and their partners. Involving the women in this first session only is intended to establish that men are responsible for their own behaviors and change; to operationalize the program contract in which expectations of contact between the group leaders and the women are defined in relation to safety needs and clear definitions of confidentiality; to establish realistic expectations of the program; and to begin skill building by providing 'time out' as a tool for beginning the change process.

The potential for generating shame inherent in this process is controlled through relying on didactic presentation and the extensive use of reframing. For example, the female leader (who conducts most of this session) reframes the change process as one requiring great courage and strength. The co-leaders make deliberate use of the gender difference to model equality, thus reinforcing related norms. For example, the didactic content outlining appropriate expectations of the group and introducing the 'time out' are outlined by the female co-leader while the male co-leader conducts the contracting process in which men are held accountable for their commitment to group and for the safety of their partners. From this point on, only the men are involved in the group.

The pre-affiliation phase extends through the second and perhaps the third session. Safety within the group, which is initially established through the introduction of norms, is reinforced by the leadership's deliberate modeling of these norms. For example, the demonstrable equality between the group leaders generates the norm of equality between members. Furthermore, when the norm is challenged through the traditional resurgence of competitiveness among men, group leaders intervene by highlighting commonality among members. Such interventions lay the groundwork for a safe environment in which shame can be experienced and tolerated.

Within this framework of safety, the group begins with an identification of individual and then group goals. The male takes the lead in this process and elicits detailed elaborations of behaviors that need to be changed. This intervention is a precursor to the confession (Wallace & Nosko, 1993) and begins to trigger both defensive scripts and the affects underlying that scripting. To avoid amplifying the defenses and heightening shame beyond the point of tolerance, the male co-leader directs this process, focusing on the cognitive dimension of goal setting while beginning to use emotional language to describe their goals. For example, as group members resist describing their violent behaviors and associated anger, the co-leaders will address how difficult it is for the men to acknowledge before others what they have done. This begins to set the stage for the therapeutic use of contagion. By then identifying common group goals, the basis for experiencing the therapeutic impact of universality is established.

To contain the affect released in the process of setting goals, the leaders deliberately shift to the cognitive task of defining anger and violence in the second part of this session. This task orientation, which is a familiar part of male socialization, is reinforced by then reviewing their experience of the 'time out,' introduced in the first session. Such a review also constitutes a skill building exercise and furthers the members' sense that anger can be controlled by identifying and monitoring their triggers to anger.

In the third session, members are invited to check-in with the group about violence related issues as they emerged in the past week. There are several purposes attached to this intervention. First, it affords men an opportunity to identify and problem solve around potentially urgent issues related to their experience of anger. Second, it provides a means for the co-leaders to monitor homework and support skill building. Third, it provides a structure through which the co-leaders can identify and challenge defensive scripts as well the emotions underlying them. The structure of the initial check-in is maintained throughout the group program. However, its quality and tone reflects the group's stage of development.

Power and Control

This phase of group process represents the members' attempt to resolve the contradiction between the group norms and their defensive scripts. Also at issue is the ambivalence group members feel in attaching to both the leadership and to one another. This crisis around attachment and interdependence generates a high degree of turbulence in this stage and is characterized by a power struggle between the group members and the leadership (Nosko & Wallace, 1988; Wallace & Nosko, 1993). The power struggle manifests through rebellion, confrontation with the group leaders, withdrawal from one another, and attempts to split the group leadership. For example, the group may attempt to devalue or disregard the female leader while attempting to induce the male leader into an alliance against the female. This often mirrors the dysfunction in their own relationships.

The power struggle may also manifest as apparent compliance with the norms of the group leaders where the language and values are mimicked by members without congruent affect. For example, a member may speak the language of responsibility by espousing guilt for his actions. On further exploration, however, rhetoric about women's rights and men's responsibilities for being non-violent may reveal itself to be disconnected from the emotions of responsibility, from the man's behaviors, and from their shame based fears of abandonment.

The successful resolution of Power and Control and passage to the next stage is dependent on the internalization of the group norms in the context of support and protection from the leadership. This is necessary to fully establish the safety needed for a grouping to mature into a group (Garland, Jones, & Kolodny, 1973), where interdependence and functional attachment prevail. Every intervention by the co-leadership is a deliberate effort to uphold and support the group's norms and values and is directed to making this transition possible. It is therefore critical that the co-leaders recognize and depersonalize this process through the use of highly supportive confrontation.

It is important to recognize that the power struggle with the co-leadership is less about who controls the group process than it is about shifting the locus of power from the individual members to the group itself. In endowing the group with power through the resolution of this stage, the men are enabled to own their power over themselves as individuals. In internalizing group norms around mutual aid, affective integrity and emotional support, the men are able to access more parts of themselves and make different choices about their lives. In other words, the leadership's goal in resolving the power struggle is to harness the power of the members to help themselves through the establishment of group. As the group as a whole resolves its defensive posture, there is a corresponding change in the defensive scripting at an individual intrapsychic level.

The beginning of the Power and Control phase tends to coincide with the introduction of "the confession" (Wallace & Nosko, 1993), in which the female co-leader directs each member's disclosure of the worst incident of relationship violence. By requiring each member to go through this experience, it imposes a structure that in turn generates process within both the group and all its members. Through public disclosure, shame is ignited; this in turn tends to activate the defensive scripts. This will manifest through intellectualization, blaming the victim, denial, silence, and anger. When the leaders prompt this process by eliciting details, safety becomes a critical group issue that is addressed by identifying and exploring the emergent defensive scripts in the here and now, by separating the individual's behaviors and affects from identity, by acknowledging the pain of disclosure, by defining public disclosure as courageous, and by supporting painful affects when they emerge. In supporting the individual's tolerance for the experience of the confession and in addressing group responses, a climate of group safety is being established. There is, therefore, an isomorphic relationship between the individual's ability to tolerate shame and that of the group. Out of this process emerges an increased capacity for mutual support and, therefore, more functional attachment behaviors.

It is also important to note that use of the confession extends over several sessions with no less than two members experiencing the process in any one session. The experience of the process changes over time as the issues evoked are confronted by the group and resolved. Thus, a confession may extend for a considerable time when the intervention is introduced and trigger Power and Control. By the last confession, several weeks later, the process may be shorter and generate the behaviors associated with the stage of intimacy.

Re-socialization in the Power and Control stage is inherent in the struggle to accept the norms and values of the group and is exemplified by the leaders through the course of the confession. The lead in "the confession" is taken by the female co-leader and inevitably produces increased challenges to her authority as members struggle with the affective consequences of confessing both before a woman and one another. The role of her co-leader is to take the lead in exploring how individuals are defending against underlying shame and in exploring how such defenses mirror the process of the group as a whole. The sexual division of labor at this point is also designed to challenge role-based expectations by casting the male as well as the female in a supportive, nurturing but challenging role.

Throughout this stage of group, sessions contain confessions in conjunction with other cognitive and skill building interventions. These are equally important given Nathanson's (1992) argument that emotion emerges out of physiological arousal followed by the cognitive phase of scripting. It is therefore equally important to address these dimensions at the same time. The shift to cognitive and skill building interventions within each session also serves to contain the intense emotions generated by the confession. This helps solidify the experience of safety in the group as it resolves Power and Control issues. In other words, by experiencing the containment in group of moving between affective and cognitive levels, there is a corresponding recognition of how the use of affect management strategies can impact on the individual's experience of anger and shame.

Interventions that accompany the use of the confession in this phase include: teaching about the interconnectedness of emotions, physiology, thoughts and behaviors; teaching self-monitoring through the introduction of scaled anger charts and logs; and teaching self-talk as a strategy of affective modulation. Members also have an opportunity to practice associated skills through resolving affective and interpersonal issues in the here and now.

Intimacy

As the members accept and internalize the group norms, cohesion, which embodies a growing sense of safety, takes hold. The sense of belonging, which involves their ownership of the group process, permits members to work with one another to provide support and to engage in constructive confrontation. This is core to the emergence of mutual aid, a process in which members become more actively involved in identifying and supporting one another in the use of different and more effective strategies for dealing with shame and its related scripts. The conditions that prevail at this stage are perfect for accessing and tolerating shame; the experience of safety and belonging that emerges out of participating in "the confession" enhances identification with the norms of the group. As we have argued previously, the norms, once internalized, detoxify shame and reduce the need to rely on "attack other" defensive scripts.

A critical backdrop to this process is the continuation of teaching and skill building exercises. This includes the presentation of didactic material on aspects of effective communication, such as rules of fair fighting (Gondolf, 1985), which are then practiced through role-plays. Also included at this time are: (1) the teaching and practicing of progressive relaxation and autogenic exercises; (2) the introduction of the Transactional Analysis metaphor of Parent, Adult and Child, which provides a tool for the identification of vulnerable emotions and the self-nurturance needed to contain and tolerate them; (3) the exploration with the men of family of origin issues related to male-female role expectations; and (4) the conduct of a visualization in which the men are led to identify vulnerable emotions and internal parental responses to the vulnerability encountered through generating the image of a sad little boy.

In Intimacy, the men are more actively engaged than in the Power and Control phase; participation is greater and more distributed as the group experiments with the use of positive behaviors, thoughts, and emotions in managing anger and shame. The group also becomes more involved in identifying alternative strategies to violence.

As the members explore alternatives to anger and violence, the group process of mutual aid and constructive confrontation engender defensive scripts and emotional responses that are recognized and labeled by the co-leaders and, increasingly, by the group members themselves. The impact of this is to heighten the capacity of members to experience and tolerate a greater variety of affective responses and to separate the fact of experiencing these emotions from shame. This enhances the members' ability to contain and manage affects associated with vulnerability (e.g., shame and sadness) without resorting to "attack other" defensive scripts.

Differentiation

Differentiation represents the point at which the group becomes self-autonomous with members directing the activities (Lang, 1979). Operationally, this means that members take the initiative for labeling and exploring affective states; they utilize the skills taught in the earlier phases of group; they demonstrate an interest in exploring family of origin issues as they relate to shaming experiences; they use the co-leaders as consultants rather than relying on them to provide content and structure; and they begin to generate their own process in accordance with the norms and values introduced earlier. The structure of group discussion thus becomes directed by the group rather than by the co-leaders with members initiating and moderating their own exchanges.

The men's enactment of the group norms consolidates the re-socialization process. In reaching this stage, the men have learned to respond to one another on a basis of equality, accept a woman in a position of power, and both acknowledge and tolerate painful emotions. Furthermore, the group's identification with these norms has a relationship with intrapsychic changes related to a modification of defensive scripting and the consequent ability to access and tolerate shame without resorting to aggression.

The role of the co-leaders shifts with the group's acceptance of responsibility for directing itself and reaching its goals. The co-leaders support this process by developing agendas for the remaining sessions in consultation with group members. Inevitably the content areas generated by the men build on and reflect earlier work reflecting the men's ownership of the group's goals.

Termination

Three to four weeks prior to termination, the co-leaders address the issue of the group's impending end. Often, this triggers a regressive process that may manifest at different intensities and in different ways by individual members. At the heart of the termination process is the members' fears of losing the relationships within the group as well as the support the group as a whole provided. The resolution of this stage is critical because the fear of loss and abandonment are critical to the dynamics of shame. Thus, this phase represents a time of consolidation in which the leaders once more become active in supporting changes made by the men to this point. The leaders assume greater control of the group's structure by presenting material on the nature of endings, predicting possible manifestations of regression, labeling defensive scripts as they reemerge, and supporting vulnerable affects. Given that for these men, the relationships formed in the group are among the most intimate experienced in their lives, it is also important to encourage an on-going connection with one another, address how they can continue the personal work begun in the group, and identify the resources available to them as they continue to work through their issues (e.g., individual therapy, couples counseling where safety is no longer an issue, other groups on related issues). Finally, in the last session the men review the goals set in the second session in order to ground them in a sense of healthy pride and to provide an experience of ending which has a positive meaning.

RESEARCH

In a pilot outcome study conducted by the Family Service Association of Metropolitan Toronto (Freeman, Lambert, & Nosko, 1994, p. 57), the model outlined above was standardized (Crosby, 1994) into an 18-week program. Thirty-six men agreed to participate in data collection on a range of instruments and were used as their own historical controls in a single case analysis. Twenty-eight of the 36 men participated in a post-test and 17 of the 28 participated in a 3-month follow-up. Only 15 female partners participated in the pre-test with 8 participating in post-test and 3 in the follow-up. Data collection was hindered by a number of practical and ethical considerations.

There was positive and statistically significant change between pre and post-tests on the verbal and physical subscales of the Conflict Tactic Scale, the Psychological Maltreatment of Women Inventory, the Rosenberg Self Esteem Inventory and the Family Assessment Measurement self and dyadic scales. Between post-test and follow-up, the positive changes were maintained but there was no further statistically significant change.

CONCLUSION

Through the course of this article, we have used affect theory to hypothesize a link between shame and anger. Within this framework, externally directed anger, which manifests as partner abuse, represents the abuser's attempt to avoid the experience of unmanageable shame. We have further argued that the link between the two affects correlates to anxious/ambivalent attachment and Borderline Personality Organization. Particular attention has been paid to understanding these relationships in the context of Affect Theory.

These hypothetical links direct the choice of therapeutic milieu (i.e., group) and within that context, determine all interventions. We have suggested that a social group work model, which incorporates focused strategies of cognitive restructuring, the structured induction of emotion, skills building, and re-socialization, is the most effective form of intervention because the evolution of group structure and process parallels the intrapsychic process of repairing the effects of toxic shame in individual men. As the group moves through stages, corresponding changes occur in the defensive strategies mobilized to protect against shame.

REFERENCES

Alonso, A., & Rutan, S. (1988). The experience of shame and restoration of self-respect in group therapy. *International Journal of Group Psychotherapy, 38*(1), 3-14.

Barnett, O. W., & Hamberger, L. K. (1992). The assessment of maritally violent men on the California Psychological Inventory. *Violence and Victims, 7*(1), 15-28.

Bergman, S. (1991). *Men's psychological development: A relational perspective.* Wellesley, MA: The Stone Center.

Bersani, C. A., Chen, H. T., Pendleton, B. F., & Denton, R. (1992). Personality traits of convicted male batterers. *Journal of Family Violence, 7*(2), 123-134.

Bowlby, J. (1988). *A secure base: Clinical applications of attachment theory.* London: Routledge.

Caesar, P. L. (1 988). Exposure to violence in the families-of-origin among wife abusers and maritally violent men. *Violence and Victims, 3*(1), 49-63.

Crosby, P. (1994). *Next steps: Working towards eliminating male violence against women: Report to funder.* Toronto: Family Service Association of Metropolitan Toronto.

Dutton, D. G. (1994a). Behavioral and affective correlates of Borderline Personality Organization in wife assaulters. *International Journal of Law and Psychiatry, 17*(3), 265-277.

Dutton, D. G. (1994b). Patriarchy and wife assault: The ecological fallacy. *Violence and Victims, 9*(2), 167-182.

Dutton, D. G. (1995). *The batterer: A psychological profile.* New York: Basic Books.

Dutton, D. G. (2002). Treatment of assaultiveness. *Journal of Aggression, Maltreatment, & Trauma, 7*(1/2), 7-28.

Dutton, D. G., Saunders, K., Starzomski, A., & Bartholomew, K. (1994). Intimacy-anger and insecure attachment as precursors of abuse in intimate relationships. *Journal of Applied Social Psychology, 24*, 1367-1386.

Dutton, D. G., & Starzomski, A. J. (1993). Borderline personality in perpetrators of psychological and physical abuse. *Violence and Victims, 8*(4), 327-337.

Dutton, D. G., & Strachan, C. E. (1987). Motivational needs for power and spouse-specific assertiveness in assaultive and non-assaultive men. *Violence and Victims 2*(3), 145-156.

Dutton, D. G., van Ginkel, C., & Starzomski, A. (1995). The role of shame and guilt in the intergenerational transmission of abusiveness. *Violence and Victims, 10*(2), 121-131.

Edelson, J., & Syers, M. (1991). The effects of group treatment for men who batter: An 18 month follow-up study. *Research on Social Work Practice, 1*(3), 227-243.

Freeman, R., Lambert, K., & Nosko, A. (1994). *Next steps: Working towards eliminating male violence against women.* Toronto: Family Service Association of Metropolitan Toronto.

Fromm, E. (1956). *The art of loving.* New York: Harper and Row.

Garland, J. A., Jones, H. E., & Kolodny, R. L. (1973). A model for stages of development in social work groups. In S. Bernstein (Ed.), *Explorations in group work* (pp. 17- 71). Boston: Milford House.

Garvin, C. (1981). *Contemporary group work.* Englewood: Prentice-Hall.

Goldberg, H. (1976). *The hazards of being male.* New York: New American Library.

Goldberg, H. (1979). *The new male: From macho to sensitive but still all male.* New York: New American Library.

Goldstein, D., & Rosenbaum, A. (1986). An evaluation of the self-esteem of maritally violent men. *Family Relations, 34*, 425-428.

Gondolf, E. (1985). *Men who batter: An integrated approach for stopping wife abuse.* Holmes Beach, Florida: Learning Publications.

Hahn, W. (1994). Resolving shame in group psychotherapy. *International Journal of Group Psychotherapy, 44*(4), 449-461.

Hamberger, L. K., & Hastings, J. E. (1986). Personality correlates of men who abuse their partners: A cross-validational study. *Journal of Family Violence, 1*, 323-346.

Harris, T. (1973). *I'm ok, you're ok.* New York: Avon Books.

Hastings, J. E., & Hamberger, L. K. (1988). Personality characteristics of spouse abusers: A controlled comparison. *Violence and Victims, 3*(1), 31-46.

Kaufman, G. (1989). *The psychology of shame.* New York: Springer.

Kaufman, G. (1992). *Shame: The power of caring.* Rochester, VT.: Schenkman Books.

Klein, A. (1972). *Effective groupwork: An introduction to principle and method.* New York: Association Press.

Kohut, H. (1978). Thoughts on narcissism and narcissistic rage. In P. Ornstein (Ed.), *The search for the self: Selected writings of Heinz Kohut, 1950-1978: Volume 2* (pp. 615-658). New York: International Universities Press.

Lang, N. (1979). Comparative examination of therapeutic uses of groups in social work and in adjacent human services professions: Part 2, the literature from 1969-1978. *Social Work with Groups 2*(3), 197-220.

Lewis, H. B. (1971). *Shame and guilt in neurosis.* New York: International Universities Press.

Lewis, H. B. (1987). Shame and the narcissistic personality. In D. L. Nathanson (Ed.), *The many faces of shame* (pp. 93-131). New York: Guilford Press.

Miller, A. (1981). *The drama of the gifted child.* New York: Basic Books.

Morrison, A. (1986). Shame, ideal self and narcissism. In A. Morrison (Ed.), *Essential papers on narcissism* (pp. 348-372). New York: New York University Press.

Morrison, A. (1987). The eye turned inward: Shame and the self. In D. L. Nathanson (Ed.), *Many faces of shame* (pp. 271-291). New York: The Guilford Press.

Morrison, A. (1989). *Shame: The underside of narcissism.* Hillsdale, N.J.: Analytic Press.

Nathanson, D. L. (1987a). A timetable for shame. In D. L. Nathanson (Ed.), *The many faces of shame* (pp. 1-63). New York: Guilford.

Nathanson, D. L. (1987b). The shame/pride axis. In H. B. Lewis (Ed.), *The role of shame in symptom formation* (pp. 183-205). Hillsdale, N.J.: Erlbaum.

Nathanson, D. L. (1992). *Shame and pride: Affect, sex and the birth of the self.* New York: W.W. Norton and Company.

Nathanson, D. L. (1994). Shame transactions. *Transactional Analysis Journal, 24*(2), 121-129.

Nosko, A., & Wallace, R. (1988). Group work with abusive men: A multidimensional model. In G. Gestel (Ed.), *Violence: Prevention and treatment in groups* (pp. 43-52). New York: The Haworth Press, Inc.

Nosko, A., & Wallace, R. (1997). Female-male co-leadership in groups. *Social Work with Groups, 20*(2), 3-16.

O'Leary, J., & Wright, F. (1986). Shame and gender: Issues in pathological narcissism. *Psychoanalytic Psychology, 3*(4), 327-339.

Osherson, S., & Krugman, S. (1990). Men, shame and psychotherapy. *Psychotherapy, 27*(3), 327-339.

Piers, G., & Singer, M. (1953). *Shame and guilt.* New York: Norton.

Retzinger, S. M. (1991). Shame, anger and conflict: Case study of emotional violence. *Journal of Family Violence, 6*(1), 37-59.

Saunders, D. (1992). A typology of men who batter. *American Journal of Orthopsychiatry, 62*(2), 264-275.

Sonkin, D. J., & Dutton, D. G. (2002). Treating assaultive men from an attachment perspective. *Journal of Aggression, Maltreatment, and Trauma, 7*(1/2), 105-133.

Stern, D. N. (1985). *The Interpersonal world of the infant: A view from psychoanalysis and developmental psychology.* New York: Basic Books.

Tolman, R., & Bennett, L. W. (1990). A review of quantitative research on men who batter. *Journal of Interpersonal Violence, 5*(1), 87-118.

Tomkins, S. (1987). Shame. In D. L. Nathanson (Ed.), *The many faces of shame* (pp. 133-161). New York: Guilford Press.

Toseland, R., & Rivas, R. (1984). *An introduction to group work practice.* New York: Macmillan.

Wallace, R., & Nosko, A. (1993). Working with shame in the group treatment of male batterers. *International Journal of Group Psychotherapy, 43*(1), 45-61.

Wright, F. (1987). Men, shame and anti-social behavior: A psychodynamic perspective. *Group, 11*(4), 238-246.

Wright, F. (1994). Men, shame and group psychotherapy. *Group, 18*(4), 212-224.

Wurmser, L. (1987). Shame: The veiled narcissism. In D. L. Nathanson (Ed.), *The many faces of shame* (pp. 64-92). New York: Guilford.

Yalom, I. (1985). *The theory and practice of group psychotherapy.* New York: Basic Books.

Dialectical Behavior Therapy in the Treatment of Abusive Behavior

Jennifer Waltz

SUMMARY. Research suggests that a subset of men who abuse their partners have characteristics associated with borderline personality disorder (BPD). Dialectical Behavior Therapy (DBT) has shown promise as a treatment for BPD, and thus may be useful for these men. This paper describes how DBT principles might be applied to address the problem of partner abuse, including discussion of why one might expect DBT to be a helpful treatment model for this population, and how implementation of the model might be designed. *[Article copies available for a fee from The Haworth Document Delivery Service: 1-800-HAWORTH. E-mail address: <docdelivery@haworthpress.com> Website: <http://www.HaworthPress.com> © 2003 by The Haworth Press, Inc. All rights reserved.]*

KEYWORDS. Dialectical Behavior Therapy, Borderline Personality Disorder, domestic violence, partner abuse

INTRODUCTION

Although a variety of advances have been made in interventions for individuals who batter their domestic partners, many who participate in

Address correspondence to: Jennifer Waltz, Department of Psychology, University of Montana, Missoula, MT 59812.

[Haworth co-indexing entry note]: "Dialectical Behavior Therapy in the Treatment of Abusive Behavior." Waltz, Jennifer. Co-published simultaneously in *Journal of Aggression, Maltreatment & Trauma* (The Haworth Maltreatment & Trauma Press, an imprint of The Haworth Press, Inc.) Vol. 7, No. 1/2 (#13/14), 2003, pp. 75-103; and: *Intimate Violence: Contemporary Treatment Innovations* (ed: Donald Dutton, and Daniel J. Sonkin) The Haworth Maltreatment & Trauma Press, an imprint of The Haworth Press, Inc., 2003, pp. 75-103. Single or multiple copies of this article are available for a fee from The Haworth Document Delivery Service [1-800-HAWORTH, 9:00 a.m. - 5:00 p.m. (EST). E-mail address: docdelivery@haworthpress.com].

http://www.haworthpress.com/store/product.asp?sku=J146
© 2003 by The Haworth Press, Inc. All rights reserved.
10.1300J146v07n01_05

such treatments continue to be abusive (Babcock, Green & Robie, under review; Dunford, 2000). Given the prevalence and consequences of this problem, exploration of new treatment approaches is warranted, in particular for men who do not improve in available treatments. Dialectical Behavior Therapy (DBT; Linehan, 1993a) offers one promising option. DBT, developed in the 1980s, was originally designed to treat individuals who are chronically suicidal and engage in self-harming behaviors. The first efficacy study of DBT included women with recent histories of self-harm, and additionally required a diagnosis of borderline personality disorder (BPD; Linehan, Armstrong, Suarez, Allmon, & Heard, 1991). DBT has subsequently been primarily associated with treatment of BPD, although it is now being applied to a range of other populations (Linehan, 2000).

Research regarding the efficacy of DBT is on-going; however, there are data from several clinical trials supporting its usefulness (Koerner & Dimeff, 2000). Linehan and colleagues (Linehan, Armstrong, Suarez, Allmon, & Heard, 1991) reported on the first randomized clinical trial (RCT) of standard DBT. The treatment lasted one year and the study utilized a treatment-as-usual (TAU) in the community control condition. The study found better results for DBT at post-test on retention in treatment, frequency of self-harm behavior, and number of days of hospitalization, all of which are the primary problems addressed in the early stages of DBT.

DBT has also been studied at other sites (Koons et al., 2001). Koons and colleagues compared standard DBT to treatment as usual (primarily cognitive-behavioral) in a Veterans Administration clinic. Subjects were 20 female veterans who met criteria for BPD. At the end of the 6-month treatment period, subjects receiving DBT showed greater decreases in depression, hopelessness, suicidal ideation and expression of anger relative to subjects in the TAU condition. This study extends findings on DBT to a population with less intense suicidality and less frequent self-harm, and, relevant to PA men, includes anger expression as an outcome variable.

DBT has begun to be applied to a broader range of clinical problems, with a number of themes common across these populations (Linehan, 2000). First, DBT is typically applied with clinical populations that are difficult to treat, or for whom traditional treatments have shown limited success. Second, the populations DBT has been adapted to generally include people experiencing problems associated with emotion dysregulation. In addition, these populations tend to have multiple diagnoses and/or life problems and high treatment drop-out rates (Linehan, 2000). Adaptations of DBT have been developed for a variety of mental health problems, including substance abuse (Dimeff, Rizvi, Brown, & Linehan, 2000), bulimia (Safer, Telch, & Agras, 2001), suicidality in adolescents (Miller, Rathus, Linehan, Wetzler, & Leigh, 1997), post-traumatic stress disorder (Becker & Zayfert, 2001) and depressed elderly patients (Lynch, 2000). There are data supporting the efficacy of DBT with some of these populations, although it does not always include RCTs (Koerner & Dimeff, 2000; Koerner & Linehan, 2000).

Clinicians and researchers working in the area of domestic violence have begun to think about using DBT with people who are violent, with some exciting work being done in this area (Fruzzetti & Levensky, 2000; McCann, Ball & Ivanoff, 2000).[1] Fruzzetti and Levensky (2000) describe an adaptation of DBT for domestic violence, and McCann et al. (2000) describe their use of DBT with people with a history of violence who are in forensic settings. To date no clinical trials have tested the efficacy of DBT to reduce violent or abusive behavior, so it is important to remain cautious about the use of DBT with this group (Scheel, 2000). Nevertheless, there are a variety of reasons to believe that DBT may be a useful treatment for partner abuse.

The purpose of this article is to provide a general description of DBT principles and interventions, and to discuss how these might be applied to address partner abuse. This chapter focuses on how standard DBT (the model tested in the original RCT) might be adapted to individuals who abuse their partners, and does not directly address treatment needs of victims, children or families. This chapter draws on the existing literature on characteristics and treatment of individuals who are abusive to their partners. The vast majority of this literature focuses on males who are abusive to female partners, which is what this chapter will focus on as well. There is a continuing need for research on partner abuse in same-sex couples. This chapter also draws on the existing literature on DBT and its applications.

Why DBT for Partner Abuse?

There are a number of reasons that DBT is attractive as a potential treatment model for partner abusive (PA) men. There is overlap in the BPD population, for whom DBT was developed, and the population of PA men. In addition, many of the difficulties faced by mental health professionals working with PA men are issues that DBT attempts to address. Following are some of the characteristics and treatment issues of

PA men that are consistent with the intended strengths of DBT as a treatment approach.

Borderline personality disorder in partner abusive men. A number of studies have found that borderline characteristics differentiate PA men from non-violent men (Hamberger & Hastings, 1991; Hastings & Hamberger, 1988), and these characteristics seem to be prominent in at least a subgroup of men who are violent to their partners (Dutton, 1995a, 1995b; Dutton & Starzomski, 1993; Gondolf & White, 2001; Waltz, Babcock, Jacobson, & Gottman, 2000). Although these studies have not typically involved diagnosis via clinical interview, they are suggestive that at least a subgroup of men who engage in partner violence have characteristics associated with BPD. In addition, a number of typologies of PA men propose that one subgroup is made up of men who have borderline characteristics (i.e., "dysphoric/borderline"; Holtzworth-Munroe & Stuart, 1994). Given that DBT was designed in part to treat individuals who meet BPD criteria, this approach may be appropriate for at least this subgroup of PA men. It is important to note that most research on DBT has included female subjects exclusively, so it remains to be seen if this approach is also effective with men.

Anger/emotion dysregulation. Consistent with one of the criterion symptoms for BPD, PA men tend to experience high levels of anger (see Schumacher, Feldbau-Kohn, Slep, & Heyman, 2001 for review). One of the primary goals of DBT is to help clients increase their ability to modulate intense negative affect, including anger. DBT targets emotion dysregulation very directly and provides a broad set of skills that help clients respond to difficult emotions more adaptively.

Multiproblem/multidiagnostic/complex treatment picture. Individuals meeting criteria for BPD often also meet criteria for one or more Axis I disorders. Similarly, at least a sizable subgroup of men seeking treatment for partner abuse experience depression (Feldbau-Kohn, Heyman, & O'Leary, 1998; Hamberger & Hastings, 1991; Hamberger, Lohr, Bonge, & Tolin, 1996; Maiuro, Cahn, & Vitaliano, 1988), substance abuse (Hotaling & Sugarman, 1998), and a variety of Axis-II related characteristics and problems (e.g., Gondolf & White, 2001; Hamberger & Hastings, 1986; Tweed & Dutton, 1998). DBT was specifically designed to treat such multiproblem/multidiagnostic individuals, and provides a set of treatment stages and targets to assist with case conceptualization, treatment planning and implementation.

Efficacy of traditional treatments limited. Both individuals meeting criteria for BPD, and people with a history of abusive behavior toward partners are difficult to treat. BPD tends to persist over time (Barasch,

Frances, & Hurt, 1985), and progress in treatment is generally slow. Men who batter their partners tend to have high recidivism rates, and treatments with broad efficacy have been elusive (Dunford, 2000). Although traditional treatments for PA men work well for some, many men continue to be violent or to engage in other abusive behaviors. DBT was specifically designed to address behaviors that are difficult to change, and to address motivational factors that interfere with change. DBT is likely to be most appropriate for those men who do not seem to benefit from traditional treatment programs.

Life-threatening behavior. Many clients in both of these populations engage in behaviors that are life-threatening, either to themselves, others or both. DBT targets life-threatening behavior as the top treatment priority, and support is provided to the therapist to pursue change in this area. Factors that maintain life-threatening behavior are carefully identified and targeted.

Therapy-interfering behavior/poor compliance. One reason standard cognitive-behavioral approaches may be less than optimally effective with both PA men and people with BPD is that compliance with treatment tends to be poor in both cases. Therapy attendance, completion of homework and collaborative behavior during sessions are often problems for both of these populations. DBT seeks to address these problems by directly targeting "therapy-interfering behavior," and by utilizing interventions to increase level of commitment to change.

High drop-out rate. Both PA men (Daly & Pelowski, 2000) and people with BPD (Kelly, Soloff, Cornelius, George, Lis, & Ulrich, 1992) have relatively high rates of drop-out from treatment. Research with PA men suggests that the multi-problem, multidiagnostic men who are less committed to change and have poorer relationships with their therapists are more likely to drop out (Rondeau, Brodeur, Brochu, & Lemire, 2001). DBT puts heavy emphasis on maintaining clients in treatment and addressing problems in the therapeutic relationship, and has been shown to have better rates of retention than TAU in the community (Linehan et al., 1991). In addition to standard DBT approaches to client retention, Dimeff, Rizvi, Brown, and Linehan (2000) have recently developed a set of "attachment strategies" for drug dependent clients with BPD who are at high risk for drop-out. The goal of these interventions is to increase the client's feeling of connection to the therapist. These or similar strategies may also be applicable to PA men.

Therapist burn-out. Mental health professionals working with both people with BPD and those working with PA men tend to experience frustration, anxiety and burn-out. DBT addresses these problems in several ways, including requiring an on-going consultation team for the therapist, providing non-pejorative ways of conceptualizing client problems, and providing a set of assumptions about patients, therapists and therapy that are designed to reduce therapist burn-out.

To what extent DBT may be appropriate for PA men who do not have borderline characteristics is less clear. In general, DBT has primarily been used to address the issues of multi-problem individuals with complicated diagnostic pictures (i.e., co-morbid Axis I and Axis II pathology). This intensive level of treatment may not be needed for PA men who fit the profile of a "family only" type, who typically do not engage in severe or frequent violence, and who tend to have minimal psychopathology (Holtzworth-Munroe & Stuart, 1994; Waltz et al., 2000) for whom traditional forms of treatment may be more appropriate.

Biosocial Theory

DBT is informed by a biosocial theory of the etiology and maintenance of borderline personality disorder; the theory was formulated by Linehan (1993a) and proposes that BPD results from a combination of biologically-based emotion dysregulation, and a particular type of interpersonal context, referred to as the "invalidating environment." The theory proposes that these two factors each influence the other in an on-going, transactional process, such that emotionally dysregulated individuals are more likely to be invalidated, and invalidation tends to increase emotion dysregulation, with the symptoms associated with BPD being the result of this process. Following is a brief review of Linehan's (1993a) theory, and discussion of how this theory may apply to PA men.

Emotion dysregulation, according to this model, involves four basic components. First, the person is more *sensitive* or reactive to events and experiences that may cause emotional responses. For example, a partner being mildly distracted may have little impact on a well-regulated person, but may set off a strong emotional response in an emotionally dysregulated individual. Second, the emotionally dysregulated person also tends to have very *intense* emotional responses. Experiencing the partner being mildly distracted not only triggers a response, it triggers a strong emotional response. The dysregulated person feels not just annoyed or impatient, but may experience intense fear, anger or rage. This intense emotional response includes the subjective experience of the emotion, the physiological arousal associated with it and other components of emotions (Linehan, 1993a). Third, once the emotionally dysregulated person is having an emotional response, it is *difficult for him to regulate* or reduce that response, including having more difficulty controlling behaviors that will decrease the emotion. For example, the person may lack the skills to self-soothe or calm himself, to focus on things that are less upsetting, or to organize himself, problem-solve or pursue obligations such as work. Finally, the dysregulated person's emotions tend to last longer than they do for others, and it takes longer for the person to return to a more neutral or calm affective state. Abusive individuals sometimes report that they became violent after a number of difficult events have happened and their anger has "built up" to an uncontrollable level. A DBT perspective would likely conceptualize this experience as reflecting an inability to return to baseline after an emotion has been triggered, leading to increased vulnerability when the next triggering event occurs.

There is evidence from a variety of sources that can be interpreted as support for the notion that men who batter their partners experience higher levels of emotion dysregulation than non-violent men. Several studies, for example, have found that PA men respond with higher levels of anger to certain types of relationship conflict scenarios than do non-violent men (Dutton & Browning, 1988; Holtzworth-Munroe & Smutzler, 1996). Dutton and Browning (1988) showed videotapes of conflictual couple interactions to PA men, and a control group of non-violent men. PA men responded to scenarios involving a wife telling her husband she was going to spend a weekend away with a friend with greater anger than did non-violent men. Holtzworth-Munroe and Smutzler (1996) similarly found that PA men responded with higher levels of anger to scenarios involving relationship conflict relative to non-violent men. Interestingly, the PA men did not report higher levels of other negative emotional responses such as sadness or fear. These studies can be interpreted as support for the notion that PA men respond to emotional stimuli with more intense responses, at least in the case of anger.

Recent psychophysiological research lends support to the notion that partner-violent individuals react more strongly to the physiological arousal associated with emotions than non-violent people (George, Hibbeln, Ragan, Umhau, Phillips, Doty, Hommer, & Rawlings, 2000). George et al. (2000) compared PA individuals (27 male and 7 female) to subjects meeting criteria for a substance abuse disorder who were non-violent, to a control group of non-violent, non-substance abusing individuals. Subjects were infused with sodium lactate at one time and a

placebo at another in a double-blind design. Sodium lactate is administered as an experimental manipulation to induce physiological symptoms associated with anxiety or panic in subjects who have panic
attacks (George et al., 2000). PA subjects reported higher levels of fear,
sense of losing control and feelings of unreality than the other two
groups of subjects. PA subjects also had significantly greater behavioral
signs of agitation, fear, panic and rage during the lactate infusion, as
rated by observers; however, PA individuals did not show significantly
greater increases in physiological measures of arousal. These results
suggest that PA individuals may respond to physiological cues of
arousal with increased levels of anxiety and agitation, possibly because
they are more sensitive to these cues, or because they fear that they will
be unable to control their emotional or behavioral responses (George et
al., 2000).

Research also supports the notion that PA men may lack emotion
regulation skills, and thus may be less able than non-violent men to regulate their negative emotions. Holtzworth-Munroe and Anglin (1991)
found that PA men generated less competent responses to scenarios depicting hypothetical relationship conflicts than did non-violent men,
when asked how they might respond to such a situation. Although this
difference could be interpreted as a lack of social or problem-solving
skills, it may also reflect an inability to regulate negative affect in order
to organize one's self to produce a skillful response. If PA men in this
study were feeling angry in response to the hypothetical conflict situation, and were unable to modulate that anger, they would be likely to
have more difficulty coming up with a reasonable solution to the situation. Taken together, these results are consistent with the notion that PA
men experience emotion dysregulation, especially with regard to anger.

Linehan's theory posits that to develop BPD, one must have not only
a biological predisposition toward emotion dysregulation, but also be
exposed to a certain type of environment, which she calls the invalidating environment (Linehan, 1993a). In invalidating families, invalidation occurs persistently and frequently. It can take many forms, but the
essence of invalidation is that the child is not treated as worthy, respected and reasonable; instead, the family communicates that the child
is unimportant, unworthy, or "crazy." (Although the "invalidating environment" is discussed here in terms of families, note that invalidation
can happen at many levels within systems, e.g., societal level or school
level).

Invalidating families do not acknowledge or accept the child's feelings or perspectives, but communicate that the way the child is respond-

ing is unacceptable or otherwise wrong or inaccurate. The child's internal states, emotions and wants may be ignored, or he may be told that he is not really feeling that way. Invalidating families generally do not provide helpful or appropriate assistance or input on how to regulate and cope with emotions. These families may emphasize having a "stiff upper lip" and "getting over it" (i.e., "acting like a man"), encouraging the child to think positively or ignore his feelings. These approaches may work for some people or in some circumstances, but for the child who is very sensitive to emotional stimuli and whose emotional responses are difficult to modulate, these approaches generally do not work well (Linehan, 1993a).

A large number of studies have investigated various aspects of the families of origin of PA men. Although none have directly assessed invalidation per se, a number of studies have assessed experiences that are likely to be related to invalidation, such as abuse in the family of origin. In a recent review, Schumacher, Feldbau-Kohn, Slep, and Heyman (2001) conclude that exposure to interparental verbal and physical abuse, and being the target of verbal or physical abuse in childhood, are consistently found to predict being violent in an adult partner relationship. Two additional family of origin variables, being rejected by one's parents and child sexual abuse, were also found to increase risk for partner violence in men, but somewhat less consistently so than exposure to verbal and physical aggression. The studies reviewed relied on retrospective self-reports of family of origin experiences. Although studies of exposure to family of origin abuse, such as those reviewed by Schumacher and colleagues, do not directly assess the experience of invalidation, on-going verbal, physical and/or sexual aggression are inherently invalidating as these experiences ignore the child's need for safety and respect. It also seems likely that other forms of invalidation occur in families experiencing abuse.

The combination of emotion dysregulation and the invalidating environment are hypothesized to interact in an on-going way, with each factor affecting the other, resulting in the problems associated with BPD (Linehan, 1993a). The dysregulated child frequently experiences intense negative emotion; however, the invalidating family responds to the child's negative affect by minimizing, ignoring, shaming or criticizing. The child therefore does not learn how to cope with his emotions. Over time, the child or adolescent in this situation may resort to more and more drastic means to cope with his emotions, such as substance abuse or self-harm. Simultaneously, his emotions, and his behavior in response to these emotions, may become more out of control. The increase in out of control behavior likely prompts further invalidation, and so on.

It is important to note that the biosocial theory informing DBT may or may not be relevant to any given man who engages in partner abuse. Although there are reasons to believe it may apply to at least a subgroup of these men, this theory was not created to explain abusive behavior in partner relationships. Some models of battering focus on the function of violence as a means of gaining power and control in relationships. Proponents of this view may argue that battering has nothing to do with poor emotion regulation capacity, but is instead used to control others. As is often the case with complex behaviors such as partner abuse, it seems likely that there are multiple factors influencing the behavior, across a variety of levels of analysis, and that these factors operate differently for different people, and across different episodes of abusive behavior. This biosocial theory may help explain some violent behavior, and be relevant for some PA men, but is not being proposed as a comprehensive theory of domestic violence.

McCann and colleagues (2000) have modified Linehan's theory for application to individuals who meet criteria for antisocial personality disorder (ASPD). McCann et al. sought to apply a DBT model in an inpatient forensic setting with a population composed largely of men with histories of violent crime. Many of the men in their population meet criteria for ASPD and/or for BPD. They felt that Linehan's biosocial theory did not adequately describe certain aspects of the clinical picture associated with ASPD. Specifically, rather than emotion dysregulation, characterized by a high level of emotional *sensitivity*, they describe ASPD men as experiencing emotional *insensitivity*, meaning that they do not identify the fact that they are experiencing an emotion until the emotion has reached a very intense level. They also describe the childhood environments these individuals were exposed to as characterized by both invalidation, and, additionally, support for violent and aggressive behavior. Such behavior is both reinforced and modeled in these families.

Theoretical Underpinnings of DBT: Behavioral Theory, Dialectics and Zen

Although primarily based on a behavioral orientation, DBT diverges from an exclusively behavioral approach in that it incorporates two other systems of thought: dialectical philosophy and zen. Each of these rich traditions informs DBT in a variety of ways. Although too complex to address in full here, both of these systems will be discussed, with emphasis on how each influences the treatment.

A dialectical philosophy holds the assumption that given a particular stance or position, truth can also be found in the opposite position (Linehan & Schmidt, 1995). It also assumes that change comes about through achieving a synthesis of these opposite positions. Rather than searching for a "right" position and a "wrong" position, a dialectical approach advocates looking for the truth that is present in each position, with change and growth emerging through that process as a synthesis arises. A dialectical approach is ideally suited to respond to the many polarities that arise in work with individuals with BPD, both in terms of their black-or-white world views, and in terms of mental health professionals' sometimes black-or-white responses to these difficult clients.

Linehan (1993a) suggests that the central dialectic in therapy with borderline clients is that of acceptance versus change. Therapeutic interventions are organized around this underlying principle, and stalemates or stuck points in therapy are evaluated in terms of how they may reflect being off-balance in the direction of acceptance, or in the direction of change. Change refers to interventions and therapeutic stances focused on promoting development of new behaviors. Traditional behavioral and cognitive-behavioral therapies focus almost exclusively on helping clients change. In DBT, acceptance refers to therapeutic interventions focused on validating the valid aspects of the client's thoughts and reactions, understanding things from his perspective and acknowledging his reality. People with BPD are often frantic to avoid or eradicate parts of their own experience, in particular painful emotions. Another aspect of acceptance in DBT is working on allowing one's self to experience reality, to simply experience one's emotions as they occur, without avoidance. DBT therapists strategically knit both change-oriented and acceptance-oriented interventions throughout treatment.

Applying a dialectical philosophy to working with PA men, several dialectical polarities emerge. One crucial dilemma is the dialectic around, on the one hand, holding the person accountable for his abusive behavior and clearly communicating the unacceptability of the behavior and the need for change, while on the other hand seeing and understanding the client's perspective, his limitations and the factors that have influenced him to be abusive. From a DBT perspective, both of these positions are valid and necessary parts of the picture. It is the case that abusive behavior is destructive, that the person must be held responsible for it and that it must change. It is also the case that the abusive person's history and context have shaped him and influenced his behavior, and that he is worthy of caring and empathy. From a DBT perspective, therapy is unlikely to be effective if the therapist neglects or ignores either side of this dialectic. Of course, these two positions can be very difficult to maintain simultaneously. The therapist may need to work on developing his/her capacity for holding onto two seemingly contradictory realities at the same time. Having a theoretical basis for understanding PA men that promotes a compassionate view of the problem may be helpful (Linehan, 1993a). Working within a consultation team that is actively involved in holding onto both of these realities may also be helpful in preventing the therapist from getting overly invested in one or the other position.

DBT also utilizes concepts from a zen philosophical tradition, which influence the flavor of the treatment in a broad way. All the specifics of how this philosophy is incorporated cannot be described here, but a general sense will be provided. A mindfulness tradition emphasizes developing an ability to directly experience one's reality without avoidance, as well as developing a stance from which to observe one's experience. Many people with BPD, like all of us, struggle to escape the reality of the suffering that is present in life, which is of course understandable; however, the struggle to escape leads to many maladaptive behaviors. In DBT, the skills of tolerating painful affect and other aspects of experience, being willing rather than willful, and learning to experience rather than avoid are integrated throughout the treatment. Clients practice skills that help them to develop an ability to *notice* and describe what they are experiencing (e.g., to notice their own emotional states, the thoughts going through their minds, their urges) (Linehan, 1993b). Many PA men have tremendous difficulty observing their own internal states, and thus have difficulty developing more adaptive ways of responding.

A mindfulness tradition informs a number of important concepts that are part of the treatment, including the notion of being "non-judgmental." A non-judgmental stance is one that focuses on the consequences of one's behavior, rather than a moralistic assessment of "good" versus "bad" (e.g., identifying the destructive consequences of violence, as opposed to identifying someone as a "bad" person because of their history of violent behavior). Clients are taught to identify judgments and to notice the impact of judgmental thinking. In addition, therapists work on developing a non-judgmental stance themselves. A non-judgmental stance means avoiding being superior or patronizing toward the client, or assuming that the client is somehow less of a person. Maintaining a non-judgmental stance toward the violent person means shifting one's focus from the "badness" of the behavior or person to instead focus on the consequences of violence: that it is harmful to others, prevents the development of healthy relationships, and creates many problems in the abusive person's life, and is therefore worth changing. It is important to be clear that being non-judgmental does not mean that the behavior is viewed as "acceptable" or "OK" in the sense that it is condoned. The point is to focus on abusive behavior as a problem to be solved, rather than focusing on a more moralistic view.

OVERVIEW OF TREATMENT

Standard DBT is a multimodal outpatient psychotherapy that provides intensive services (i.e., individual psychotherapy, group skills training, phone consultation for the client); however, this model is based on a set of principles that can be applied in a variety of treatment settings. In addition to being principle-driven, DBT utilizes a stage model of treatment. Each stage has a set of hierarchically arranged treatment targets representing the client problems that are addressed at that stage. Some of the basic DBT principles that guide the structure of DBT programs will be described here.

From a DBT perspective (Linehan, 1993a), there are five basic components that are essential to the change process for individuals meeting criteria for BPD, and for comprehensive DBT programs to function well. The first function is the development of new, more adaptive behaviors that are currently outside the client's repertoire. There is an assumption in DBT that people in this population lack the skills they need to behave more adaptively, so instruction in new skills is an essential aspect of treatment. New skills are most often taught in a group skills training format. Second, there is also an assumption that there are generally many obstacles to utilizing these new skills, and these obstacles must be addressed. Factors such as lack of motivation, intense emotions that make using skills difficult, or relationships or other life circumstances can all interfere with change. In DBT, these types of obstacles are usually addressed in individual psychotherapy. Third, generalization of new skills to a variety of contexts is essential, but often requires specific support. Many clients have difficulty generalizing new behaviors to their day-to-day lives; DBT addresses this problem through between-session phone consultation with a therapist or skills coach, milieu treatment, via homework assignments and other interventions that promote generalization. Fourth, DBT is a team approach and makes the assumption that working with extremely difficult client populations requires the support and input of a team, as opposed to a single practitioner working in isolation; therefore, team consultation is also an essential function. Finally, DBT provides for a "structuring the environment" function; this function involves a team member or administrator having sufficient control over the treatment setting that the resources and processes needed to conduct DBT can be accessed.

DBT is a stage model of treatment, including pre-treatment and stages one through four. Pretreatment and Stage 1 have been more elaborately developed and tested than Stages 2 through 4, and are the primary focus of this article. Stage is determined by the problems the client is experiencing that need to be addressed in treatment, and each stage includes a set of hierarchically organized treatment targets or problems that are the focus for change at that stage. The purpose of the treatment target hierarchy is, at the broadest level, to assist the clinician in developing a conceptualization of the client, and at the more concrete level, in deciding what to focus on in a given session or interaction with the client. Clients with borderline characteristics often have numerous difficult problems happening at once, as well as frequent crises. DBT provides guidelines regarding when addressing certain targets should be adhered to strictly (i.e., when life-threatening behavior has occurred) versus when flexibility is expected. The targets help insure that issues that are difficult to address (such as abusive behavior) do get focused on in the session, but the guidelines are not to be used rigidly.

The pre-treatment stage is for clients who have yet to commit to changing targeted behaviors (e.g., self-harm, violence), have yet to commit to therapy, and/or have committed at some point but are no longer committed. At this stage, the therapist orients the client to treatment by explaining how DBT is conducted and what he can expect if he decides to participate. The therapy also focuses on increasing the client's level of commitment.

Commitment to change is often a major problem for people with violent behavior. Many abusive clients enter therapy under court referral, and are likely to be working at a pre-treatment level, in which they are not committed to therapy or to changing abusive behaviors. The DBT therapist in this situation focuses on the pre-treatment target of increasing level of commitment, before trying to achieve other goals. DBT includes a variety of strategies used for increasing the client's level of commitment, which would be used at this point in the therapy process. For example, the therapist may have the client explore the pros and cons of stopping abusive behavior versus continuing to be abusive. The therapist may explore any areas of the client's life that he *does* want to change and then link those goals to reducing abusive behavior (i.e., stopping violence in the service of having a more satisfying relationship with one's partner). The therapist is likely to try to build on any commitment the client is willing to make, and to reinforce him for small commitments, while attempting to shape him into larger commitments.

When to move from pretreatment to Stage 1 can be a difficult decision that involves an important dialectic. On the one hand, Stage 1 work is impossible if the client has absolutely no commitment to change. It is not reasonable to attempt Stage 1 treatment if the client expresses no interest in changing his behavior. On the other hand, blaming others, minimizing and denying are often viewed as hallmarks of the behavior of PA men; it does not make sense to expect the client to be one hundred percent committed to change before working on violence. Consequently, the DBT therapist must make a decision about what level of commitment is sufficient to proceed from pretreatment into Stage 1, balancing both sides of this dialectic. Work on commitment level is likely to continue intermittently during Stage 1, as the client's level of commitment waxes and wanes.

It is important to note that DBT is a voluntary treatment; for individuals who are mandated into treatment, it is important that they still have the opportunity to opt into or out of DBT. This is sometimes accomplished by having two programs available–a DBT approach and some other treatment approach. McCann et al. (2000) provide a useful discussion of approaches to working with involuntary patients.

Once at Stage 1, the primary goals become establishing a strong therapeutic relationship, developing safety in the person's life, and learning important skills to deal with intense emotions and relationship difficulties. The specific treatment targets are, in order: (1) suicidal and other life-threatening behaviors; (2) therapy-interfering behaviors; (3) quality-of-life interfering behaviors (e.g., homelessness, lack of employment, or substance use); and (4) increasing skills (Linehan, 1993a).

The therapy is structured around these treatment targets such that, if a top treatment target behavior has occurred since the previous session (e.g., the person has been violent or engaged in parasuicide), it is a focus of the session. If no life-threatening behavior has occurred, the therapist turns the focus to any behaviors on the part of the client that are interfering with the process of therapy (therapy-interfering behavior). The third highest priority is then quality-of-life interfering behaviors, which include any problems that significantly interfere with the client's quality of life, such as substance abuse, lack of employment or adequate housing, or unaddressed medical problems. Finally, the therapist includes teaching and coaching on DBT skills throughout. Although these targets are arranged hierarchically, in practice a given session often includes some focus on all of the top targets. As noted by Fruzzetti and Levensky (2000), even if a client has not specifically been violent since the previous session, other violence-relevant target behaviors are likely to be a focus, such as urges to be violent and verbal abuse.

Therapy-interfering behavior of the client refers to problematic behaviors, such as not completing homework, missing or coming late to sessions, or any other behavior that interferes with therapeutic progress. In addition, Linehan (1993a) also includes behaviors that have a negative impact on the therapist, such as behaving abusively toward the therapist, or more subtle behaviors that reduce the therapist's desire and motivation to work with the client. With clients who have significant relationship problems, it is crucial that the therapist and client work on their relationship, and the client's behavior that affects the relationship, so that the therapist-client team is able to maintain a good connection and be motivated to work together. In DBT, therapy-interfering behavior is ideally addressed directly but nonjudgmentally, with the therapist both calling attention to the behaviors, and then working with the client on how to change them. Therapy interfering behaviors of the therapist are also viewed as very important, and are most often addressed within the context of the consultation team.

Stage 1 also addresses significant quality of life interfering behaviors, such as substance abuse, homelessness, unemployment, dysfunctional health-related behaviors, and so on. These are organized hierarchically in terms of their relationship to the higher level targets, such that any quality of life interfering behavior that contributes to the client engaging in suicidal or violent behavior would likely be a high target. DBT uses a variety of standard cognitive-behavioral and problem-solving approaches to address quality of life targets.

In developing new forms of DBT to address the needs of other treatment populations, DBT therapists and researchers often develop a more detailed set of targets relevant to the problems of that population (Linehan, 2000). For example, in a version of DBT developed for substance abusers, substance abuse is the top quality-of-life interfering behavior. In addition, a more detailed set of targets relevant to substance abuse is also used (Dimeff et al., 2000), including behaviors such as "keeping options to use drugs open" (e.g., by staying in contact with your dealer). Having such a list of violence-relevant target behaviors may also be helpful, and would likely include such behaviors as destroying property, verbal abuse, out-of-control anger, urges to be violent, and so on. Self-monitoring of violent and abusive behaviors, as well as these violence-relevant targets may be useful in determining the focus of sessions. Clients may be reluctant, embarrassed or unwilling to self-monitor and report abusive behavior. If so, this would be targeted as a therapy-interfering behavior.

Once Stage 1 issues have been addressed, the person advances to Stage 2, in which they focus on post-traumatic stress issues. This is not to say that these issues are ignored at Stage 1; however, they are not addressed via re-experiencing/exposure interventions until safety and skills are well-established. Finally, if they choose to, the person moves into the more advanced stages of therapy that focus on individual goals (e.g., for career, education, or relationships), building of self-respect (Stage 3) and a capacity for true joy and connection (Stage 4).

INTERVENTIONS

DBT interventions embody the central dialectic of the treatment: acceptance versus change (Linehan, 1993a). Change-oriented interventions focus on eliciting, teaching and developing new behaviors. Acceptance-oriented strategies focus on acceptance of reality as it is, acknowledgment of what is and validation of the client. Although it is not possible to describe all of the therapeutic interventions that are a part of DBT here, some primary ones will be discussed. The implications of applying these interventions to aggressive and abusive behavior will be explored.

Orienting and Commitment

DBT begins with orientation to the treatment and a focus on the client's commitment to changing targeted behaviors and to participating in treatment. Orienting involves describing and explaining what the treatment is about and how it works. The client is told what he can expect from the therapist, and what will be expected of him if therapy is pursued. Orienting strategies are used throughout treatment, in particular when a new intervention or goal is being introduced. As with cognitive-behavioral therapies more generally, DBT assumes that clients can more actively participate in treatment if they are informed about what it involves. Orienting with abusive clients would include explanation of the fact that one purpose of the therapy is to stop abusive behavior. They would be given information about what is meant by abusive behavior, and given an explanation of how abusive behavior develops and is maintained. From a DBT perspective, this explanation would likely include some emphasis on emotion dysregulation and the effects of the invalidating environment. It may also incorporate other research findings on the development and maintenance of abusive behavior.

Therapy also begins with the client being asked to make a commitment to whatever goals are being established, such as stopping abusive behavior and participating in therapy. Continuing with DBT would not be viewed as appropriate if the client has absolutely no interest in changing abusive behavior, although this lack of commitment could be the focus of "pretreatment" intervention. Commitment strategies are used in the eliciting and strengthening of commitment, with the goals being that the client be realistic about what he is agreeing to, making as firm a commitment as possible, and committing in a way that is most likely to promote keeping the commitment.

Validation

At the most fundamental level, validation in DBT is the therapist communicating to the client "that her responses make sense and are understandable" (Linehan, 1993a, p. 222). As described earlier, many people with BPD have extensive histories of *invalidation*, having been told that their reactions are unreasonable, that they are just "too sensitive," or that the way they are reacting to events is inappropriate. Validation in therapy helps the client come to trust his own responses more, to feel understood and connected, and to gain a better understanding of what normative responses are.

An important component of validation is that it involves "confirming" a person's experience, as opposed to being complimentary (Linehan, 2001). For example, telling someone they have done a good job when they firmly believe they have not is actually invalidating. In addition, the DBT therapist strives to only validate that which is valid, rather than to be universally validating. Valid responses include those that are normative, make sense given the circumstances, or make sense given the person's goals (Linehan, 2001). For example, getting angry when one's partner criticizes harshly may be valid in the sense that most people would react that way; however, responding by hitting the partner is not valid if the goal is to improve the relationship.

The DBT therapist searches for client responses that can be validated. Validating various experiences and emotions that lead up to violence is often important (Fruzzetti & Levensky, 2000). For example, as noted by Fruzzetti and Levensky, the therapist would likely communicate that it makes sense that the client feels fear and sadness when his partner threatens to leave, since most people feel those emotions when the loss of an important relationship seems likely. Finding things to validate can be particularly difficult with abusive clients. Much of their experience of the violence may be outside the realm of what should reasonably be validated. For example, the client may think that the victim "deserved" to be hit or that his violent behavior was "her fault." The therapist needs to consider a variety of factors in choosing what to validate, including in what sense the behavior is "valid" (i.e., in terms of past learning, being a normative response that most people would experience, or moving one in the direction of one's goals) (Linehan, 1997). Some behaviors may make sense (be valid) in terms of the client's history, but not in terms of the client's goals. For example, it may make sense that a client is violent if he was physically abused and emotionally neglected in childhood, witnessed violence between his parents, never learned skills to cope with anger, and is now in a conflictual relationship (Fruzzetti & Levensky, 2000). On the other hand, violence is not valid in terms of reaching one's goals, if those goals include having a good relationship with a partner, staying out of jail, etc. The therapist should also carefully consider whether the validation is likely to reinforce that particular behavior in a problematic way.

Behavioral and Solution Analysis

One of the most central strategies of DBT is behavioral analysis (BA; Linehan, 1993a). It is crucial that therapists doing DBT have a thorough understanding of basic behavioral principles and interventions, including behavioral analysis. A brief description will be provided here.

In behavioral analysis, a problematic behavior (which could include thinking, feeling, overt behavior or some combination) is analyzed in terms of the precipitants leading up to it and the events that follow. The first step is identifying what the problematic behavior is, being as behaviorally specific as possible. The therapist and client then talk through very specifically the events, thoughts, feelings and behaviors that led up to the problematic behavior, and follow this through to include an analysis of the events that followed, with particular attention to the consequences of the problematic behavior. Behavioral analyses in DBT tend to emphasize the occurrence of emotions and emotion dysregulation, as these tend to be a primary target for intervention (Fruzzetti & Levensky, 2000).

The therapist uses his/her knowledge of the client and the client's history to develop hypotheses about what factors might be influencing the client. This includes the use of "insight strategies" (Linehan, 1993a). Insight strategies involve noting connections and patterns. For example, the therapist may focus on how certain events or emotions often lead to the client responding in a particular way. The therapist may also focus on in-session behavior, for example, commenting on how the client responds to the therapist. The goal is to develop an understanding of what events, thoughts and emotions trigger problem behaviors, and what consequences are present that may be maintaining these behaviors, in order to identify places to intervene.

Applying DBT to the problem of eliminating violent and abusive behavior would likely include heavy use of behavioral analysis. A therapist working with a PA man would conduct behavioral analyses of past instances of violent and/or abusive behavior, in order to formulate an understanding of what variables are influencing the behavior. The first step would be to identify the specific violent/abusive behaviors being targeted. This is particularly important because the client's conception of what constitutes violent and abusive behavior may be different than the therapist's. For example, threatening one's partner with a raised fist, without actually hitting her, may be considered abusive by the therapist, but not by the client. Self-monitoring of the behaviors of interest is likely to be useful. In the case of low base rate behaviors (e.g., a PA man who is only infrequently violent), it may be particularly useful to monitor related behaviors such as level of anger, thoughts about being abusive, urges to be abusive, and so on. Behavioral analyses can then be done on these target-relevant behaviors (Fruzzetti & Levensky, 2000).

As described earlier, the behavioral analysis should be a very detailed, step-by-step description of the events leading up to the violence/abuse, the actual violent/abusive behaviors and the consequences. Fruzzetti, Saedi, Wilson, Rubio, and Levensky (1999) have developed a semi-structured interview, the Domestic Violence Interview (DVI), which guides the interviewer through a behavioral analysis of violent or aggressive behavior (Fruzzetti & Levensky, 2001). The analysis should begin as early in the chain of events as necessary (e.g., when the client first noticed himself becoming angry, agitated or upset, or when stressful things first started affecting him). Although each person is unique, some common factors that may be identified through behavioral analysis of abusive behavior will be described. These factors are then targeted for intervention through a solution analysis.

One factor that can contribute to problematic behavior is that the person may be lacking the skills needed to behave more adaptively. For example, the abusive person may lack self-observation skills crucial to noticing that he is becoming angry; he may lack assertiveness skills with his partner (Dutton & Strachan, 1987; O'Leary & Curley, 1986); he may lack skills to soothe or calm himself or he may lack skills to express emotions other than anger. Any of these behavioral deficits may increase the risk for violence, and would direct the therapist to working on increasing skills in these areas. In DBT, if a skills deficit appears to be contributing to the problem, the intervention of choice is skills training. The therapist works with the client to learn the needed new behaviors, and to apply those in the relevant contexts.

Violent and abusive behavior can also be maintained by reinforcing consequences. The violence or abuse may be reinforced by the PA man getting his way in an argument, by the partner stopping some aversive behavior or by the reduction of a state of negative affect or arousal following violent behavior. All of these scenarios are familiar to professionals who work with PA men. It may be difficult to think of a case where violent or abusive behavior did not seem to be reinforced in some way, at least in the short term. One reason these consequences of violent behavior are powerful is that they are usually very immediate.

If violent or abusive behavior is being reinforced, one approach is to attempt to change the contingencies so they no longer support this behavior. This type of intervention is referred to as "contingency management." Obviously this is a difficult task since the therapist does not have control over all the contingencies. The use of arrest is an example of using punishment to decrease violent behavior. In the absence of direct control over contingencies, the therapist may help the client get more in touch with the broader range of consequences of both his abusive and more adaptive behavior. Highlighting the longer-term negative consequences of violence may be useful. Self-monitoring of times when the client had the urge to be abusive but was not can provide opportunities for the therapist to give or highlight reinforcing consequences of non-abusive behavior. The difficulties with controlling consequences also suggest the importance of concentrated work earlier in the chain of events leading up to violence, to prevent its occurrence whenever possible (Fruzzetti & Levensky, 2000).

Sometimes maladaptive behaviors occur because the individual's engagement in more adaptive behavior is blocked by strong emotions, such as fear, guilt or anxiety. They may know what to do, and could actually do the behavior if they were not fearful or guilty, but are blocked by those emotions. For example, an abusive person may want to ask for something from his partner, but feel afraid and avoid doing it. The fear and frustration about not being able to make a request may lead to anger and then abusive behavior. In DBT, the intervention of choice in situations where emotions like fear, guilt or shame are blocking adaptive behavior is the behavioral technique of exposure. The word "exposure" refers to the person being exposed to, or in the presence of, the feared stimulus. This can be done through imagery, or in vivo. Exposure-based techniques are widely used in the treatment of PTSD and a variety of other anxiety-related disorders. By way of example, if a PA man who is a war combat survivor has an intense fear reaction to some stimulus, he may then have a secondary emotional response of anger, and become violent. In addition to other interventions, exposure to the combat-related traumatic cues may reduce the fear response, and decrease the likelihood of violence.

Finally, problematic behavior may be influenced or maintained by clients' beliefs or cognitions. If the behavioral analysis suggests that the client's beliefs or thoughts play a role in maintaining the behavior, cognitive-based interventions may be useful. This could include a range of interventions used in cognitive-behavioral therapies, such as self-monitoring of cognitions, examining evidence for the cognitions, and developing challenges for maladaptive cognitions.

Irreverent and Reciprocal Communication Styles

DBT therapists utilize stylistic strategies to guide some specific aspects of how they interact with clients. These stylistic strategies must be adapted to fit with a given therapist's style; however, they can be very useful in responding to some of the more difficult elements of treating individuals with BPD. These two styles, irreverent and reciprocal communication, provide two sides of a dialectic, one end representing warmth and responsiveness, the other end representing confrontation and desynchrony (Linehan, 1993a).

The reciprocal style involves expressing warmth, connection and caring. It also includes use of self-disclosure. Two types of self-disclosure are used in DBT: disclosures about the therapist's reactions to the client, and disclosures about the therapist's use of skills, approach to problems, or other forms of modeling. Self-disclosure is carefully used for the client's benefit, not to inappropriately meet the therapist's own needs. DBT therapists use self-disclosure to give the client feedback about how the client is affecting the therapist or about how he is coming across, particularly when the client engages in therapy-interfering behaviors. DBT takes the stance that the therapist's reactions and feelings can provide essential feedback to the client, allow him to learn about his impact on others and provide opportunity for crucial processing of the therapeutic relationship.

The irreverent communication style is, as the name implies, a style that involves taking an outrageous position, being deadpan or off-beat, or taking things to an extreme. It is not disrespectful or cynical, but is often humorous. This style is used to help the client see when he is being extreme, to lighten things up or to get things moving beyond a stuck point. It is used to get the client's attention, or to shake things up when they are bogged down or stuck, in particular when the client is stuck in some rigid or extreme way of thinking.

DBT Skills Training

The teaching of skills is an integral part of DBT. The particular skills taught are divided into four types: core skills, emotion regulation skills, distress tolerance skills and interpersonal effectiveness skills (Linehan, 1993b). These skills are based on the assumption that difficulty tolerating and modulating painful affect often leads to the other behavioral problems experienced by emotionally dysregulated clients. The skills are also organized around the central acceptance-change dialectic. Clients practice both learning to change their emotional states, and learning to tolerate and be in the presence of painful emotions, without engaging in maladaptive behaviors in response to those emotions (e.g., drug use, self-harm or violence).

The core skills of DBT are based on eastern philosophy and meditative practices. They include learning to observe and describe one's thoughts and emotions, and practicing "mindfulness." Many of us spend a great deal of our time doing one thing, while thinking about several others, barely aware of what we are doing in the moment. Mindfulness involves remaining focused on "one thing at a time." It is the practice of taking control of where one focuses one's attention. Emotion regulation skills involve learning about what emotions are and how they operate, how to be less vulnerable to negative emotions and how to change negative emotional states. For example, clients learn that behaving consistent with an emotion (e.g., being passive when depressed, or aggressing when angry) tends to increase or prolong that emotion, whereas acting opposite to an emotional state (e.g., being active when depressed, being gentle or calm when angry) tends to decrease the emotion.

Distress tolerance skills involve learning to tolerate negative emotions in order to get through difficult situations, without doing something destructive. For example, clients learn skills such as how to distract, to self-soothe, to think through the pros and cons of sticking with whatever they are working on, and so on. These strategies are not designed to change or resolve the situation, but simply to help the client get through difficult or emotionally painful moments. Finally, interpersonal skills, focused primarily on appropriate assertiveness, are taught. Interpersonal situations are broken down into a number of different components, such as determining what your goals are in the situation: maintaining a positive relationship, getting what you want, and/or maintaining a sense of self-respect. Clients use homework practice and worksheets to work through various interpersonal situations, and are coached in group on ways to apply better interpersonal skills, including how to ask for things effectively, how to be direct and persuasive without alienating others, how to validate others, and so on.

Recent attempts to adapt DBT skills training to the treatment of domestic violence (Fruzzetti & Levensky, 2000) and other aggressive behavior (McCann, Ball, & Ivanoff, 2000) have included several additions and changes to the standard DBT skills package. First, a psychoeducational component on violence and abuse is likely to be helpful. Standard DBT skills groups begin with an orientation that includes a description of BPD and a description of the biosocial theory underlying DBT. A group for partner abusive men might include a psychoeducational component describing what violence and abuse are, and, from a DBT perspective, might also describe the roles of emotion dysregulation and other BPD-related problems in violent and abusive behavior. Other relevant theory and research data on domestic violence may also be provided.

Fruzzetti and Levensky (2000) describe the addition of a new module in their domestic violence treatment program, which focuses on teaching validation skills. This module instructs clients in how to validate both themselves and others. One of the goals of this module is to increase clients' levels of empathy. The skills taught in this module include "(a) understanding the forms and functions of validation (including empathy) and invalidation, (b) specific skills to identify targets (e.g., emotions, opinions, effective behaviors) for understanding and validation, (c) empathy and validation practice, and (d) the verbal and communication skills to validate others effectively" (p. 442). The practice of validation and empathy is extended to understanding and validation of victim's reactions to aggressive behavior. McCann et al. (2000) similarly added a goal of "increasing mindfulness of empathy and consequences to others" (p. 451) to their skills training program.

In addition, McCann et al. (2000) revised their skills training program after extensive consultation with a group of consumers with antisocial personality disorder who reviewed the standard DBT skills package. They concluded that their inpatient forensic population would benefit from a skills module focused on "increasing emotional attachment." To this end, they have introduced skills designed to "increase awareness of commonality of experience; increase behaviors that cause others to feel cared about; understand the reinforcers of attachment and detachment; discover and create a social support system" (p. 452). Patients are encouraged to engage in "random acts of kindness," with the goal of increasing feelings of caring for others, and ultimately feelings of attachment to others.

Finally, McCann et al. (2000) also developed a skills module they call "Crime Review," which is designed for participants who have successfully completed the other skills training modules. The goals of the Crime Review module are to increase empathy and to identify factors that contributed to violent behavior. Patients complete behavioral analyses of the violent behavior which led to their incarceration, including discussion of specifically what they did, how it affected the victim, a relapse plan and a plan for making repair. Patients present the review of their violent behavior in a systematic, structured fashion and receive feedback.

Consultation Group

The consultation team is designed to help members stay on track with the dialectics of treatment. The consultation team provides a place for team members to express their feelings about the work they are doing and to get validation and support; however, the team must provide more than just support to be effective. DBT teams also provide constructive input and feedback about the therapist's work, help team members maintain a non-pejorative stance toward clients, and stay on track with doing the best possible treatment.

Team dynamics and the maintenance of a strong team are crucial to the success of a DBT program. In the service of helping teams function well, the DBT model provides a set of assumptions about patients, therapists and therapy, and a set of agreements for consultation team members (Linehan, 1993a). For example, team members agree to do their best to be non-defensive, and to recognize that mistakes are expected. Team members agree to attempt to find the least pejorative, least blaming explanation for clients' behavior. The team is charged with helping each therapist recognize when a client's behavior is pushing the therapist beyond his/her limits, and to problem-solve ways to address such therapy-interfering behavior. In addition, the team points out any therapy-interfering behavior of the therapist, and helps the therapist find ways to deal with it.

The consultation team component of DBT has clear and direct application to the treatment of abusive people. The need for support and consultation for therapists in working with this population is clear. In addition, the role of the consultation team in maintaining a dialectical stance, and avoiding getting polarized in a destructive way, is also essential when treating abusive individuals. Maintaining a dialectical stance and avoiding black or white thinking while working with abusive individuals is probably one of the most difficult therapeutic tasks clinicians face. A strong team can be very helpful in that arena.

CONCLUSION

It is clear from the description provided here that a standard form of DBT adapted directly for treatment of PA men is likely to be more resource intensive than a typical group treatment approach, since it provides both individual psychotherapy, group skills training and phone consultation to the client. Currently available resources in many programs may make providing this form of DBT impossible. One solution is to develop criteria that can be used for selecting a subgroup of clients to be eligible for DBT. These might include high levels of emotion dysregulation, borderline characteristics, or high risk for continued violence and/or treatment drop-out. Alternatively, the standard form of DBT might be modified to meet all five functions, but do so in a less resource-intensive manner, such as addressing obstacles to change in a group that utilizes behavioral analyses, rather than doing this in individual therapy.

NOTE

Although conceived independently, this chapter converges with the thinking of Fruzzetti and Levensky (2000) and McCann, Ball, and Ivanoff (2000) in a number of areas, and diverges in others. For example, the rationale for applying DBT to address domestic violence provided here is similar to that described by Fruzzetti and Levensky (2000), as are a number of the recommendations about how to apply the model. Some of the unique treatment developments made by these two teams are discussed in this article, but we recommend their papers to the interested reader for more comprehensive descriptions of their innovative approaches. Readers primarily interested in the application of DBT to address domestic violence are referred to Fruzzetti and Levensky (2000). Readers interested in the application of DBT to individuals with antisocial personality disorder or antisocial characteristics, or to work with forensic populations, are encouraged to read McCann, Ball, and Ivanoff's (2000) paper on this topic.

REFERENCES

Babock, J. C., Green, C. E., & Robie, C. (under review). Does batterer treatment work?: A meta-analytic review of domestic violence treatment outcome research.

Barasch, A., Frances, A. J., & Hurt, S. W. (1985). Stability and distinctness of borderline personality disorder. *American Journal of Psychiatry, 142*, 1484-1486.

Becker, C. B., & Zayfert, C. (2001). Integrating DBT-based techniques and concepts to facilitate exposure treatment for PTSD. *Cognitive and Behavioral Practice, 8*, 107-122.

Daly, J. E., & Pelowski, S. (2000). Predictors of dropout among men who batter: A review of studies with implications for research and practice. *Violence & Victims, 15*, 137-160.

Dimeff, L., Rizvi, S. L., Brown, M., & Linehan, M. M. (2000). Dialectical behavior therapy for substance abuse: A pilot application to methamphetamine-dependent women with borderline personality disorder. *Cognitive and Behavioral Practice, 7*, 457-468.

Dunford, F. W. (2000). The San Diego Navy Experiment: An assessment of interventions for men who assault their wives. *Journal of Consulting and Clinical Psychology, 68*, 468-476.

Dutton, D. G. (1995a). *The batterer: A psychological profile.* New York: Basic Books.

Dutton, D. G. (1995b). Male abusiveness in intimate relationships. *Clinical Psychology Review, 15*, 567-581.

Dutton, D. G., & Browning, T. J. (1988). Concern for power, fear of intimacy and aversive stimuli for wife assault. In G. Hotaling, D. Finkelhor, J. T. Kirkpatrick, & M. A. Straus (Eds.), *Family abuse and its consequences: New direction in research* (pp. 163-175). Newbury Park, CA: Sage.

Dutton, D. G., & Starzomski, A. J. (1993). Borderline personality in perpetrators of psychological and physical abuse. *Violence & Victims, 8*, 327-337.

Dutton, D. G., & Strachan, C. E. (1987). Motivational needs for power and spouse-specific assertiveness in assaultive and nonassaultive men. *Violence and Victims, 2*, 145-156.

Feldbau-Kohn, S., Heyman, R. E., & O'Leary, K. D. (1998). Major depressive disorder and depressive symptomatology as predictors of husband to wife physical aggression. *Violence & Victims, 13,* 347-360.

Fruzzetti, A. E., & Levensky, E. R. (2000). Dialectical behavior therapy for domestic violence: Rationale and procedures. *Cognitive and Behavioral Practice, 7,* 435-447.

Fruzzetti, A. E., Saedj, N., Wilson, M. E., Rubio, A., & Levensky, E. R. (1999). *Domestic Violence Interview Manual.* Reno, NV: University of Nevada.

George, D. T., Hibbeln, J. R., Ragan, P. W., Umhau, J. C., Phillips, M. J., Doty, L., Hommer, D., & Rawlings, R. R. (2000). Lactate-induced rage and panic in a select group of subjects who perpetrate acts of domestic violence. *Biological Psychiatry, 47,* 804-812.

Gondolf, E. W., & White, R. J. (2001). Batterer program participants who repeatedly reassault: Psychopathic tendencies and other disorders. *Journal of Interpersonal Violence,* 361-380.

Hamberger, K., & Hastings, J. (1991). Personality correlates of men who batter and nonviolent men: Some continuities and discontinuities. *Journal of Family Violence, 6,* 131-147.

Hamberger, L. K., & Hastings, J. E. (1986). Personality correlates of men who abuse their partners: A cross-validation study. *Journal of Family Violence, 1,* 323-341.

Hamberger, L. K., Lohr, J. M., Bonge, D., & Tolin, D. F. (1996). A large sample empirical typology of male spouse abusers and its relationship to dimensions of abuse. *Violence and Victims, 11,* 277-292.

Hastings, J., & Hamberger, K. (1988). Personality characteristics of spouse abusers: A controlled comparison. *Violence and Victims, 3,* 31-48.

Holtzworth-Munroe, A., & Anglin, K. (1991). The competency of responses given by maritally violent versus nonviolent men to problematic marital situations. *Violence and Victims, 6,* 257-269.

Holtzworth-Munroe, A., & Smutzler, N. (1996). Comparing the emotional reactions and behavior intentions of violent and nonviolent husbands to aggressive, distressed and other wife behaviors. *Violence & Victims, 11,* 319-339.

Holtzworth-Munroe, A., & Stuart, G. L. (1994). Typologies of male batterers: Three subtypes and the differences among them. *Psychological Bulletin, 116,* 475-497.

Hotaling, G. T., & Sugarman, D. B. (1986). An analysis of risk markers in husband to wife violence: The current state of knowledge. *Violence and Victims, 1,* 101-124.

Kelly, T., Soloff, P. H., Cornelius, J., Goerge, A., Lis, J. A., & Ulrich, R. (1992). Can we study (treat) borderline patients? Attrition from research and open treatment. *Journal of Personality Disorders, 6,* 417-433.

Koerner, K., & Dimeff, L. A. (2000). Further data on dialectical behavior therapy. *Clinical Psychology: Science and Practice, 7,* 104-112.

Koerner, K., & Linehan, M. M. (2000). Research on dialectical behavior therapy for patients with borderline personality disorder. *Psychiatric Clinics of North America Special Issue: Borderline Personality Disorder, 23,* 151-167.

Koons, C. R., Robins, C. J., Tweed, J. L., Lynch, T. R., Gonzalez, A. M., Morse, J. Q., Bishop, G. K., Butterfield, M. I., & Bastian, L. A. (2001). Efficacy of dialectical behavior therapy in women veterans with borderline personality disorder. *Behavior Therapy, 32,* 371-390.

Linehan, M. M. (1993a). *Cognitive behavioral therapy of borderline personality disorder.* New York: Guilford.

Linehan, M. M. (1993b). *Skills training manual for treating borderline personality disorder.* New York: Guilford.

Linehan, M. M. (1997). Validation and psychotherapy. In A. Bohart & L. Greenberg, (Eds.), *Empathy reconsidered: New directions in psychotherapy* (pp. 353-392). Washington, D.C.: American Psychological Association.

Linehan, M. M. (2000). Commentary on innovations in Dialectical Behavior Therapy. *Cognitive and Behavioral Practice, 7,* 478-481.

Linehan, M. M., Armstrong, H. E., Suarez, A., Allmon, D., & Heard, H. L. (1991). Cognitive-behavioral treatment of chronically parasuicidal borderline patients. *Archives of General Psychiatry, 48,* 1060-1064.

Linehan, M. M., & Schmidt, H. III. (1995). The dialectics of effective treatment of borderline personality disorder. In W. O. O'Donohue & L. Krasner (Eds.), *Theories in behavior therapy: Exploring behavior change* (pp. 553-584). Washington, D.C.: American Psychological Association.

Lynch, T. R. (2000). Treatment of elderly depression with personality disorder comorbidity using dialectical behavior therapy. *Cognitive and Behavioral Practice, 7,* 468-477.

McCann, R. A., Ball, E. M., & Ivanoff, A. (2000). DBT with an inpatient forensic population: The CMHIP Forensic Model. *Cognitive and Behavioral Practice, 7,* 447-456.

Maiuro, R., Cahn, T., & Vitaliano, P. (1988). Anger, hostility, and depression in domestically violent versus generally assaultive men and nonviolent control subjects. *Journal of Consulting and Clinical Psychology, 56,* 17-23.

Miller, A. L., Rathus, J. H., Linehan, M. M., Wetzler, S., & Leigh, E. (1997). Dialectical behavior therapy: Adaptations and new applications. *Cognitive and Behavioral Practice, 7,* 420-425.

O'Leary, K. D., & Curley, A. D. (1986). Assertion and family violence: Correlates of spouse abuse. *Journal of Marital and Family Therapy,* 281-289.

Rondeau, G., Brodeur, N., Brochu, S., & Lemire, G. (2001). Dropout and completion of treatment among spouse abusers. *Violence & Victims, 16,* 127-143.

Safer, D. L., Telch, C. F., & Agras, W. S. (2001). Dialectical behavior therapy for bulimia nervosa. *American Journal of Psychiatry Special Issue, 158,* 632-634.

Scheel, K. R. (2000). The empirical basis of Dialectical Behavior Therapy: Summary, critique and implications. *Clinical Psychology: Science and Practice, 7,* 68-86.

Schumacher, J. A., Feldbau-Kohn, S., Slep Smith, A. M., & Heyman, R. E. (2001). Risk factors for male-to-female partner physical abuse. *Aggression & Violent Behavior, 6,* 281-352.

Tweed, R. G., & Dutton, D. G. (1998). A comparison of impulsive and instrumental subgroups of batterers. *Violence & Victims, 13,* 217-230.

Waltz, J., Babcock, J., Jacobson, N. S., & Gottman, J. M. (2000). Testing a typology of batterers. *Journal of Consulting and Clinical Psychology, 68,* 658-669.

Treating Assaultive Men
from an Attachment Perspective

Daniel J. Sonkin
Donald Dutton

SUMMARY. This chapter explores the relationship between attachment theory and treatment of perpetrators of domestic violence. First, the authors present a brief overview of attachment theory. This is followed by a discussion of how domestic violence research findings suggests that attachment theory is a good paradigm to understanding the phenomenon of intimate violence. Lastly, the authors describe the elements of attachment-oriented psychotherapy as they might apply to working with perpetrators of domestic violence. *[Article copies available for a fee from The Haworth Document Delivery Service: 1-800-HAWORTH. E-mail address: <docdelivery@haworthpress.com> Website: <http://www.HaworthPress.com> © 2003 by The Haworth Press, Inc. All rights reserved.]*

KEYWORDS. Attachment theory, attachment, psychotherapy, domestic violence, perpetrator treatment

Address correspondence to: Daniel J. Sonkin, PhD, Independent Practice, 1505 Bridgeway Suite 105, Sausalito, CA 94965 (E-mail: daniel@daniel-sonkin. com); or Donald Dutton, PhD, Professor of Psychology, University of British Columbia, 2136 West Mall, Vancouver V6T 1Y7 (E-mail: dutton@interchange.ubc.ca).

[Haworth co-indexing entry note]: "Treating Assaultive Men from an Attachment Perspective." Sonkin, Daniel J., and Donald Dutton. Co-published simultaneously in *Journal of Aggression, Maltreatment & Trauma* (The Haworth Maltreatment & Trauma Press, an imprint of The Haworth Press, Inc.) Vol. 7, No. 1/2 (#13/14), 2003, pp. 105-133; and: *Intimate Violence: Contemporary Treatment Innovations* (ed: Donald Dutton, and Daniel J. Sonkin) The Haworth Maltreatment & Trauma Press, an imprint of The Haworth Press, Inc., 2003, pp. 105-133. Single or multiple copies of this article are available for a fee from The Haworth Document Delivery Service [1-800-HAWORTH, 9:00 a.m. - 5:00 p.m. (EST). E-mail address: docdelivery@haworthpress.com].

http://www.haworthpress.com/store/product.asp?sku=J146
© 2003 by The Haworth Press, Inc. All rights reserved.
10.1300J146v07n01_06

In a landmark series of studies entitled *Attachment and Loss*, Bowlby (1969, 1973, 1980) outlined a remarkable theory that posited that early attachment had sociobiological significance and constituted a powerful human survival motive. The theory has implications for anger in interpersonal relationships and for the seemingly irrational outburst that accompany real or imagined separation. Primary attachment (usually to the mother[1]) is governed by three important principles: first, alarm of any kind, stemming from any source, activates an attachment survival system in an infant that directs and motivates it to seek out soothing physical contact with the attachment figure. Second, when activated, only physical attachment with the attachment figure will terminate it. Third, when the system has been activated for a long time without soothing and termination, angry behavior appears; if soothing and protection is not eventually found, the system can then become suppressed. Bowlby reported observations he made of young children (15-30 months) separated for the first time from their mothers. He witnessed a three phase behavioral display: anger, despair, and detachment. He concluded from these observations that the primary function of anger was to generate displays that would lead to the return of the absent mother. Anger is thus an attempt to recapture the object that can soothe tension and anxiety at a developmental stage where the child cannot yet self soothe through signaling the mother that she is wanted and/or needed. Anger is an emotion "born of fear" of loss. Dysfunctional anger, occurring later in adult affectional bonds, was defined as anger that distanced the attachment object instead of bringing (her) closer.

Subsequent empirical studies by Ainsworth and her colleagues (1978) showed that different "attachment styles" existed for infants. Initially these were classified as "secure," anxious-avoidant, and anxious-ambivalent. A fourth category emerged in their research that was eventually called disorganized. Subsequent terms for the three insecure patterns were dismissing, preoccupied, and fearful (see Figure 1). The pre-occupied and fearful types sought attachment but experienced anxiety as a consequence of attachment. Also, both experienced anxiety at the disappearance of the mother and were difficult to soothe upon reunion. The fearful children were particularly ambivalent upon reunion with their attachment figure, both approaching and avoiding contact. Dutton cites Bowlby (1969) as describing these children as "arching away angrily while simultaneously seeking proximity" (Dutton, 1995, p. 113) when re-introduced to their mothers. Interestingly, although the avoidant or dismissing children seemed content in the absence of their attachment figure and not

FIGURE 1. The Development of Attachment

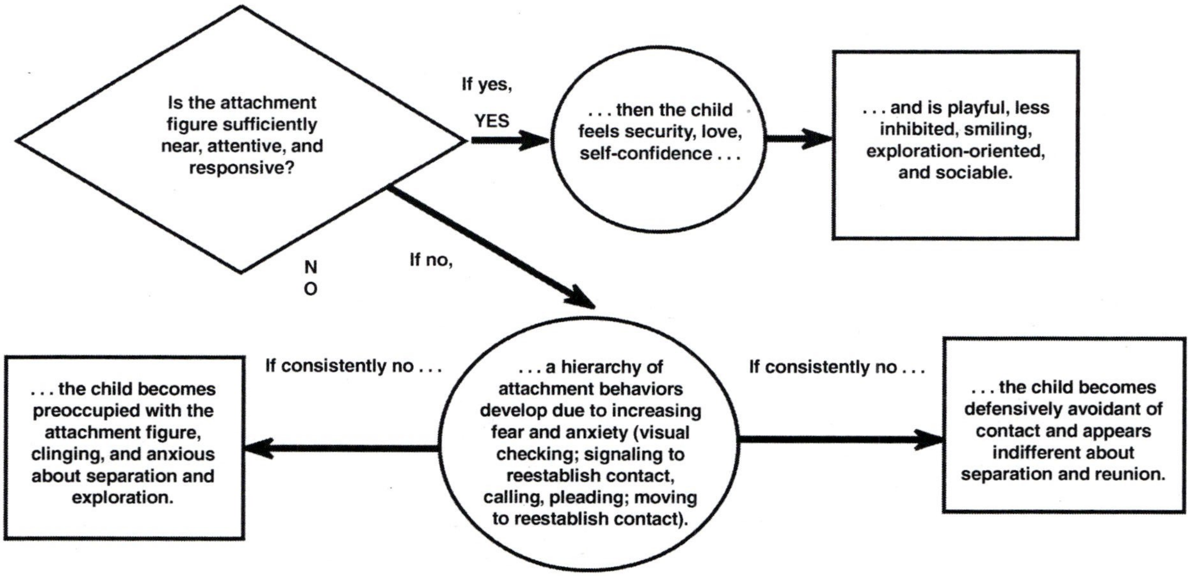

Is the attachment figure sufficiently near, attentive, and responsive?

If yes, YES

... then the child feels security, love, self-confidence ...

... and is playful, less inhibited, smiling, exploration-oriented, and sociable.

NO

If no,

... a hierarchy of attachment behaviors develop due to increasing fear and anxiety (visual checking; signaling to reestablish contact, calling, pleading; moving to reestablish contact).

If consistently no ...

... the child becomes preoccupied with the attachment figure, clinging, and anxious about separation and exploration.

If consistently no ...

... the child becomes defensively avoidant of contact and appears indifferent about separation and reunion.

particularly interested in reconnecting upon reunion, when physiological measures were taken, these children were quite anxious during separation, but somehow learned to repress their feelings (Karen, 1977).

In 1987, Hazan and Shaver published a landmark study that showed that adult "attachment styles" resembled infant attachment styles. (The spate of research that emerged on adult attachment styles is too voluminous to review here; however, the interested reader is referred to Karen (1977) or Sperling and Berman (1994) for a discussion on the history of attachment theory.) Assessment of adult attachment can be done through interviews (Main & Goldwyn, 1998), projective tests (West & George, 1999) or self reports (see http://psychology.ucdavis. edu/Shaver/lab.html). Sperling and Berman (1994) define adult attachment as "the stable tendency of an individual to make substantial efforts to seek and maintain proximity to and contact with one or a few specific individuals who provide the subjective potential for physical and/or psychological safety and security" (p. 8).

One of ways attachment styles have been deconstructed involves what are called *representational models* of self and other (Bartholomew & Horowitz, 1991). Each of these representations is a network of beliefs and expectancies about how the relationship will function. It is a cannon of attachment theory that these representational models are internalized through the attachment process. They include positive and negative views of self, expectancies about what will be received from another and generalized projections about relationship outcome. Bartholomew (1990) systematized these into a 2×2 arrangement for each of four attachment styles, each having a positive or negative self-concept and expectation of another (via relationships). These beliefs present another aspect of attachment that is open to therapeutic intervention. In Bartholomew's schema, Preoccupied attachment styles have negative self-images, while Dismissing attachment styles have negative other images. Fearful attachment styles have both negative self and other images. Fearful attachment styles also expect the worst from an intimate relationship but need such a relationship to heal their damaged self-image. Hence, they are thrown into an ambivalent double avoidance (aloneness versus engulfment) that may serve as the basis for borderline alternation (see Dutton, 1998).

Dutton, Saunders, Starzomski, and Bartholomew (1994) attempted to relate attachment style in adults to abusive behaviors. In a sample of 120 men in treatment for wife assault and 40 demographically matched controls, they assessed men's attachment style using a self report measure called the Relationship Style Questionnaire (Griffin &

Bartholomew, 1994) and abusiveness through wives' reports using the Psychological Maltreatment of Women Inventory (PMWI; Tolman, 1989). A Fearful attachment style in the male perpetrator was highly related to abusiveness, correlating +.46 with the Domination/Isolation subscale of the PMWI, and +.52 with the Emotional Abuse subscale. These relationships were highly significant. To a lesser extent, an attachment style called Preoccupied also correlated significantly with abuse. Fearfully attached men also reported high levels of chronic anxiety and anger. Bartholomew, Henderson, and Dutton (2001) also found that women in shelters escaping abusive relationships could be classified with Preoccupied (53%) or Fearful (35%) attachment styles. These styles were related to the woman's difficulty in leaving the relationship.

Dutton (1998) described what he called the "abusive personality," a constellation of psychological traits that, when assessed in males, are highly related to partners' reports of abusiveness. Fearful attachment was an important component of this personality constellation and, according to Dutton, directed the anger to an intimate target. Men whose violence was predominantly or exclusively in intimate relationships probably have an attachment disorder. This disorder may be related to personality disorder diagnoses such as Borderline or Dependent personality; however, it has an attachment aspect to its origin and plays itself out in intimate relationships. Dutton has suggested that such men have both a public and private (intimate) personality that may be quite dissimilar.

Typically, batterer treatment has not included specific work on attachment (but see Coleman, 2002 and Leisring et al., 2002), yet therapists regularly hear of delusional construals of or pre-occupation with the spouses' behavior (deemed "conjugal paranoia"). For example, one of the authors (Don Dutton) had a client who was convinced that his wife was having an affair when he found "a key with a man's name on it" (the key manufacturer). Many batterers present as cold, unemotional, and non-empathetic, similar to persons with avoidant attachment and those suffering from psychopathy. Likewise, it is common for batterers to show patterns of approach/avoidance as seen with disorganized attachment and borderline personality disorder. Spousal homicide committed by males is frequently in response to real or perceived abandonment (Dutton & Kerry, 1999). Browning and Dutton (1986) obtained pronounced anger/arousal responses in batterers who witnessed a videotape depiction of an "abandonment" (a woman unilaterally deciding to visit another city with female friends and join a woman's consciousness-raising group). Their anger/arousal scores were significantly higher than control groups of men, and were especially pronounced on this "abandonment" scenario. The relationship between fear of abandonment and rage thus appears strong in this group of partner abusive men. The conversion of fear to rage could occur because the latter is more consistent with male sex role conditioning. Regardless, the confrontation of this emotional contribution to abuse deserves therapeutic attention.

These data suggest that incorporating attachment theory into batterer treatment is well founded. First, it can enable batterers to perceive a broader pattern in their reactions to loss and separation in their intimate relationships. Second, this theory supports the prevailing notion that clients need to learn emotion self-regulation during periods of attachment-anxiety. Third, attachment theory suggests that through altering the internal working models of self and other the client can break a perceptual mold in which attachment-anxiety is reduced to either distancing, clinging, or approach/avoidance.

THEORY TO PRACTICE: ATTACHMENT THEORY INFORMED PSYCHOTHERAPY

Although psychotherapy with adults from an attachment perspective is still in early development, some significant clinical ideas and applications exist. Some clinical scholars have incorporated attachment theory into other theories (Masterson & Klein, 1995; Schore, 1994), which has served to enhance general psychoanalytic theory and practice. However, other psychoanalytically oriented theorists have criticized this theory based on its interpersonal versus intrapsychic focus and the categorical, mutually exclusive attachment categories (Fonagy, 1999). To date, there exists little (Slade, 1999) or no specific models of attachment theory informed psychotherapy with adults. It is beyond the scope of this chapter to debate the strengths and weaknesses of attachment theory as it applies to psychotherapeutic intervention, but regardless of the final outcome of such a debate, Arietta Slade sums up the controversy by stating, "In essence, attachment categories do tell a story. They tell a story about how emotion has been regulated, what experiences have been allowed into consciousness, and to what degree an individual has been able to make meaning of his or her primary relationships" (p. 585). Given this perspective, let's first look at the road map Bowlby has laid out when applying his theory to clinical practice.

Bowlby explicitly saw the therapist as a surrogate mother who encouraged the client to explore the world from a secure base he or she creates. In the context of therapeutic work with individuals, Bowlby (1988) defined five tasks:

1. Create a safe place, or Secure Base, for client to explore thoughts, feelings and experiences regarding self and attachment figures;
2. Explore current relationships with attachment figures;
3. Explore relationship with psychotherapist as an attachment figure;
4. Explore the relationship between early childhood attachment experiences and current relationships; and
5. Find new ways of regulating attachment anxiety (i.e., emotional regulation) when the attachment behavioral system is activated.

Each of these five tasks is described in detail below.

Creating a Secure Base

The primary task that Bowlby states as necessary to addressing attachment in psychotherapy is the development of the secure base. In this section, we will define the secure base, and discuss its development and function in the therapeutic relationship.

What Is a Secure Base?

In order to understand Bowlby's concept of the secure base in psychotherapy, one must look at how this is developed between the mother and child. The infant's inability to communicate in adult terms makes parenting a challenging task. Parents (and mothers in particular) must develop skills in empathy and attunement in order to understand the needs of the developing child. An attuned mother (or father) can tell the difference between a full diaper cry, a hungry cry, and a tired cry. Even if they can't tell the exact difference, they are quick to assume that the baby is distressed and in need of some form of caretaking, and if in their response one strategy does not work, they quickly employ another. Compare this to an insensitive or misattuned parent, who either ignores that child's needs altogether, considers the crying a problem and loses sight of the underlying needs, or is overwhelmed by the baby's needs.

The attachment behavioral system, according to Bowlby, however, does not just activate when the child is hungry or needs a diaper change.

The attachment system activates when there is fear or vulnerability for some reason. Perhaps the baby heard a loud noise or woke up in the dark. These experiences activate the attachment system, which serves to motivate the infant to seek protection from threatened danger. The infant is like, as Cassidy (1999) describes, a heat-seeking missile, looking for an attachment object (typically the parent) that is sufficiently near, available, and responsive. When this attempt for protection is met with success, the attachment system de-activates, the anxiety is reduced, the infant is soothed, and play and exploration can resume. When these needs are not met the infant experiences primal anger accompanied by extreme arousal and terror. These reactions, according to Bowlby, set a template for later adult reactions to abandonment.

The parental caretaking system compliments the infant's attachment behavioral system. It is the caretaking system that responds with the goal being to protect and reassure in order to reduce the child's anxiety. Behaviors that can accomplish this goal can range from the practical (e.g., putting the child down for a nap, or feeding or removing a child from a dangerous or frightening situation) to the more complicated process of mirroring the child's inner life in words that help the child to learn self-reflection and understanding. For example, for the two-year-old who is involved in a full-fledged tantrum, the parent may reflect the child's feelings (e.g., "you must be so tired," or "I know it hurts when I say no sometimes"). As the child gets older, this mirroring process becomes more complex reflecting the child's more sophisticated understanding of their feelings, needs, and relationships.

No parent always knows how to respond, or even how to respond constructively. Misattunements are an inevitable part of the parenting process. This is beneficial for the child, because if a child grew up with a perfectly attuned parent, they would not be prepared for the vicissitudes of life. They would be sadly disappointed to discover that other people in the world did not provide the same sensitivity as their mother or father. Mis-attunements are opportunities for the child to develop realistic expectations about the world in response to their needs. These mis-attunements and attunements are also an opportunity for parents to help children learn about the give and take of relationships. Through the rupture and repair process, children learn about how people become intimate in spite of differences and conflict. They develop a sense of poignancy and tolerance for the ambiguities of intimate relationships.

This process of the activated attachment behavioral system and the complimentary caretaking system helps to create the secure base necessary for healthy development, exploration, and play. According to

Bowlby's theory, this healthy developmental process gets derailed when the parental caretaking system is not adequately or appropriately near, attentive, or responsive to the child's attachment behavioral system.

The Secure Base in Psychotherapy

The parent who provides a secure base for their child through attunement, sensitivity, caring, setting limits, and teaching helps the child to learn to soothe the anxiety generated by the activated attachment system, and hence return to exploration and play. It is through this exploration and play process that the child is developing a sense of self. In the case of psychotherapy, the clinician is the caretaking figure who likewise provides a secure base so that the client's attachment system is sufficiently deactivated and the client is free to explore and play. In therapy, however, the exploration is the inner world of feelings, thoughts, and experiences, and the play is, for example, trying on new identities and responses to stress and conflict.

Developing a secure base in psychotherapy would be very easy if it were as simple as therapists being available, attentive, responsive, and attuned. Unfortunately, it is not so elementary (see Wallace & Nosko, 2002). What is interesting about psychotherapy is that, like the strange situation (Ainsworth et al., 1978), it too creates a degree of emotional stress, can be threatening emotionally to clients, and can be detected by observing the coherence of the client's stories about their attachment experiences (Main & Weston, 1981). Sitting in the room with a stranger and talking about emotionally laden material can be quite anxiety provoking and likely to activate the attachment behavioral system right from the start of therapy. Unlike the infant whose attachment experiences are not yet solidified into firmly established working models of self and others, the adult client has already developed a response set to stress and vulnerability within the interpersonal context. That set, depending on the attachment style, will be similar to responses to other interpersonal relationships in their life, behaviors that contribute to problems that they are seeking help for in the first place. Those attachment behaviors may be obvious, but can also be so subtle that the therapist will not recognize that they are present and interfering with the change process. So on one hand the client is seeking help, yet on the other hand the client's attachment behavioral system may be the very thing that presents obstacles to actually receiving assistance from the therapist.

Research in domestic violence suggests that male batterers represent all three insecure attachment classes: avoidant, pre-occupied, and disorganized or fearful (Holtzworth-Monroe et al., 2000). Each form of insecure attachment has particular defense mechanisms as a method of coping with attachment anxiety. Batterers with an avoidant style present as disconnected emotionally, lacking empathy, cold, and uninterested in intimate relationships. They can vacillate between being distant and cut-off emotionally to critical and controlling. These clients need to incorporate an emotional soundtrack, as one client put it, into their life. Batterers with a pre-occupied style try to please others in order to receive approval. They can present as extremely self-controlled except when experiencing loss anxiety, when they can become extremely clingy and angry. When experiencing emotion, these clients are overwhelmed by their attachment needs and are often unable to contain themselves. Unlike their avoidant counterparts, these clients need cognitive structures necessary to contain their intense emotional reactions. The fearful, or disorganized, batterer can manifest elements of both the avoidant and pre-occupied batterers. They experience attachment anxiety, and fear of rejection or being hurt if they are too close and anxiety if they are too distant. Like the disorganized children in the strange situation, these clients do not have an organized strategy for dealing with attachment anxiety. Dutton (1998) has written extensively about the fearful/disorganized or borderline batterer.

How the therapist proceeds in the early stages of therapy with domestic violence clients is critical to the creation of the secure base. If the therapist fails to notice the client's strategies and their psychological function, the therapist's responses will most probably confirm the client's inner working models of self and others and reinforce the attachment behavioral system as it currently manifests. However, if the therapist responds with empathy and attunement, two things can happen. First, the client gets a different experience of him/herself. The attuned therapist, like the attuned parent, will look beyond the client's response set and help them recognize their unconscious motivations, needs, and emotions. The therapist also helps the client view their response set (attachment behaviors) from a different perspective–how they undermine their getting their needs met in interpersonal relationships. This rudimentary process is the beginning of the client altering their inner working models of self.

The second possible outcome of therapist empathy and attunement is that the client experiences the therapist in a positive way, in that they feel understood, seen, and cared for by the therapist. When the client feels understood and not judged, that experience in and of itself can be relieving and soothing, thereby beginning to alter their inner working models of others. These processes, feeling understood and recognizing underlying needs and feelings, is the rudimentary beginning of the creation of a secure base in psychotherapy, a necessary first step in the process of altering the attachment behavioral system so that it is not likely to wreak havoc in interpersonal relationships.

However, like parenting in the real world, even the most sensitive and talented therapists are not always going to be perfectly attuned; therefore, clients are likely to experience ruptures in this state of understanding and perfect attunement by the therapist. Like with the developing child, these ruptures are not only inevitable but necessary to the process of therapy and the development of a more adaptive attachment behavioral system. We will discuss these opportunities later in the section on utilizing the therapeutic relationship to effect change.

However, most batterers present in therapy with severe acting-out problems. These can range from physical or non-physical abuse towards their family members or others to substance abuse, missing sessions, hostility toward the therapist, or other oppositional behavior. The therapist is confronted with the following dilemma. On one hand, the client requires understanding and support for the pain they are experiencing that leads to these behaviors. On the other hand, continued acting-out will interfere with the client benefiting from the therapeutic experience. Therefore, a combination of interpretation, which is necessary to facilitate the development of a secure base with the therapist, and confrontation, which is also necessary in setting limits on the self or other destructive acting-out behaviors, is needed.

An Empirical Description of Secure Base Priming

The idea of creating a secure base in psychotherapy sounds good, but is this a real concept or just another variation of the therapeutic alliance? Researchers in adult attachment have been able to empirically test the notion that creating a secure base experience for individuals may temporarily alter an individual's inner working models of others and therefore change behaviors or emotional states. The idea of "secure base priming" has been gaining attention in the adult attachment literature. Mario Mikulincer and Phil Shaver (2001) examined the effects of secure base priming on intergroup bias. They hypothesized that having a secure base could change how a person appraises threatening situations into more manageable events without activating insecure attachment-like behaviors such as avoidance, fear, or preoccupation. They utilized a series of well-validated secure base priming techniques (described below) that have appeared to create in subjects a sense of security one would find in individuals who would otherwise be assessed as having a secure attachment style. These techniques were quite creative and had powerful effects on subjects.

One group was primed using subliminal presentation of words that exemplify a secure schema (e.g., love, support) within a word relation task (Arndt, Greenberg, Pyszczynski, & Solomon, 1997). This is not unlike the therapist who gives verbal as well as non-verbal messages to clients communicating support, caring, and empathy. In another study, participants performed a guided imagination task in which they visualized an interpersonal episode containing the prototypical if-then sequence of the secure base schema (Mikulincer & Arad, 1999). This method seemed close to the process of helping clients imagine a situation with positive outcomes, such as one used by cognitive-behaviorists called rehearsals with a positive outcome. What would it be like if they got the love and support that they deserve? The third priming technique was Baldwin, Keelan, Fehr, Enns, and Koh Rangarajoo's (1996) visualization task, in which participants visualized a real person who served as a secure base for them. Here again, it is not unusual to ask clients to talk about positive experiences in their life, or for the client to report thinking about the therapist (or another positive attachment figure such as a peer in the batterer's group) outside of the session as a means to self-soothe, feel reassured, or bolster confidence.

In all five of these studies, those subjects exposed to secure base priming acted in the experimental condition similar to securely attached individuals who did not receive priming but were nevertheless exposed to similar conditions assessing intergroup bias. The authors suggest that secure base priming enhances motivation to explore by opening cognitive structures and reducing negative reactions to out-group members or to persons who hold a different world view. The observed effects of secure base priming may reflect cognitive openness and a reduction in dogmatism and authoritarianism (Mikulincer & Shaver, 2001). Other similar studies have found that secure base priming will have a positive effect on cognitive and affective states (Mikulincer, 1998). Although these studies are not meant to be applied to clinical situations, they have powerful implications for the clinical setting. Aspects of the psychotherapy process are similar to these descriptions of secure base priming and through that process clients may begin to change their internal representations of self and others or attachment styles.

Exploring Current Relationships with Attachment Figures

As the therapy proceeds and the therapist works to create the secure base environment, Bowlby's second task eventually begins to become a focus of the psychotherapy: exploring current relationships with attachment figures. These attachment figures include family members, friends, relatives, partners, and spouses. Here the client is exploring patterns in their close relationships, while the therapist is listening for patterns of relating that suggest secure or insecure attachment patterns, and if the latter, which particular insecure attachment style. The exploration of these relationships helps the therapist understand the client's attachment style as it manifests in the significant relationships of his or her life. Research suggests that people may demonstrate different attachment styles in different relationships (Feeney, 1999). This makes a certain amount of sense. Since the attachment system is closely tied to the attachment figure's caretaking system, then how the attachment figure responds to the client will in part determine the client's response to attachment system activation. In addition, in adult relationships (unlike a child-mother relationship) both adults are acting in the capacity of caretaker and seeking attachment for their own needs. This fact is likely to complicate the issue of stability of attachment style within differing contexts.

It is not completely clear how attachment style correlates with the issue of personality disorders (Dozier, Stovall, & Albus, 1999). It is generally thought that people suffer from one personality disorder rather than multiple personality disorders. Neither attachment theory or the empirical literature on personality disorders can say they have spoken the final word on this issue. What is seen clinically, however, is that people do seem to have consistent core issues, but these issues may manifest differently in different contexts. Like attachment relationship dynamics, personality disorders are likely to manifest differently depending on the context or relationship. It is believed that attachment styles are not so much categorical as much as degrees; hence, different client-attachment figure relationships are likely to evoke different degrees of insecurity. For example, one relationship may generate a mild avoidant response by the client, whereas another relationship may evoke an extreme avoidant reaction. Even in the same relationship, different degrees of avoidance or anxiety may be evoked depending on the situation. The same can be said about personality disorders. Therefore, determining the attachment style of a particular client is only part of the goal of this process; more importantly, assessment is also done on how the attachment system is being activated with the client in a particular relationship or context.

Domestic violence perpetrating clients spend a great deal of time talking about their experiences with the partner they have abused. The tendency to focus on the relationship or partner is great in this population. These clients grew up in families where the attachment figure was not sufficiently present, attentive, or responsive; therefore, a great deal of personal energy was expended focusing on the attachment figure–are they present? Are they going to respond positively? Are they even going to know what I need? These same questions are evoked in their adult relationships, either consciously or unconsciously. Directing the clients to their inner experience is key to turning this pattern of externalizing behavior to one of personal awareness and responsibility. Because so much focus in traditional domestic violence treatment is on anger management and power and control dynamics, therapists do not pay enough attention to the client's inner psychological experience of relationships. Here attachment theory can enhance the current domestic violence treatment paradigms. By exploring the unconscious internal working models of self and other, clients can begin to understand why they may have the difficulties in regulating affect or why they experience a need to control others as a means to regulate attachment-related affect.

Exploring the Relationship Between Early Childhood Attachment Experiences and Current Relationships

An important and necessary aspect of psychotherapy from an attachment perspective is the exploration of early childhood experiences and their effect on the inner experience of self and others. Those experiences with caregivers formed the representational models of self and others from which the client views self and the significant attachment relationships in their life. Although Bowlby's description of this process seems primarily cognitive in nature, there is a significant emotional component to this task of psychotherapy. In many cases, domestic violence perpetrators present with unresolved trauma, loss, and other emotionally laden relationship experiences that must be worked through cognitively, emotionally, and physically. Victims of physical, sexual, and psychological maltreatment will experience a range of emotional reactions to this exploration process from depression to rage. The therapist must be willing to work these painful minefields with the client. Much has been written on addressing childhood abuse in psychotherapy (e.g., Herman, 1992; Van der Kolk, McFarlane & Weisaeth, 1996), a topic that is beyond the scope of this paper. But even with clients whose experiences would not be classified as "abuse," painful recollections of subtle and no-so-subtle rejections and misattunements by parents evoke powerful feelings of sadness, loss, and anger. Research in domestic violence treatment outcomes suggests that some perpetrators may need to address unresolved trauma before, or at least concurrently to, addressing violent acting-out behavioral patterns.

An important part of this process involves the exploration of the representational models of self and attachment figures that resulted from these experiences with the goal being to reappraise them and restructure them in light of the understanding and insight gleaned from this process. Most often children's strategy for dealing with unpleasant experiences is to put them out of mind. In psychotherapy, the client can revisit these experiences but with the benefit of having an adult mind that can understand the reasons for their experiences and how they affected them psychologically. Where the therapist has the most leverage in assisting the client in changing these representational models is through new relational experiences that the client has in therapy with the therapist him/herself. The goal of this historical exploration is helping the client to be less "under the spell" of historical experiences with attachment figures. In doing so, current relationships with attachment figures will be less charged.

Another important aspect of this process is to explore the more pathological aspects of insecure attachment. Jealousy in batterers was first described by Walker (1979) and reiterated in Sonkin, Martin, and Walker (1985). It was described as taking the form of frequent questioning of whom a spouse has been with or where she has been, accusations of her attraction to other men, and suspiciousness that she is being flirtatious with other men. In extreme cases, this serves as a motive for "pseudo-incarceration," the literal isolation and confinement of the woman to the home and monitoring of her phone contacts. It can also involve frequent phone calls to her place of work and insistence upon picking her up from work. Duluth Model "explanations" for these behaviors has been to label them as "Power and Control." Dutton (1998) pointed out that the use of power and control was relationship-specific to batterers, and that people exercise control most when they are anxious and afraid. The control of batterers is exercised because of a fear, the same anger "born of fear" that Bowlby described. Because men often look to external causes of their discomfort, they assuage the fear and anxiety within themselves by controlling their partner, who is the perceived source of their anxiety.

Although insight into attachment patterns is an important task in treating male batterers from an attachment perspective, the strong agent of change in this form of psychotherapy is the development of new strategies for coping with attachment related anxiety. On a practical level, one immediate therapeutic objective is developing the ability to recognize an anxious reaction to loss and the ability to self-soothe. However, because this ability should have developed through sensitive attunement by the attachment figure as a child, it now must also be learned through the attunement of an attachment figure such as a therapist. The therapist must be that soothing voice until the client learns to find that voice within him or herself.

In an group psychotherapy format, this could be established through the introduction of a topic such as "fear of losing her," in which "abandonment" scenarios are described (e.g., you call and she's not home, she's late returning from work or shopping, or she pursues a job or hobby that takes more of her time). It is possible to have men generate loss-fear diaries the same way they would generate anger diaries. A discussion of the timing and frequency of daily contact might help establish a pattern: Who initiates the contact? Is it by phone? How frequently does it occur? What are the reactions to a failure to establish contact?

In a more unstructured domestic violence therapy, the client will eventually bring in material where attachment or separation anxiety has been triggered and the therapist can be a soothing voice with a more objective perspective that helps the client learn to do similarly for him or herself. It is also possible to structure systematic desensitization exercises to loss-fear in the same fashion as any other fear based cognitive-behavioral intervention (e.g., fear of flying), where an anxiety gradient is established with the most fear-inducing scenarios at the top, less serious at the bottom. The client then visualizes the less serious scenarios and is taught relaxation techniques to extinguish the anxiety at the lower levels. When these are mastered, the therapist proceeds to a more anxiety-producing level.

Clulow (2001) discussed working with insecure attachment in a couples therapy context. In this context the focus is on establishing a secure base in the couples relationship. Although couples therapy is not advisable in some domestic violence situations, attachment theory can provide a valuable perspective to understanding and treating domestic violence with couples as well as individual or groups.

The secure base relationship creates the safe container from which representational models of the client and his attachment figures can be explored. Bowlby (1988), in one of his last papers, outlined this surrogate task as follows:

> A therapist applying attachment theory sees his role as being one of providing conditions in which his client can explore his representational models of himself and his attachment figure with a view to reappraising and restructuring them in the light of the new understanding he acquires and the new experiences he has in the therapeutic experience. (p. 138)

> The therapeutic alliance appears as a secure base, an internal object as a working, or representational, model of an attachment figure, reconstruction as exploring memories of the past, resistance as a deep reluctance to disobey the past orders of parents not to tell or not to remember. (p. 151)

Exploring the Relationship with the Psychotherapist

In any ongoing psychotherapeutic process, the client may begin to consciously or unconsciously view the therapist as an attachment figure (Farber, Lippert, & Nevas, 1995). If this indeed occurs, there is a great possibility that the attachment behavioral system will activate at various points in the therapy process. Although talking about events and relationships outside of therapy is helpful, therapy from an attachment perspective must include, at some point, a discussion of the attachment dynamics between the therapist and the client–Bowlby's third task for the attachment informed psychotherapist. Psychotherapy may be viewed as common place for many people who have participated in the process, particularly for therapists who live and breathe the profession. However, for most domestic violence clients, the act of entering a therapist's office and disclosing private thoughts and feelings is likely to raise a degree of attachment-related anxiety. Therefore, it is important that therapists pay close attention to their client's verbal and non-verbal behaviors from the moment they make contact to begin to hypothesize how their particular attachment behavioral system is activated.

Most clients rarely readily admit to having feelings about their therapist, or at least being in therapy. Their rational mind takes over and they tell themselves, "Of course I feel comfortable with my therapist," or "Why would I be here if I didn't feel comfortable?" In reality, however, it would be considered highly problematic if the client only had positive feelings while in therapy. Not all clients will be able to directly confront their feelings about the therapy and therapist early in the therapeutic relationship. Individuals with some attachment styles are not likely to admit that the relationship is significant, let alone admit that they have deep emotional reactions to the therapist. Just as differential diagnosis guides the clinician about treatment planning and pacing, so does understanding a client's particular attachment style inform the attachment-oriented psychotherapist about how and when to address the therapeutic relationship with a particular client.

Addressing the therapeutic relationship from an attachment perspective is important for a number of reasons. First, it is through the intimate relating that occurs within the clinical hour that there is the opportunity to explore and hopefully change the representational models that determine a client's attachment style. Second, working with the client when feelings arise in therapy helps him/her find ways of regulating attachment anxiety and patterns of avoidance when attachment system is activated. Viewing attachment from the perspective of anxiety and avoidance (Hazan & Shaver, 1987) suggests that changing attachment styles involves the client learning to regulate attachment anxiety and/or finding other means of expressing attachment needs other than through avoidance. Lastly, there is some evidence that long term psychotherapy can affect the neuro-circuitry that gives rise to attachment related representations as well as emotion regulation (Perry, 1995; Vaughan, 1997).

Regulating Attachment Anxiety When Attachment System Is Activated

As mentioned above, the activation of the attachment behavioral system in the therapeutic hour can be the most effective way to address attachment anxiety with the client. The distancing of the dismissing attachment style, the pleasing and idealizing behaviors of the preoccupied attachment style, and the erratic dependency and distancing of the fearful attachment style will eventually manifest in therapy in subtle and no-so-subtle ways. When the therapist develops a secure base relationship with the client and the client has some of the above mentioned insight into his/her attachment relationships, the ground is set to address these behaviors as they manifest in the relationship with the therapist. Through both the interpretation and confrontation of these behavioral manifestations of the activated attachment system, the client can learn to face the pain and vulnerability that underlie these defenses. This approach also allows the clients to be understood and supported by the therapist, and eventually develop within themselves new skills in self-soothing, reassurance, and relaxation. The net result is the client is able to reduce the reactivity and sensitivity to perceived cues of threatened safety or protection.

Much of what's published in the domestic violence field speaks to this task of the attachment-oriented therapist. Education, cognitive interventions, and behavioral therapy all focus their efforts at assisting the client (or student in the case of educational based programs) in learning new methods of coping with anger, conflict, or any emotionally difficult situations. Although some programs address childhood abuse issues (Bowlby's fourth task), it has been promulgated by leaders in the domestic violence field that it is more effective to focus on the here and now and less on childhood abuse experiences, which can be addressed later in the treatment process. This mythology seems to contradict research that suggest otherwise (Saunders, 1996). Saunders found that some batterers may actually improve faster by focusing on childhood abuse issues earlier in psychodynamically oriented treatment. Additionally, Dutton's (1998) research on male batterers suggests that for a significant percent of men, childhood trauma has led to borderline personality organization. Thus, it appears that addressing childhood abuse issues is a necessary element of the treatment process. Although cognitive and behavioral interventions are an important element in domestic violence treatment, they clearly are not sufficient given the fact that a significant percentage of persons who complete domestic violence treatment do seem to re-offend. In addition, even though physical rates of violence do significantly decrease post treatment, psychological or non-physical violence do persist at relatively high rates (Rosenberg, 2001). Dutton (1998) found a 21% arrest rate for an eleven-year follow-up, with partner interview violence rates at approximately 16%. These data suggest that at least 20% of persons completing treatment will re-offend. Higher rates of physical and non-physical violence have been found in other studies (Gondolf, 1997).

Taken together, this data suggests that the treatment programs developed to date may still be missing important elements necessary to long term cessation of physical and non-physical abuse. Cognitive and behavioral interventions are necessary but not sufficient for long-lasting, successful treatment. Treatment of domestic violence from an attachment-informed perspective may include the missing elements that can ultimately lead to lasting change with clients, manifested not only by the cessation of violence but also by a significant change in their experience of close relationships in general.

Dutton's research suggests that batterers will present with all three types of insecure attachment styles in similar frequencies (Dutton, Saunders, Starzomski, & Bartholomew, 1994). However, Fearful, and to a lesser extent Preoccupied, styles are correlated with partner's reports of abuse. These findings suggest that the subcategories/typologies of batterers are sufficiently different enough to justify therapists approaching treatment from an assessment based perspective, as opposed to using a cookie-cutter approach to treatment whereby all batterers are treated as if their violence has a single origin or etiology. In addition, studies on drop-out rates of individuals in domestic violence treatment (Daly & Pelowski, 2000) suggest that one factor, psychopathology, may be related to this phenomenon. Therapists who begin to recognize that they will need to vary their conceptualization and intervention with different clients may be able to reduce the drop-out rates in their treatment program. Attachment informed psychotherapy recognizes that different attachment styles may need different therapeutic conceptualizations and interventions (Slade, 1999).

THE ASSESSMENT OF ADULT ATTACHMENT STATUS

Numerous measures of adult attachment have been developed over the past ten years each with their own strengths and weaknesses (Crowell & Treboux, 1995). Generally, these measures fall into two categories: self-completed questionnaires (questions or statements responded to with a Likert-type scale) and those administered by a trained evaluator. We would like to discuss three of these instruments because each one deconstructs attachment somewhat differently, and we believe that each method has clinical relevance to treating domestic violence clients.

The Adult Attachment Interview. Main and Goldwyn (1998) developed the Adult Attachment Interview (AAI), as system based on the structural qualities of narratives of early experiences. The interview consists of eighteen questions about childhood experiences with attachment figures. The trained evaluator is not so much interested in the content, as much as the coherence of the interviewee's narrative. Arieta Slade (1999) explains Main's definition of coherence as the following:

> For Main, the capacity to represent past experiences in a coherent and collaborative fashion is the most significant and compelling aspect of adult security, and is clearly the most predictive of infant

security. A coherent interview is both believable and true to the listener; in a coherent interview, the events and affects intrinsic to early relationships are conveyed without distortion, contradiction or derailment of discourse. The subject collaborates with the interviewer, clarifying his or her meaning, and working to make sure he or she is understood. Such a subject is thinking as the interview proceeds, and is aware of thinking with and communicating to another; thus coherence and collaboration are inherently intertwined and interrelated. (p. 580)

While autonomous individuals value attachment relationships and are able to integrate memories into a coherent narrative, insecure individuals are poor at integrating memories of experience with the meaning of that experience. Those persons classified as having a dismissing attachment style tended to deny negative memories, and idealize early relationships. Their stories were very brief, general, and often full of contradictory data (e.g., describing negative experiences but talking about the parent in a positive light). Preoccupied individuals tend to be preoccupied with childhood attachment experiences, often still complaining of childhood slights, echoing the protests of the resistant infant. Their stories are often long and grammatically entangled with vague usages ("dadadadada," or "and that"). Unresolved individuals give indications of significant disorganization in their attachment relationship representation via either semantic or syntactic confusions in their narratives concerning childhood trauma or a recent loss (Fonagy, 1999). These individuals show striking lapses in monitoring of reason or discourse (George, Kaplan, & Main, 1996).

The relevance of the AAI to clinical work with batterers is that clinicians can listen to their client's narratives from the beginning of treatment so as to begin to form hypotheses about attachment status. Additionally, as the narratives begin to evidence certain forms of incoherence, the clinician can also strategize treatment interventions that specifically address the client's defensive patterns that have led to the particular form of incoherence. For example, for the avoidant or dismissing client who presents little data, idealizes their attachment experiences, and is unable to express affect, the therapist can begin to formulate strategies that help draw out the client's story, listen for inconsistencies in their recollections of childhood experiences and begin to point them out, and slowly help the client connect with the emotional track of their narratives. The pre-occupied client, whose narratives are convoluted and saturated with uncontained affect about attachment experiences, will need to learn how to better self-soothe so that their narratives will have a certain degree of objective distance or cognitive structures that contain the appropriate degree of affect. With the fearful or disorganized batterer, the therapist will need to address the early childhood trauma experiences, whose resultant repressed affect leads to dissociation and other forms of maladaptive emotion regulation. When treating domestic violence perpetrators, it would be our hope that as the client learns more about himself and his attachment relationships and becomes more effective at modulating attachment anxiety, his/her narratives will become more coherent.

Experiences in Close Relationships Questionnaire. Brennan, Clark and Shaver (1998) developed the Experiences in Close Relationships (ECR) questionnaire, a self-report measure that assesses adolescent and adult romantic-attachment orientations (secure, anxious, and avoidant– the three patterns identified by Ainsworth, Blehar, Waters, & Wall, 1978 in their studies of infant-caregiver attachment). They deconstruct attachment on two continuums: anxiety (need for approval, preoccupation with relationships, fear of being abandoned) and avoidance (discomfort with intimacy and closeness). Persons with low anxiety and low avoidance are within the secure range. Those with high anxiety and low avoidance are within the preoccupied range, while those with low anxiety and high avoidance are within the dismissing range. Finally, persons with high anxiety and high avoidance are within the fearful range. Clients can fill out the 36 questions fairly quickly. The client is asked to read each statement and answer to what degree it reflects how they see themselves. They can even take the test online and receive the results immediately (http://www.geocities.com/research93/). Unlike the AAI, the ECR scores the person in degrees of avoidance and anxiety, and therefore is somewhat less categorical in nature.

The Relationship Questionnaire. Another self-report adult attachment measure is the Relationship Questionnaire, developed by Bartholomew and Horowitz (1991). This measure, although similar in form to Brennan, Clark and Shaver's (1998), conceptualizes attachment in terms of internal working models of self and others. This deconstruction of attachment is based on Bowlby's (1973, 1979) original conceptualization of attachment. Bartholomew provides two theoretically unrelated dimensions giving four quadrants or categories. Positive working models of the self and positive working models of others give rise to the secure attachment status. Negative working models of the self and positive working models of others give rise to the preoccupied attachment status, while positive working models of the self and negative working models of others give rise to the dismissing attachment status. Finally, negative working models of both the self and others give rise to the fearful attachment status.

Understanding attachment from the internal working model perspective helps to explain many of the behaviors evident in perpetrators of domestic violence. The pre-occupied client who is trying to please or receive validation from the therapist, or his partner, is avoiding experiencing the sense of defective self or self-hatred that would result from focusing on himself. Addressing issues of self-esteem is critical with this client, whereas the avoidant client has learned to protect himself from others by distancing and may experience his partner or the therapist as intrusive and/or controlling and may act out violently or aggressively in retaliation. An important issue being discussed among researchers developing these methods of measuring or identifying attachment styles is the notion of categorical typologies versus dimensions of security or insecurity. In the real world, clients present with varying degrees of mental illness. Therefore, it would be expected that attachment status would be no different. The strength of the ECR and the Relationships Questionnaire is their use of the Likert-type scales that allow respondents to rate themselves in degrees of similarity or dissimilarity to each attachment related statement, rather than the categorical nature of the AAI.

Discussion of Adult Attachment Measures. Each of these models of adult attachment (coherence, anxiety/avoidance, and internal working models of self/others) can be useful in understanding psychotherapy with perpetrators of domestic violence. Although there is considerable overlap in how each of these attachment categories manifest interpersonally, they each suggest unique treatment goals. Based on the AAI, the goal of therapy is helping the client reduce their anxiety sufficiently to reconstruct a coherent narrative of their attachment-related experiences, both in the past as well as currently. As Jeremy Holmes (2001) suggests (2001), attachment based psychotherapy is a process of story-making and story-breaking. One needs to break the rigid, unemotional, and unrelated story of the avoidant individual and create a story with greater emotional content, better balance of positive and negative experiences, and a more descriptive and realistic narrative description of relationships. With the pre-occupied individual, one must break the emotional dysphoria by creating one that is also infused by logic and perspective and balance of affect and reflective understanding.

Similarly, the Brennan, Clark, and Shaver (1998) model suggests that by learning to self-soothe attachment anxiety and find other mechanisms besides avoidance to deal with the fear and vulnerability that can be activated within close relationships, clients can begin to develop more secure relationship experiences. The Bartholomew and Horowitz (1991) model suggests that working more on improving self esteem and reassessing feelings of distrust and fear of others will ultimately allow the client to experience relationships from a secure perspective. There is some question as to whether or not Bowlby's concept of "internal working models" is the same as attachment styles described in the current literature. At a recent meeting of the American Psychological Association, Adult Attachment Discussion, the issue of working models attachment styles or attachment representations were explored among researchers in the field and the following was noted (Adult Attachment Lab website, 1998):

> There was some initial disagreement over the use of the terms "working models," "attachment styles," and "attachment representations." It was generally agreed that the term "attachment style" is best reserved for describing observable or manifest patterns of behavior, and the term "working models" is best reserved for describing the latent mental structures giving rise to variability in attachment styles.
>
> It was suggested that the concept of working models is of relatively little use in describing the psychological dynamics of attachment because the concept brings to mind conscious-evaluative belief systems (positive/negative models of self/others) operating with little input from motivational and defensive goals or overlearned strategies of behavioral and emotional regulation. In contrast, but also speaking to the limitation of the concept of working models, it was suggested that the concept was broad enough to refer to both declarative and procedural aspects of cognition and behavioral/emotional regulation.
>
> It was generally agreed that the concept of working models is most useful when referring to organized strategies for regulating emotion, attention, and behavior with respect to attachment concerns. It was also suggested that a number of social-cognitive techniques exist that can be exploited to investigate the procedural and unconscious aspects of working models.

Main (1999) notes that there is research that suggest there are in fact neurological correlates to internal working models as either neurological circuits or patterns that are ingrained from experience or a function of working memory. In either case, understanding the neurological basis of internal representations of self and others may be an important element to understanding attachment patterns in children and adults.

CONCLUSIONS

Psychotherapy with perpetrators of domestic violence from an attachment perspective involves creating a secure base environment so that clients can explore their current and past attachment relationships within the safety of the therapeutic relationship. Safety is critical, because many insecure batterers have experienced tremendous loss, hurt, and disappointments within their close relationships; they therefore enter therapy with fears and anxiety about opening up to someone who is perceived as having power over them. This is particularly true for the court-mandated client, where the therapist may indeed have a great deal of influence over their criminal justice experience. For these reasons, creating a secure base environment is a critical first step to achieving therapeutic goals, such as learning emotional self regulation or resolving childhood trauma. Another critical element to attachment oriented psychotherapy with perpetrators of domestic violence is the "not-one-size-fits-all" maxim. Different attachment styles need different interventions and approaches. The batterer with the overly structured dismissing attachment style needs to connect to their emotional life and acknowledge the importance of attachment in their lives. They need to learn that attachment relationships do not need to be exploitative, hurtful, controlling, or rejecting. The batterer with the preoccupied attachment style needs structures necessary to contain their emotional reactivity in attachment interactions, while learning greater self-sufficiency and less dependency on attachment figures for self-definition and security. The batterer with the fearful attachment style likewise needs to heal the split that exists within them from childhood trauma and losses so that they can both learn to self-soothe their attachment anxiety through means other than avoidance or pushing others away through anger and violence.

Using the therapeutic relationship (or peer relations when utilizing a group intervention modality) is the most powerful means to highlighting attachment behavioral system patterns in psychotherapy. Through these in-the-moment experiences, therapists can help raise the client's awareness of these patterns, but most importantly strategize more adaptive responses to attachment anxiety. This process takes therapists out of their heads and challenges them to work within the here and now with clients. Quick thinking, self-awareness, and sensitive attunement to the client are critical to making use of these "now-moments" (Stern, 1998). Making use of them on a continual basis gives the client the message that he/she and the therapist can go to that frightening place of emotions and the meaning of intimacy.

Because domestic violence clients are a heterogeneous population, clinicians are likely to encounter all three insecure attachment styles. An assessment of the client's attachment status is necessary to understand how the client's attachment behavioral system activates and the mechanisms they use to cope with the anxiety associated with attachment. Understanding the client's attachment status helps us to form some hypotheses about the etiology of the client's violence. Psychotherapy offers the domestic violence client the opportunity to learn more adaptive methods of regulating attachment anxiety, reevaluate internal models of self and others, and experience intimate relationships (with the therapist or fellow group members) in new and positive ways. Through long term exposure to these therapeutic experiences, changes in the internal working models and attachment style is not only possible but inevitable.

Although John Bowlby began his work on attachment theory over fifty years ago, there are still varying ideas about how one approaches psychotherapy from an attachment perspective. Unlike most clinical theories, attachment theory has had the benefit of more than forty years of empirical research before discussions even began on the clinical applications to adult psychotherapy. So as the clinical application of this theory evolves, clinicians will have at their disposal a continually growing body of empirical data that will hopefully meld with clinical experience. Through a positive attachment between clinicians and academics, the application of this theory will unfold in the years to come.

NOTE

From his early writings, Bowlby used the terms "principal attachment figure" or "mother figure" rather than the word "mother." This usage underscored his belief that although the principal attachment figure is often the mother, it may also be another person (such as father or grandparent). For the purposes of this paper, we shall use the term "principal attachment figure" keeping in mind that although for most of our patients this is the biological mother, it is not necessarily so.

REFERENCES

Adult Attachment Lab. (1998). *Notes from the Adult Attachment Discussion Session* at the 1998 meeting of the American Psychological Association. Retrieved March 17, 2002, from http://psychology.ucdavis.edu/Shaver/apasum.html.

Ainsworth, M. D. S., Blehar, M. C., Waters, E., & Wall, S. (1978). *Patterns of attachment: A psychological study of the strange situation.* Hillsdale, N.J.: Erlbaum.

Arndt, J., Greenberg, J., Pyszczynski, T., & Solomon, S. (1997). Subliminal exposure to death-related stimuli increases defenses of the cultural worldview. *Psychological Science, 8,* 379-385.

Baldwin, M. W., Keelan, J. P. R., Fehr, B., Enns, V., & Koh Rangarajoo, E. (1996). Social-cognitive conceptualization of attachment working models: Availability and accessibility effects. *Journal of Personality and Social Psychology, 71,* 94-109.

Bartholomew, K. (1990). Avoidance of intimacy: An attachment perspective. *Journal of Social and Personal Relationships, 7,* 147 -158.

Bartholomew, K., Henderson, A., & Dutton. D. G. (2001). Insecure attachment and abusive intimate relationships. In C. Clulow (Ed.), *Adult attachment and couple psychotherapy* (pp. 43-61) Taylor & Francis: Philadelphia.

Bartholomew, K., & Horowitz, L. M. (1991). Attachment styles among young adults: A test of a four category model. *Journal of Personality and Social Psychology, 61*(2), 226-244.

Bowlby, J. (1969). *Attachment and loss: Vol. 1. Attachment* (2nd Ed). London: Hogarth Press.

Bowlby, J. (1973). *Attachment and loss: Vol. 2. Separation.* New York: Basic.

Bowlby, J. (1980). *Attachment and loss: Vol. 3. Loss, sadness, and depression.* New York: Basic Books.

Bowlby, J. (1988). *A secure base: Clinical applications of attachment theory.* London: Routledge.

Brennan, K. A., Clark, C. L., & Shaver, P. R. (1998). Self-report measurement of adult attachment: An integrative overview. In J. A. Simpson & W. S. Rholes (Eds.), *Attachment theory and close relationships* (pp. 46-76). New York: Guilford Press.

Browning, J. J., & Dutton, D. G. (1986). Assessment of wife assault with the conflict tactics scale: Using couple data to quantify the differential reporting effect. *Journal of Marriage and the Family, 48,* 375-379.

Cassidy, J. (1999). The nature of the child's ties. In J. Cassidy & P. R. Shaver (Eds.), *Handbook of attachment: Theory, research, and clinical applications* (pp. 355-377). New York: Guilford Press.

Clulow, C. (2001). *Adult attachment and couple psychotherapy.* Brunner- Routledge: London.

Coleman, V. E. (2002). Treating the lesbian batterer: Theoretical and clinical considerations. A contemporary psychoanalytic perspective. *Journal of Aggression, Maltreatment, and Trauma, 7*(1/2), 159-205.

Crowell, J. A., & Treboux, D. (1995). A review of adult attachment measures: Implications for theory and research. *Social Development, 4,* 294-327.

Daly, J. E., & Pelowski, S. (2000). Predictors of dropout among men who batter: A review of studies with implications for research and practice. *Violence and Victims, 15*(2), 137- 160.

Dozier, M., Stovall, K. C., & Albus, K. (1999). Attachment and psychopathology in adulthood. In J. Cassady & Phillip Shaver (Eds.), *Handbook of attachment theory: Research and clinical implications* (pp. 497-519). Guilford: New York.

Dutton, D. G. (1998). *The abusive personality*. Guilford: New York.

Dutton, D. G., & Kerry, G. (1999). Modus operandi and personality disorder in incarcerated spousal killers. *International Journal of Law and Psychiatry, 22*(3-4), 287-300.

Dutton, D. G., Saunders, K., Starzomski, A. J., & Bartholomew, K. (1994). Intimacy-anger and insecure attachment as precursors of abuse in intimate relationships. *Journal of Applied Social Psychology, 24,* 1367-1386.

Farber, B., Lippert, R., & Nevas, D. (1995). The therapists as attachment figure. *Psychotherapy, 32*(2), 204-212.

Feeney, J. (1999). Adult romantic attachment and couple relationships. In J. Cassidy & P. R. Shaver (Eds.), *Handbook of attachment: Theory, research, and clinical applications* (pp. 355-377). New York: Guilford Press.

Fonagy, P. (1999). Psychoanalytic theory from the viewpoint of attachment theory and research. In J. Cassidy & P. R. Shaver (Eds.), *Handbook of attachment: Theory, research, and clinical applications* (pp. 355-377). New York: Guilford Press.

George, C., Kaplan, N., & Main, M. (1996). *Adult Attachment Interview Protocol* (3rd Ed.) Unpublished manuscript, University of California at Berkeley.

Gondolf, E. (1997). Patterns of reassault in batterer programs. *Violence and Victims 12*(4), 373-387.

Hazan, C., & Shaver, P. (1987). Conceptualizing romantic love as an attachment process. *Journal of Personality and Social Psychology, 52,* 511 -524.

Herman, J. L. (1992). *Trauma and recovery.* New York: Basic Books.

Holmes, J. (2001). *In search of the secure base.* London: Routledge.

Holtzworth-Monroe, A., Meehan, J., Herron, K., Rehman, U., & Stuart, G. (2000). Testing the Holtzworth-Monroe and Stuart (1994) batterer typology. *Journal of Consulting and Clinical Psychology, 68*(6), 1000-1019.

Griffin, D., & Bartholomew, K. (1994). Metaphysics of measurement: The case of adult attachment. In K. Bartholomew & D. Perlman (Eds.), *Advances in personal relationships, Vol. 5: Attachment processes in adulthood* (pp. 17-52). London: Jessica Kingsley.

Karen, R. (1977). *Becoming attached: Unfolding the mystery of the mother-infant bond and its impact on later life.* Warner Books: New York.

Leisring, P. A., Dowd, L., & Rosenbaum, A. (2002). Treatment of partner aggressive women. *Journal of Aggression, Maltreatment, & Trauma, 7*(1/2), 257-277.

Main, M. (1999). Attachment theory: Eighteen points with suggestions for future studies. In J. Cassidy & P. R. Shaver (Eds.), *Handbook of attachment: Theory, research, and clinical applications* (pp. 355-377). New York: Guilford Press.

Main, M., & Goldwyn, R. (1998). *Adult attachment classification system.* Unpublished manuscript. University of California: Berkeley, CA.

Main, M., & Weston, D. (1981). Quality of attachment to mother or father: Related to conflict behavior and the readiness for establishing new relationships. *Child Development, 52,* 932-940.

Masterson, J. F., & Klein, R. (Eds.). (1995). *Disorders of the self: New therapeutic horizons.* New York: Bruner Mazel.

Mikulincer, M. (1998). Adult attachment style and affect regulation: Strategic variations in self-appraisals. *Journal of Personality and Social Psychology, 75*, 420-435.

Mikulincer, M., & Arad, D. (1999). Attachment, working models, and cognitive openness in close relationships: A test of chronic and temporary accessibility effects. *Journal of Personality and Social Psychology, 77*, 710-725.

Milkulincer, M., & Shaver, P. (2001). Attachment theory and intergroup bias: Evidence that priming the secure base schema attenuates negative reactions to out-groups. *Journal of Personality and Social Psychology, 81*, 97-115.

Perry, B. (1995). Incubated in terror: Neurodevelopmental factors in the "Cycle of Violence." In J. D. Osofsky (Ed.), *Children, youth and violence: Searching for solutions* (pp. 124-148). Guilford: New York.

Rosenberg, M. (2001). Domestic violence in Sonoma County: An outcome study of court- mandated offenders. Unpublished manuscript.

Schore, A. N. (1994). *Affect regulation and the origin of the self : The neurobiology of emotional development.* Erlbaum: Hillsdale, N.J.

Slade, A. (1999). Attachment theory and research: Implications for the theory and practice of individual psychotherapy with adults. In J. Cassidy & P. R. Shaver (Eds.), *Handbook of attachment: Theory, research, and clinical applications* (pp. 355-377). New York: Guilford Press.

Saunders, D. (1996). Feminist-cognitive-behavioral and process-psychodynamic treatments for men who batter: Interaction of abuser traits and treatment models. *Violence and Victims, 11*(4), 393-414.

Sonkin, D. J., Martin, D., & Walker, L. E. A. (1985). *The male batterer: A treatment approach.* New York: Springer Publications.

Sperling, M. B., & Berman, W. H. (1994). *Attachment in adults: Clinical and developmental perspectives.* Guilford: New York.

Stern, D. (1998). The process of therapeutic change involving implicit knowledge: Some implications of developmental observations for adult psychotherapy. *Infant Mental Health Journal, 19*, 300-308.

Tolman, R. M. (1989). The development of a measure of psychological maltreatment of women by their male partners. *Violence & Victims, 4*(3), 159-177.

Van der Kolk, B., A., McFarlane, A. C., & Weisaeth, L. (Eds.). (1996). *Traumatic stress: The effects of overwhelming experience on mind, body, and society.* New York: The Guilford Press.

Vaughan, S. (1997). *The talking cure: Why traditional talking therapy offers a better chance for long-term relief than any drug.* New York: Owl Books.

Walker, L. E. A. (1979). *The Battered Woman.* Harper & Row: New York.

Wallace, R., & Nosko, A. (2002). Shame in male spouse abusers and its treatment in group therapy. *Journal of Aggression, Maltreatment, & Trauma, 7*(1/2), 47-74.

West, M., & George, C. (1999). Violence in intimate adult relationships: An attachment theory perspective. *Attachment and Human Development, 1*, 137-156.

Stopping Wife Abuse
via Physical Aggression Couples Treatment

Richard E. Heyman
Karin Schlee

SUMMARY. The purpose of this article is to provide an overview of an empirically tested program for physical aggression: Physical Aggression Couples Treatment (PACT). Although we do not advocate standard "marital therapy" when there is ongoing husband-to-wife interspousal aggression, we present the rationale for, description of, and empirical support for a conjoint treatment approach to wife abuse abatement. *[Article copies available for a fee from The Haworth Document Delivery Service: 1-800-HAWORTH. E-mail address: <docdelivery@haworthpress.com> Website: <http://www.HaworthPress.com> © 2003 by The Haworth Press, Inc. All rights reserved.]*

Address correspondence to: Richard E. Heyman, PhD, Department of Psychology, State University of New York at Stony Brook, Stony Brook, NY 11794-2500 (E-mail: Richard.Heyman@Stonybrook.edu).

The authors wish to dedicate this paper to the memory of their colleague Peter Neidig. Peter was to be a contributor to this paper, but died before the writing commenced. His influence has an obvious, and profound, impact on the work that is described in this paper. The authors would also like to acknowledge the influence of K. Daniel O'Leary and Dina Vivian. The ongoing debates about the etiology and treatment of wife abuse have contributed immeasurably to the ideas discussed in this paper.

This paper was supported by NIMH grant R01MH42488.

[Haworth co-indexing entry note]: "Stopping Wife Abuse via Physical Aggression Couples Treatment." Heyman, Richard E., and Karin Schlee. Co-published simultaneously in *Journal of Aggression, Maltreatment & Trauma* (The Haworth Maltreatment & Trauma Press, an imprint of The Haworth Press, Inc.) Vol. 7, No. 1/2 (#13/14), 2003, pp. 135-157; and: *Intimate Violence: Contemporary Treatment Innovations* (ed: Donald Dutton, and Daniel J. Sonkin) The Haworth Maltreatment & Trauma Press, an imprint of The Haworth Press, Inc., 2003, pp. 135-157. Single or multiple copies of this article are available for a fee from The Haworth Document Delivery Service [1-800-HAWORTH, 9:00 a.m. - 5:00 p.m. (EST). E-mail address: docdelivery@haworthpress.com].

http://www.haworthpress.com/store/product.asp?sku=J146
© 2003 by The Haworth Press, Inc. All rights reserved.
10.1300J146v07n01_07

KEYWORDS. Physical Aggression Couples Treatment (PACT), conjoint treatment, communication, couples, outcome research, safety, gender-specific treatment, feminist/social learning treatment

Several years ago, the first author co-wrote a clinical paper entitled "Is There a Place for Conjoint Treatment of Couple Violence?" (Vivian & Heyman, 1996). The title reflected an ongoing controversy within the batterer treatment community. Some believe that battering should only be treated via single sex groups; indeed, such advocates have succeeded in some U.S. states in proscribing conjoint treatment if there is any evidence of battering.

Although we certainly do not advocate conjoint treatment for all aggressive men, neither do we believe that it is wise to prohibit it. There is no single "batterer" profile (Holtzworth-Munroe & Stuart, 1994) and there is no single approach that will be the treatment of choice for all men under all circumstances. To advocate otherwise is a political, not a therapeutic, stance.

The purpose of this paper is to provide an overview of an empirically tested program for physical aggression: Physical Aggression Couples Treatment (PACT). The name of the program was chosen purposefully to indicate that although the format is conjoint, our program is not standard marital therapy. *We do not advocate "marital therapy" when there is ongoing husband-to-wife aggression.* Our program is designed with the sole purpose of eliminating physical and psychological aggression in the home. Thus, the conjoint treatment approach is merely a vehicle to accomplish the same goal as other abuse abatement programs.

Why use a conjoint approach? This chapter will describe the rationale for PACT and review research evaluating that rationale. We will then provide a brief overview of how we assess and treat couples in which there is ongoing husband-to-wife aggression. Finally, we provide research supporting the efficacy of PACT in treating aggressive men. Readers interested in a more detailed description of the program can refer to Heyman and Neidig (1997).

THERAPEUTIC RATIONALE

PACT is an expanded version of Neidig's Domestic Conflict Containment Program (DCCP; Neidig & Friedman, 1984). The initial version of PACT was used in a treatment study (O'Leary, Heyman, & Neidig, 1999) comparing PACT to gender specific groups (i.e., men's and women's groups). Although PACT, like most treatments for battering, was administered in a group format, we are increasingly modifying and enriching it for use with individual couples (e.g., Vivian & Heyman, 1996).

Neidig developed DCCP after studying wife abusive members of the U.S. military and concluding that wife abuse was "linked to specific, measurable skill deficits in the areas of anger control, stress management, and communication. The violence typically occurred in the context of a dysfunctional relationship during periods of high stress" (Neidig & Friedman, 1984, p. 1). DCCP grew out of behavioral approaches to anger (e.g., Ellis, 1977; Novaco, 1975) and marital therapy (e.g., Jacobson & Margolin, 1979; Stuart, 1980). Like many behavioral marital therapists, Neidig's approach was heavily influenced by systems theorists such as Bateson, Haley, and Watzlawick.

Rationale of DCCP

DCCP's rationale is as follows: Most acts of physical aggression in intimate relationships occur in the context of an argument between partners (Dobash & Dobash, 1984). Conflict escalates until one or both partners strike the other. According to principles of systems theory, one must be cognizant of the concept of *circular causality*: each spouse's behavior is both a response to the partner's behavior and a stimulus for the partner's subsequent response. That is, most spouses punctuate conflicts as follows: partner's behavior → my behavior. Systems approaches suggest the following: partner's behavior → my behavior → partner's behavior → my behavior, etc.

DCCP holds each spouse solely responsible for his or her own choice to use violence. However, both partners play a role in conflict escalation; therefore, *either* can take actions to reduce the likelihood of violence. Special care must be taken when explaining circular causality to avoid the implication that the woman can prevent the violence by being non-conflictual; this is the very belief that aggressors (and at times, society as a whole) use to excuse violence. Rather, to reduce the risk of violence, both partners must accept the responsibility for managing their own anger and take steps to eliminate their own use of violence.

With circular causality at the core of DCCP's rationale, the goal of treatment is to make partners more skillful at defusing conflict before it reaches the point of psychological or physical aggression. DCCP uses three approaches: (1) increase awareness about aggression (e.g., definition of psychological, physical, and sexual abuse; description of Walker's [1979] cycle of abuse); (2) increase anger management skills (e.g., time out, recognition of anger-provoking thoughts via the Antecedent-Belief-Consequence cognitive model); and (3) improve communication skills.

The principles of the program are explained to participants during session one (see Heyman & Neidig, 1997). These principles are as follows: (1) the primary goal of the program is to eliminate violence in the home; (2) although anger and conflict are normal elements of family life, violence within the family is never justified; (3) we learn to be violent and we can learn to be non violent. Violence is a choice; (4) abusive behavior is a relationship issue in which each partner must be responsible for his or her own behavior. The consequences of violence are serious for all members of the family; (5) abusiveness is a desperate, but self-defeating, effort to change the relationship; and (6) abusiveness tends to escalate in severity and frequency if not treated.

DCCP differed from most treatment approaches for battering (i.e., men's programs) in Neidig's insistence that perpetrator/victim distinctions are a "therapeutic dead end" (Neidig & Friedman, 1984, p. 4). DCCP adopts a "no blame" policy similar to that described by Geffner, Mantooth, Franks, and Rao's (1989):

> [C]linicians actively work to have both partners accept responsibility for their own behavior . . . The counselors have used 'no blame' to build an alliance and trust in the counseling environment. The 'no blame' approach further suggests that counselors are nonpunitive and do not seek to punish the violent man. We are adamant about our belief that counselors should not become punishing agents. . . . [W]hen each is held accountable in a nonblaming manner by the counselors and their partners, the bonding and trust tends to increase, and the therapy process is enhanced. (pp. 118-119)

Neidig's overall stance can be called "gender neutral" in that his "no victims or villains" approach tends to de-emphasize the physical and cultural differences in the meaning and effects of aggressive behavior toward the spouse. Those adopting a gender neutral approach sometimes cite nationally representative questionnaire findings that demonstrated that husbands and wives are equally physically aggressive (e.g.,

Steinmetz, 1987; Straus & Gelles, 1990). Further, more recent observational findings documented that destructive couple conflict and mutual verbal aggression are among the strongest correlates of couple violence (see Weiss & Heyman, 1997).

This viewpoint is sharply contrasted with that of feminists, who identify the problem as being husband-based and related to issues of gender socialization, patriarchy, power, coercive control, and male psychopathology (e.g., Bograd, 1990; Yllö, 1993). In the most extreme version of this view, all couple approaches to treating violence are considered dangerous and antithetical to feminist principles (i.e., implicitly blames the woman for her husband's violence, puts the women at risk for further violence, encourages the woman to change when it is the man who must change).

Our work has evolved from Neidig's original positions. We agree that blaming clients is a therapeutic dead end. However, we recognize that although women may be involved in interpersonal processes leading to couple violence, they (a) are more likely to be the predominant victims when considering injury and psychological impact (e.g., Cascardi, Langhinrichsen, & Vivian, 1992; Stets & Straus, 1990); and (b) have less power at all levels of society.

PACT attempts to be "gender sensitive" in that we increasingly assess and emphasize the gender differences in the effects and meaning of anger and aggression. Our work has been influenced tremendously by our collaboration with Dina Vivian, with whom we have attempted to assess couple violence "in context," that is, according to its multiple dimensions (i.e., severity, frequency, psychological impact, and resulting injuries) and forms (i.e., psychological, physical, and sexual; Cascardi et al. 1992; Cascardi & Vivian, 1995; Vivian & Langhinrichsen-Rohling, 1994). This work (see Vivian & Heyman, 1996 for a summary) found that, in the majority of *marital therapy* seeking clients, both spouses report engaging in aggressive acts; however, wives suffer the worst consequences. Wives, compared with their husbands, (a) report being the target of more psychological aggression and coercion (including sexual coercion); (b) are more likely to use severe physical aggression in the context of self-defense; and (c) are less likely to use physical aggression to get their way. Furthermore, there are distinct subgroups of aggressive clinic couples based on the frequency and severity of each partner's violence (Vivian & Heyman, 1995; Vivian & Langhinrichsen-Rohling, 1994): (a) *Mild Bidirectional*–About one-half of marital clinic couples report low frequency of mild aggression (e.g., pushes, grabs, slaps) committed by both husband and wife, with wives often reporting more negative psychological impact from the violence than do husbands; (b) *Moderate* and (c) *Severe Wife Victimization*–Between 30%-40% of cases report high levels of husband → wife aggression and much lower levels of wife → husband aggression; and (d) *Moderate/Severe Husband Victimization*–small subgroup of couples report higher levels of husband victimization. Severe wife victimizers (group c) are poor candidates for PACT, as the descriptions of their aggressive incidents typically have little to do with *couple* conflict, but seem more rooted in the man's extreme power and control tactics. Thus, these spouses are more similar to those treated in typical batterer programs and women's shelters and thus are more appropriately referred for such services.

Feminist-Social Learning Perspective

PACT can most correctly be described as a feminist-social learning approach to ending wife abuse. We agree with Neidig's position that it is important to understand the couple context of violence (i.e., the factors that precede it, maintain it, and reinforce it); yet it is important to look at the social context in which marriage itself is embedded. This context is characterized by gender inequalities at all levels of society. Husband → wife aggression represents (and perpetuates) the most extreme imbalance of power between genders.

Ganley (1989) outlined nine facets of an integrated feminist/social learning approach to aggression. We will revisit each of Ganley's points (in italics), and comment on their implications for the design of PACT.

1. *"[Aggression] is conceptualized as behavior taking place in an interpersonal context but having multiple determinants: individual, interpersonal, and social. These multiple determinants stem from both the current and the historical experiences of the [aggressive man]."* (p. 218)

2. *Interventions must address all determinants of aggression.*

We believe that for many, but not all, couples, when treating a "behavior that takes place in an interpersonal context" it is important to have both members of this interpersonal system present. The design of PACT emphasizes the individual and interpersonal aspects of wife abuse. The first half of the program focuses on individual (intrapersonal) factors (i.e., learning histories, individual anger control, abuse-promoting beliefs), whereas the second half focuses on interpersonal factors (communication, problem resolution, increasing positive activities). Social factors are interwoven throughout the program (e.g., during the abuse awareness section, negotiating an equitable marriage contract). We are in the process of piloting a new version of PACT that increases the emphasis on how social factors (e.g., male power) affect risk.

3. *Aggression continues because it works. Rewards are sometimes intrapersonal and sometimes interpersonal.*

PACT principle five states "abusiveness is a desperate, but self-defeating, effort to change the relationship." The program is founded on the social-learning premise that aggression continues because it works. The man must learn other methods that work, and we believe that this is often best accomplished with both partners developing new, more effective, and more just ways of dealing with each other.

4. *Aggression is a product of interpretations about the partner's behavior rather than by the behavior itself.*

The defining feature of social learning models is that our cognitions determine the meaning of behaviors in our social milieu. The intrapersonal section of PACT focuses on these interpretations (or "hot thoughts") and how they maintain anger and increase the risk for abusiveness. Because this section is intrapersonal, it is not necessary to have both partners present. We are now testing an alternative version of PACT that conducts the first half of the program with separate sessions for men and women, bringing the interpersonal system together only for the interpersonal sections of the program.

5. *Treatment of husband → wife aggression must include the husband.*

We would, of course, concur. In addition, we believe that for couples in the "mild bidirectional" and "moderate wife victimization" groups, treatment of husband → wife aggression would ideally also include the wife.

6. *The goals of intervention are (a) to stop all aggression (physical, psychological, and sexual); and (b) to foster a relationship based on equality, rather than an abuse of power.*

These are, in a nutshell, the goals of PACT.

7. *The therapist must define what aggression is and confront the aggressor when it is occurring, model and teach nonaggressive strategies, and reinforce nonaggressive behavior.*

The sequential progression of PACT (definition/awareness, intrapersonal anger control, interpersonal communication [emphasizing equality and respect]) meets Ganley's charge. Again, we would emphasize the advantage, when teaching nonaggressive *interpersonal* strategies, to have the interpersonal system in the room at the same time.

8. *Therapists must extend their efforts to foster nonviolence to contexts outside of the therapy room.*

Although this recommendation obviously takes a variety of forms depending on the setting, our center at Stony Brook has been deeply involved in the following activities: training of wife abuse researchers and therapists; dissemination of wife abuse research findings, both in professional journals and in more mainstream media; abuse prevention programs in high schools; treatment of abuse in marriages; and abuse prevalence assessment and prevention program implementation with the U.S. military.

9. *The safety of the victim is paramount.*

As will be discussed later, we will not employ conjoint treatment with severe wife victimization couples. Instead, we refer such couples to our county batterers program. Any program that treats wife abuse must make the safety of the victim paramount; we do not believe, nor has our research shown, that conjoint treatment of abuse violates this central tenant.

EMPIRICAL SUPPORT FOR PACT'S RATIONALE

Prevalence of Aggression in Couples Seeking Marital Therapy

Although battering that arouses community intervention (via arrest and/or shelter) is the most salient form of wife abuse, the most common form is aggression within intact marriages where *neither person defines physical aggression as a problem.* Within a clinic population seeking standard marital therapy, 71% of the couples reported physical aggression in their marriage in the prior year (Cascardi et al., 1992; O'Leary, Vivian, & Malone, 1992). Although the majority were experiencing mild forms of aggression (push, grab, shove, etc.), 34% of the husbands were classified as severely aggressive and 13% of the abused wives sustained substantial injuries (e.g., broken bones/teeth or injury to sensory organs). Interestingly, almost none were seeking treatment specifically for the physical aggression; most identified other marital problems as their presenting concern. Despite the presence of aggression, these couples were committed enough to their marriage to seek couples therapy.

The disparity between percentages of couples experiencing marital aggression and those reporting or identifying it as a marital problem is noteworthy. A recent study (Ehrensaft & Vivian, 1996) explored reasons for this phenomenon using some of the same couples from the study by Cascardi and colleagues (1992). The top three reasons for not reporting were (1) "It is not a problem" (29%); (2) "It is unstable/ infrequent" (26%); and (3) "It is secondary or caused by other problems" (22%). Although spouses may choose not to report aggression due to social desirability, a perhaps stronger influence is the spouses' subjective definition of aggression (Ehrensaft & Vivian, 1996). Some spouses do not seem to consider their own acts, be they mild or more severe, to fall into the general category of aggression (even if they would define the same act as aggression if committed by someone else). This concurs with other findings that both spouses report more partner-to-self aggression than they do self-to-partner aggression (Browning & Dutton, 1986; Gelles, 1979). Taken as a whole, these findings imply that the marital therapy office may be an important site for catching and treating cases involving physical aggression, despite the couple's failure to self-identify it as a marital problem. Clearly, couples experiencing aggression present to conjoint therapy at a relatively high rate. Treatment models like PACT are highly palatable to these couples because PACT provides treatment in the conjoint format requested by the couple. PACT is also often palatable to the practitioner because it focuses on the aggression problem prior to other marital presenting problems.

Not only do couples presenting for general marital therapy report aggression, but couple conflicts also appear to be at the heart of the majority of abuse precipitators. As noted in the rationale section, aggression typically occurs within an interpersonal context. Recent research has focused on a qualitative evaluation of the use and occurrence of aggression between spouses. According to Cascardi and Vivian (1995), who interviewed over 200 aggressive couples seeking marital therapy, violence generally grows out of conflict in which each spouse "actively contributes–albeit not necessarily symmetrically–to the escalation of violence" (p. 282). This interview data are corroborated by observational studies discussed below. Given that most couples label their marital problem as a communication deficit and that aggression often stems from verbal conflict, conjoint treatment focusing on aggression is an "easy-sell." From a feminist perspective, "communication problems are an unintended result of violence-promoting gender-based struggles" (Vivian & Heyman, 1996, p. 30). Conjoint feminist social-learning approaches allow for contextual factors involved in the escalation of conflict to violence to be the focus of treatment with both spouses. Importantly, Cascardi and Vivian (1995) also reported that "psychologically abusive/coercive behaviors may be a crucial antecedent to marital violence" (p. 282). However, when husbands were interviewed individually, they tended to minimize their use of these tactics. Thus, only by having both spouses present can a therapist more accurately assess the role each spouse plays in the escalation of conflicts and the factors contributing to the use of aggression.

Communication of Aggressive Couples

A burgeoning area of research has evolved comparing the observed interactions of physically aggressive couples and nonaggressive couples (including nondistressed couples). Aggressive spouses display more overall hostility than nonaggressive couples (Burman, John, & Margolin, 1992; Burman, Margolin, & John, 1993; Cordova, Jacobson, Gottman, Rushe, & Cox, 1993; Margolin, John, & Gleberman, 1988; Margolin, John, & O'Brien, 1989). Aggressive couples are also more likely to show negative reciprocity patterns (e.g., Burman et al., 1992, 1993; Cordova et al., 1993). Furthermore, abused wives clearly engage in high levels of verbal hostility and reciprocity (i.e., respond with hostility to husbands' hostility), contrary to the clinical descriptions of battered women (e.g., Walker, 1979). Although complaints arising from disempowerment appear to be a strong contributor to such negativity (Vivian, Langhinrichsen-Rohling, & Heyman, in press), the results converge on a picture of high degrees of mutual verbal combat (and little placating) in the marriages of moderately to severely abusive couples.

In conclusion, the observational literature supports the contention that aggressive couples have communication deficits. The general finding that both spouses are hostile during conflicts argues for clinical attention to both spouses when intact couples seek treatment. However, as Vivian and colleagues' work demonstrates, sensitivity to gender issues is critical to understanding *why* husbands and wives are hostile. The data would support the rationale for conjoint approaches only if such treatments are sensitive to gender inequalities and struggles.

ASSESSMENT

Because we do not believe conjoint treatment is appropriate for every couple requesting this format, the assessment process is one of the most critical steps when providing couples treatment for aggression. In our program, separate interviews with each spouse are conducted to assess carefully several factors related to treatment assignment. These interviews have two foci: assessing factors related both to the marital relationship and the individual.

First and foremost, a thorough evaluation of the aggressive episodes is necessary. This was assessed in several ways. Each spouse completed the Modified Conflict Tactics Scale (Neidig & Friedman, 1984; an expanded version of Straus' [1979] Conflict Tactics Scale), which requires a report on self and partner aggression. Next, in an oral interview each spouse was asked to estimate the overall frequency of aggressive episodes in the past year. Studies of couples' voluntary reporting of aggression (e.g., Ehrensaft & Vivian, 1996; O'Leary et al., 1992) found there to be differential reporting between these two techniques and thus concluded that both are necessary to get a full picture of the extent and frequency of the aggression.

In the oral interview, each spouse discussed, in detail, the most severe and the three most recent episodes in the past year. Factors such as injury, need for medical attention, intentional and causal attributions, and police involvement were directly assessed. Since this treatment focuses on the cessation of aggression, at least two aggressive episodes in the past year must be reported to qualify for the program. Couples with lower levels of aggression do not generally identify this as a problem and will not find the target of intervention to be well-matched to their needs. However, exclusionary criteria for couples on the severe end of the continuum are also necessary.

Several factors related specifically to the aggression indicated whether the couple was appropriate for a conjoint format:

1. *Severity of aggression*–If aggression was extreme in frequency or severity, the wife's safety became the immediate focus of intervention. Couples in this situation were referred to community agencies more suitable to their needs. Interestingly, very few couples who volunteered reported severe levels of aggression. It may be that the more severely aggressive couples naturally seek other forms of intervention.

2. *Injury or hospitalization*–If the wife reported that she had sustained injuries serious enough for her to have sought medical care, the couple was referred to other modes of intervention.

3. *Husbands' admission of aggression*–For the sake of group cohesion, participants must share the goals of the group and the program. Cases in which the husband denied his use of aggression were deemed inappropriate for this format of intervention.

4. *Wife's fear of husband*–It was important to ensure that both partners were comfortable with the presence of the spouse in sessions. Thus, it is necessary for wives to feel able to disclose information and participate in group activities. If the wife reported fearfulness of participating in group sessions with the husband present or of increased aggression as a result of participating, the couple was given referrals.

Several other factors were assessed to determine the appropriateness of conjoint therapy for aggression. First, the couple must be married and living together. A number of activities are suggested for the week between sessions to improve anger control and enhance couple interactions. Couples not cohabitating are unable to practice frequently the necessary skills and activities. Obviously, the more severe cases in which the couple is not cohabitating because the wife has found a safer living arrangement or has acquired an order of protection against the husband would not meet this criterion. Second, each spouse's individual functioning should be assessed. As with most forms of group therapy, it is important to insure that the individual does not present with competing problems that may interfere with reaching the group's goals. A full Structured Clinical Interview of the DSM III-R (SCID), including the supplementary module for Posttraumatic Stress Disorder, was administered to each spouse individually. Exclusionary criteria at this phase of assessment included: (1) a current substance abuse diagnosis, (2) the presence of psychotic symptoms, or (3) any diagnosis of psychopathology deemed to be severe enough to interfere with successful participation in the group (e.g., bipolar disorder, schizophrenia). Finally, the husbands' past history of aggression in contexts other than their marital relationship was assessed. Men who have a pattern of violent or criminal behavior in a variety of contexts (with co-workers, friends, or strangers) are not considered to be appropriate for this mode of treatment.

For those cases in which severity and frequency of aggression, injury or hospitalization and wives' fearfulness were approaching an extreme level or warranted exclusion from the program, a final step was added to the interview. Wives were individually introduced to safety planning and were provided with help-seeking resources (e.g., hotlines, shelters). In some situations, depending on the wife's feedback, interviewers also brought both partners together at the close of the assessment to discuss the use of a time-out procedure.

DESCRIPTION OF TREATMENT

We have already discussed the main goals and core components of our treatment of aggressive couples in great detail. Heyman and Neidig (1997) discussed PACT when conducted in groups. Vivian and Heyman (1996) discussed our more feminist-oriented version of conjoint treatment for individual couples. Both papers include treatment transcripts. Thus, in this chapter we will only briefly outline the key objectives of the 14 sessions of the program. Table 1 provides a session-by-session summary of PACT program content.

Intrapersonal Sessions (1-7)

Our clinical belief is that spouses must learn to identify and manage their anger before it will be beneficial to focus on their marital conflicts. Thus, the first half of the program focuses on intrapersonal skills by: (a) emphasizing self-responsibility for one's own conflict behaviors; (b) guiding spouses through a heightened discrimination of their anger responses; (c) implementing a contract for nonviolent conflict management (i.e., time out); (d) teaching spouses how to identify and cope with anger provoking cognitions; and (e) exploring the effects of stress and Type-A personality behaviors on spouses' coping abilities (c.f., Dutton, 2002).

Session 1: Introducing the program and Disclosing past aggression. The objectives of the first session are to: (a) establish the fact that the participants are there because of their past violent behavior; (b) foster a sense of personal responsibility for their own violent behavior; (c) reduce resistance and denial; (d) explain the objectives, structure, and rationale of the program; and (e) encourage realistic grounds for optimism. In the second half of session 1, each couple is asked to describe their most recent episode of physical violence. The intent of this portion of Session 1 is the following: (a) to clarify that it is the violent behavior that resulted in their selection for the program; (b) to highlight that the program's goal is the elimination of future incidents; (c) to share this common concern; and (d) to assess and to reinforce their acceptance of personal responsibility for the violent behavior. Personal responsibility is emphasized by asking questions such as "What do you think you did that made the situation worse?"

Session 2: Cycle of violence and Discriminating different levels of anger. We introduce Walker's (1979) three phase model of battering (tension building, abusive incident, remorse) as a framework for under-

TABLE 1. Session by Session Summary of PACT

Session	Content
Session 1	Introducing the program; Recounting violent incident
Session 2	Cycle of violence; Discriminating different levels of anger
Session 3	Discriminating different levels of anger (cont.), Time Out procedures
Session 4	Cognitive-Behavioral (ABC) Model of anger
Session 5	Anger control techniques; Challenging hot thoughts
Session 6	Stress-Abuse connection; Irrational beliefs
Session 7	Midterm Progress Evaluation; Review
Session 8	Communication principles and skills; Positive behaviors
Session 9	Gender differences in communication; Expressing feelings; Empathy
Session 10	Assertion versus aggression; Equality in rights and decision making
Session 11	Conflict escalation process; Principles of conflict containment
Session 12	Dirty fighting techniques
Session 13	Sex; Jealousy; Expanding social support network
Session 14	Wrap-up; Maintaining gains; Expressive versus instrumental violence

standing the processes that set the stage for and result in physical aggression. Session 2 introduces the systemic idea of mutual and circular causality of couple conflict. Prior to this, spouses typically believe that they are reacting to the partner's provocative behavior, and that the responsibility for reducing conflict lies in the partner. By realizing that they are both provoking and being provoked, spouses understand that they must take responsibility for reducing their own conflict escalating behaviors. This is the core construct on which the program is built. It is critical to reiterate, during the presentation of the model, the program principle that each partner is solely responsible for his/her aggression. Although each partner can take steps to reduce the likelihood of conflict escalation, the use of violence is a personal choice and not the result of provocation.

During the second half of this session, we use the short film, *Deck the Halls* (O.D.N. Productions, 1981), to provide a memorable stimulus for discussing both the context of aggression and the affective, behavioral, and cognitive precipitants of abuse. Through discussion, we highlight (a) the concept that anger is not an on/off toggle switch, but rather exists on a continuum; and (b) that conflict escalates sequentially to the point of violence and that spouses have ample warning of the changes in their thinking, feeling, and acting.

Session 3: Discriminating different levels of anger (cont.) and Time Out procedures. For homework between sessions 2 and 3, participants map out their own affective, behavioral, and cognitive changes as anger escalates. Once participants can recognize their own anger cues, they are ready for the first anger management strategy: Time Out. The six steps of time out (self-watching, signaling for time out, acknowledging the part-ner's signal, separating, cooling off, returning) are outlined for the group and discussed.

Session 4: Cognitive-behavioral (ABC) model of anger. Session 4 is devoted to introducing the cognitive-behavioral model of anger and an-ger control. Affective, behavioral, and cognitive anger cues, which were first explored in the previous session, are reviewed. Participants are then introduced to the idea that anger requires cognitive mediation (as was dis-cussed in the rationale section of this chapter). Participants typically be-lieve that events cause their anger; the program introduces the model that events cause thoughts that cause anger. Finally, six types of cognitive dis-tortions are covered as a means of identifying distortion. Couples practice challenging these distortions in the next session.

Session 5: Anger control techniques and Challenging hot thoughts. Once participants recognize anger cues, they are typically eager to begin modifying their anger responses. Four steps are presented: (a) recognize anger signs; (b) pause (i.e., counting to ten, repeating anger control re-minders, deep breathing, and thought stopping); (c) decide what to do; and (d) control thinking. The second two steps receive the most attention in this session. The discussion about "deciding what to do" centers on the function of anger and violence (e.g., making someone shut up or do things your way). Participants explore whether the ends or the means (or both) are maladaptive, and practice more constructive alternatives. The last step, "controlling your thinking," involves participants taking exam-ples of their hot thoughts and generating alternative cool thoughts.

Session 6: Stress-abuse connection and Irrational beliefs. Much of this session is spent solidifying the cognitive anger control strategies from the previous session. At this point we commonly address participant questions such as, "I have no problem identifying my hot thoughts. But what do you do if they're right?" We are likely to agree with the participant's perception that the thought seems to fit at the time. However, we then help them recognize how maladaptive the thoughts are. Thus, quite a bit of work is still necessary before participants are as comfortable with their cool thoughts as they are with their hot ones. The leader also attempts to derive some of the underlying beliefs that guide their hot thoughts and bring them into open discussion. This is accomplished through the kind of Socratic questioning familiar to cognitive therapists. The objective of the remainder of session 6 is to explore the relationship between stress and violence and to introduce some stress management strategies.

Session 7: Midterm Progress Evaluation and Review. Session 7 is the mid-program self-evaluation and review.

Interpersonal Sessions (8-14)

At this point spouses should have rudimentary abilities to (a) use Time-Out; (b) understand the definition of physical and psychological aggression and the cyclical pattern of aggression found in many marriages; and (c) take responsibility for their own anger response and manage it appropriately. At this point many couples believe that they have learned to use the "brakes," but that they have not resolved the conflicts that led them to seek treatment. Thus, although most couples feel positive about their increased ability to control arguments, they are actively pressing for some time to resolve their problems.

Session 8: Communication principles and skills and Positive behaviors. The objective of this session is to introduce some basic principles of communication and to review some basic communication skills. The final segment of session 8 is devoted to increasing positive interaction. As with most discordant couples, participants often report that they derive little pleasure from their relationships and neglect to do most of the activities that made their courtship fun. Increasing these positive behaviors directly increases their marital satisfaction and indirectly makes compromise and conflict management more appealing.

Session 9: Gender differences in communication, Expressing feelings, and Empathy. Work on communication from session 8 continues in session 9. The goal of the remainder of the session is to explore gender-related differences in the participants' communication skills. Areas such as asking permission, decision making, request making, talking about problems, and seeking and sharing information are discussed. Because many (if not most) aggressive men have difficulty identifying and/or expressing their feelings, an exercise is devoted to this skill. This leads to a discussion of the difference between primary emotions (like sadness or anxiety) and secondary emotions (like anger) (c.f., Greenberg & Johnson, 1988) and the impact each has on a partner during a conflict. Although this concept requires a bit of practice during the group, it can be a very powerful exercise as wives say that they would respond much better to husbands expressing hurt or disappointment rather than anger.

Session 10: Assertion versus aggression and Equality in rights and decision making. The first half of this session is devoted to the difference between assertion (standing up for your own rights without violating the rights of others) and aggression (enforcing your own rights or will without regard for the rights of others). The second half of the session has participants complete a "Marriage Bill of Rights." In this exercise, both people respond to a list of behaviors (e.g., the right to be treated with respect, the right to express opinions, the right to come and goes as you please) with one of the following choices: "the husband only has this right," "the wife only has this right," "we both have this right," or "neither has this right." Although this straightforward exercise will not work miracles for highly controlling men, it does result in spirited discussions, with couples agreeing with each other far more than they disagree. A similar exercise is conducted on decision making rights.

Session 11: Conflict escalation process and Principles of conflict containment; Session 12: Dirty fighting techniques. Now that participants have obtained a modest degree of anger control proficiency, have begun trying to unearth their communication skills, and are reconsidering their rights and responsibilities in the marriage, the next two sessions are aimed at consolidating these gains. The goal of session 11 is to emphasize a "team" approach to conflict containment and resolution (see Baucom & Epstein, 1990; Markman, Stanley, & Blumberg, 1994 for additional material on standard behavioral couples therapy approaches in this regard). Session 12 continues to focus on conflict containment with a humorously presented workbook exercise on "Dirty Fighting Techniques" (e.g., blaming, using money, being sarcastic). Although entertaining, participants are sometimes rattled by how many of these techniques they employ. The typical result is a strengthened commitment to "play by the book," and the remainder of the session can be used to continue practicing conflict resolution.

Session 13: Sex, Jealousy, and Expanding social support network. The goal of session 13 is to bring up three interrelated topics: sex, social support networks, and jealousy. See Heyman and Neidig (1997) for a discussion of how these topics are addressed.

Session 14: Wrap-up, Maintaining gains, and Expressive versus instrumental violence. Among the final goals of session 14 are to (a) recognize the achievements of the group; (b) anticipate the consequences of conflict; (c) make commitments for additional change; and (d) provide a forum for airing feelings about termination. Included in this session is a violence contingency contract, in which participants list the concrete steps they will take should violence occur again (e.g., call Time Out, separate and cool down).

EMPIRICAL EVALUATION OF PACT'S EFFICACY

The Stony Brook Wife Abuse Treatment Project aimed to compare the effectiveness of two modes of treatment for spouse abuse. We hypothesized that both PACT and Gender Specific Treatment (GST) effectively reduce physical aggression, but that PACT would result in better gains on marital adjustment, communication, and psychological aggression. At one year, we predicted significantly higher relapse in physical aggression for those who received GST. Complete results can be found in O'Leary et al. (1999).

As hypothesized, physical aggression (both mild and severe) at posttreatment significantly decreased according to both husbands' and wives' reports. This "no difference" finding between couples and gender-specific approaches to wife abuse treatment has been found in two other studies using programs similar to PACT but with participants mandated to treatment, not volunteers (Brannen & Rubin, 1996; Dunford, 2000).

Furthermore, in both groups, husbands and wives scored significantly higher on marital adjustment and on positive feelings about the spouse at posttreatment than at pretreatment. They also scored significantly lower on measures of psychological aggression and on maladaptive beliefs (that spouses cannot change and that all disagreement is destructive). There were no differential effects for format of treatment.

At posttreatment, husbands reported significant increases in taking responsibility for their own aggression and significant decreases in placing responsibility for their own aggression on their wives. Wives significantly decreased taking responsibility for the husbands' aggression.

O'Leary et al. (1999) summarized the main findings as follows:

> With a sample of volunteer, intact couples, we found that commonly expressed fears about conjoint treatment by some who work with court mandated men (e.g., Adams, 1988; McMahon & Pence, 1996) did not apply to our setting. For example, compared to wives in gender specific treatment, wives in the conjoint treatment were not fearful of participating with their husbands, were not fearful during the sessions, did not blame themselves for the violence, and were not put at an increased risk for violence during the program. (p. 498)

Assessed one year later, husbands' physical aggression (both mild and severe) was significantly reduced, according to husbands' and wives' reports. Both husbands' and wives' marital adjustments were still significantly higher than at pretreatment, and husbands' psychological aggression was significantly reduced. Contrary to our hypotheses, both programs worked equally well.

Consumer satisfaction was high for both groups. At post assessment and one-year follow-up, participants were very highly satisfied (average of 8 on a 9 point scale) with both treatments (e.g., how interesting the group was, relevance of program, personality of therapist, skills of therapist, how much their concerns or goals were met by program). At follow-up, however, PACT participants rated their "interest and involvement in the program" as significantly higher than GST participants. Spouses also reported feeling slightly to moderately better (6 to 7 on a 9 point scale) at controlling anger, at self-control and accepting responsibility for their own actions, in their ability to contain conflict, and in their ability to refrain from using verbal aggression. Spouses rated themselves moderately better (7 on a 9 point scale) at curtailing mild and severe physical aggression.

Two limitations were noted (see O'Leary et al., 1999, for a more expansive discussion). First, the drop out rate in this study was 47%. This rate is similar to that often reported in the batterers treatment literature and is perhaps not surprising for a treatment that was offered only in a less-preferred format (groups), conducted on Tuesday nights only, and focused on a problem (aggression) that most participants believed to be of secondary importance (nearly all couples wanted free couples therapy). Second, the aggression cessation rate of 26% at one-year follow-up may be lower than that found in programs with court-mandated men.

In summary, both groups appear to be successful in reducing physical aggression and in improving the marital quality of participants. Furthermore, some of these effects (including the significant reduction, but not elimination, of the intensity and frequency of aggression) continued one year following treatment. In general, participants who completed the program appeared to be pleased with the treatment they received. However, most GST participants wanted to add to their treatment a component that focused specifically on their couple issues following 14 weeks of gender specific treatment.

FUTURE DIRECTIONS IN PACT

Several states in the U.S.A. have adopted policies proscribing couples treatment when there is aggression. How this affects a treatment specifically for spouse abuse that nevertheless uses a conjoint format (i.e., PACT) is unclear. Obviously, therapists need to be aware of the legal and ethical regulations in their area. Spouse abuse is a highly political area and therapists considering employing PACT should familiarize themselves with the controversies in this field (e.g., Caesar & Hamberger, 1989; Gelles & Loseke, 1993; Yllö & Bograd, 1988).

We are in favor of a format that combines gender specific treatment and PACT. Many therapists believe that men must participate in individual therapy before they are ready for conjoint sessions. Although this belief seems reasonable, it has not been empirically tested. In conducting the O'Leary et al. (1999) study, we noticed that, in PACT groups, a husband's failure to master strategies in the initial half of the program would interfere with his ability to focus more directly on communication enhancement, problem solving, and insight into the problems.

In conclusion, we have presented the rationale for a conjoint approach to treating wife abuse, some data supporting that rationale, the content of our program, and some data supporting its effectiveness. That PACT is as effective as single-sex groups indicates that, at least for intact couples, either approach may be successful. Such research does not inform clinicians about which treatment would best suit a particular case. We can point to many couples who would not be appropriate for a conjoint approach. However, many couples would like this approach. It is especially sensible when the couple presents for standard marital therapy and the clinician discovers the presence of aggression. Despite the controversy over conjoint approaches, we are happy to have had this opportunity to present the rationale and data supportive of its judicious use.

REFERENCES

Adams, D. (1988). Treatment models of men who batter: A profeminist analysis. In K. Yllö & M. Bograd (Eds.), *Feminist perspectives on wife abuse* (pp. 176-199). Newbury Park, CA: Sage Publications.

Baucom, D., & Epstein, N. (1990). *Cognitive-behavioral marital therapy*. New York: Brunner-Mazel.

Bograd, M. (1990). Why we need gender to understand human violence. *Journal of Interpersonal Violence, 5*, 132-135.

Brannen, S. J., & Rubin, A. (1996). Comparing the effectiveness of gender-specific and couples groups in a court mandated spouse abuse treatment program. *Research on Social Work Practice, 6*, 405-424.

Browning, J., & Dutton, D. (1986). Assessment of wife assault with the Conflict Tactics Scale: Using couple data to quantify the differential reporting effect. *Journal of Marriage and the Family, 48*, 375-379.

Burman, B., John, R. S., & Margolin, G. (1992). Observed patterns of conflict in violent, nonviolent, and nondistressed couples. *Behavioral Assessment, 14*, 15-37.

Burman, B., Margolin, G., & John, R. S. (1993). America's angriest home videos: Behavioral contingencies observed in home reenactments of marital conflict. *Journal of Consulting and Clinical Psychology, 61*, 40-50.

Caesar, P. L., & Hamberger, L. K. (1989). *Treating men who batter: Theory, practice, and programs*. New York: Springer.

Cascardi, M., Langhinrichsen, J., & Vivian, D. (1992). Marital aggression: Impact, injury and health correlates for husbands and wives. *Archives of Internal Medicine, 152*, 1178-1184.

Cascardi, M., & Vivian, D. (1995). Context for specific episodes of marital violence: Gender and severity of violence differences. *Journal of Family Violence, 10*, 265-293.

Cordova, J. V., Jacobson, N. S., Gottman, J. M., Rushe, R., & Cox, G. (1993). Negative reciprocity and communication in couples with a violent husband. *Journal of Abnormal Psychology, 102*, 559-564.

Dobash, R. E., & Dobash, R. P. (1984). The nature and antecedents of violent events. *British Journal of Criminology, 24*, 269-288.

Dunford. F. W. (2000). The San Diego Navy Experiment: An assessment of interventions for men who assault their wives. *Journal of Consulting and Clinical Psychology, 68*, 468-476.

Dutton, D. G. (2002). Treatment of assaultiveness. *Journal of Aggression, Maltreatment, & Trauma, 7*(1/2), 7-128.

Ellis, A. (1977). *How to live with–and without–anger*. New York: Thomas Crowell.

Ehrensaft, M. K., & Vivian, D. (1996). Spouses' reasons for not reporting existing marital aggression as a marital problem. *Journal of Family Psychology, 10*, 443-453.

Ganley, A. L. (1989). Integrating feminist and social learning analyses of aggression: Creating multiple models for intervention with men who batter. In P. L. Caesar & L. K. Hamberger (Eds.), *Treating men who batter: Theory, practice, and programs* (pp. 196-235). New York: Springer.

Geffner, R., Mantooth, C., Franks, D., & Rao, L. (1989). A psychoeducational, conjoint therapy approach to reducing family violence. In P. L. Caesar, & L. K. Hamberger (Eds.), *Treating men who batter: Theory, practice, and programs* (pp. 103-133). New York: Springer.

Gelles, R. J. (1979). *Family violence.* Beverly Hills, CA: Sage.

Gelles, R. J., & Loseke, D. R. (Eds.) *Current controversies on family violence.* Newbury Park, CA: Sage Publications.

Greenberg, L. S., & Johnson, S. M. (1988). *Emotionally focused therapy for couples.* New York: Guilford.

Heyman, R. E., & Neidig, P. N. (1997). Physical aggression treatment in a couples format. In W. K. Halford & H. J. Markman. (Eds.), *Clinical handbook of couples relationships and couples interventions* (pp. 589-617). New York: Wiley.

Holtzworth-Munroe, A., & Stuart, G. L. (1994). Typologies of male batterers: Three subtypes and the differences among them. *Psychological Bulletin, 116,* 476-497.

Jacobson, N. S., & Margolin, G. (1979). *Marital therapy.* New York: Brunner/Mazel.

Margolin, G., John, R. S., & Gleberman, L. (1988). Affective responses to conflictual discussion in violent and nonviolent couples. *Journal of Consulting and Clinical Psychology, 56,* 24-33.

Margolin, G., John, R. S., & O'Brien, M. (1989). Sequential affective patterns as a function of marital conflict style. *Journal of Social and Clinical Psychology, 8,* 45-61.

Markman, H., Stanley, S., & Blumberg, S. L. (1994). *Fighting for your marriage.* San Francisco: Jossey-Bass.

McMahon, M., & Pence, E. (1996). Replying to Dan O'Leary. *Journal of Interpersonal Violence, 11,* 452-455.

Neidig, P. H., & Friedman, D. H. (1984). *Spouse abuse: A treatment program for couples.* Champaign, IL: Research Press.

Novaco, R. W. (1975). *Anger control.* Lexington, MA: Lexington Books.

O.D.N. Productions (Producer). (1981). *Deck the halls* [Motion picture]. (Available from O.D.N. Productions, PO Box 128, Seaside Heights, NJ 08751).

O'Leary, K. D., Heyman, R. E., & Neidig, P. H. (1999). Treatment of wife abuse: A comparison of gender-specific and couples approaches. *Behavior Therapy, 30,* 475-505.

O'Leary, K. D., Vivian, D., & Malone, J. (1992). Assessment of physical aggression against women in marriage: The need for a multimodal assessment. *Behavior Assessment, 14,* 5-14.

Steinmetz, S. K. (1987). Husband Battering. In V. B. Van Hasselt, R. L. Morrison, A.S. Bellack, & M. Hersen (Eds.), *Handbook of family violence* (pp. 233 - 246). New York: Plenum Press.

Stets, J. E., & Straus, M. A. (1990). Gender differences in reporting marital violence and its medical and psychological consequences. In M. A. Straus & R. J. Gelles, (Eds.), *Physical violence in American families* (pp. 151-165). New Brunswick, NJ: Transaction Publishers.

Straus, M. A. (1979). Measuring intra family conflict and violence: The Conflict Tactics (CT) Scales. *Journal of Marriage and the Family, 41,* 75-88.

Straus, M. A., & Gelles, R. J. (1990). *Physical violence in American families: Risk factors and adaptations to violence in 8,145 families.* New Brunswick: Transaction Publishers.

Stuart, R. B. (1980). *Helping couples change: A social learning approach to marital therapy.* New York: Guilford Press.

Vivian, D., & Heyman, R. E. (1995, July). Marital violence in clinic couples: Typologies based on a "contextualized/gender sensitive" assessment. In A. Holtzworth-Munroe (chair), *Subtypes of batterers and violent couples.* Symposium conducted at the 4th International Family Violence Research Conference, Durham, NH.

Vivian, D., & Heyman, R. E. (1996). Is there a place for conjoint treatment of marital violence? *In Session, 2,* 25-48.

Vivian, D., & Langhinrichsen-Rohling, J. (1994). Are bidirectionally violent couples mutually victimized? A gender-sensitive comparison. *Violence and Victims, 9,* 107-124.

Vivian, D., Langhinrichsen-Rohling, J., & Heyman, R. E. (in press). The Thematic Coding of Dyadic Interactions (TCDI): Observing the context of couple conflict. In P. K. Kerig, & D. H. Baucom (Eds.), *Couple observational coding systems.* Mahwah, NJ: Lawrence Erlbaum Associates.

Walker, L. E. (1979). *The battered woman.* New York: Harper and Row.

Weiss, R. L., & Heyman, R. E. (1997). Couple interaction. In W. K. Halford & H. J. Markman (Eds.), *Clinical handbook of couples relationships and couples interventions* (pp. 13-41). New York: Wiley.

Yllö, K. A. (1993). Through a feminist lens: Gender, power, and violence. In R. J. Gelles & D. R. Loseke (Eds.) *Current controversies on family violence* (pp. 47-62). Newbury Park, CA: Sage Publications.

Yllö, K. A., & Bograd, M. (1988). *Feminist perspectives on wife abuse.* Newbury Park, CA: Sage Publications.

TREATMENT
OF SPECIAL POPULATIONS

Treating the Lesbian Batterer:
Theoretical and Clinical Considerations–
A Contemporary Psychoanalytic Perspective

Vallerie E. Coleman

SUMMARY. The phenomenon of lesbian battering challenges mainstream assumptions about battering and defies traditional ways of defining and understanding domestic violence. This article identifies and illuminates variables critical to understanding and treating lesbian batterers. In particular, intrapsychic factors in the treatment of lesbian batterers are considered via an integration of the theoretical constructs of personality development with attachment theory, state and affect regulation, shame, pathological vindictiveness, and variables specific

Address correspondence to: Vallerie E. Coleman, 3231 Ocean Park Boulevard, Suite 205, Santa Monica, CA 90405-3232.

[Haworth co-indexing entry note]: "Treating the Lesbian Batterer: Theoretical and Clinical Considerations–A Contemporary Psychoanalytic Perspective." Coleman, Vallerie E. Co-published simultaneously in *Journal of Aggression, Maltreatment & Trauma* (The Haworth Maltreatment & Trauma Press, an imprint of The Haworth Press, Inc.) Vol. 7, No. 1/2 (#13/14), 2003, pp. 159-205; and: *Intimate Violence: Contemporary Treatment Innovations* (ed: Donald Dutton, and Daniel J. Sonkin) The Haworth Maltreatment & Trauma Press, an imprint of The Haworth Press, Inc., 2003, pp. 159-205. Single or multiple copies of this article are available for a fee from The Haworth Document Delivery Service [1-800-HAWORTH, 9:00 a.m. - 5:00 p.m. (EST). E-mail address: docdelivery@haworthpress.com].

http://www.haworthpress.com/store/product.asp?sku=J146
© 2003 by The Haworth Press, Inc. All rights reserved.
10.1300J146v07n01_08

to lesbian domestic violence. Finally, two case examples and treatment considerations are discussed. *[Article copies available for a fee from The Haworth Document Delivery Service: 1-800-HAWORTH. E-mail address: <docdelivery@haworthpress.com> Website: <http://www.HaworthPress.com> © 2003 by The Haworth Press, Inc. All rights reserved.]*

KEYWORDS. Lesbian battering, domestic violence, attachment theory, affect regulation, shame, pathological vindictiveness, psychoanalytic theory, borderline personality disorder, narcissistic personality disorder

I think that once hitting starts, a barrier is broken that afterwards is too easily crossed. What was once unthinkable behavior is no longer. Once hitting starts, it's like taking something precious and valuable and smashing it on the ground, and seeing it lying there broken and knowing it can never be repaired. (Lisa, 1986, p. 38)

What possesses a woman to cross that barrier–to hit, smash, cut, kick, rape, humiliate, degrade, threaten, or kill the woman she professes to love? To acknowledge the phenomenon of lesbian battering shatters mainstream assumptions about battering as a man's province, and about women's incapacity for this type of violence. As a result, there has been a tendency for society as well as clinicians to deny or minimize the existence of violence between women (Coleman, 1994). In order to understand lesbian battering and provide effective treatment for lesbian batterers, clinicians must have (1) an understanding of lesbians as individuals and as partners in relationship, (2) a conceptualization of personality development, and (3) knowledge of those critical factors that may predispose lesbian women to batter their partner.

The need for such awareness is underscored by Wise and Bowman's (1997) findings in a study that compared graduate-level counseling students' (48 women, 23 men) responses to a heterosexual (violent male) and a lesbian domestic violence scenario. The researchers used a two-paragraph vignette depicting a domestic violence incident in which the female victim is left bleeding and has a black eye. The scenario was the same for all participants, with the exception of the sexual orientation of the victim/client and the gender of the batterer; half of the sample randomly received the heterosexual scenario and the other half the lesbian scenario. The researchers found that lack of training regarding lesbian battering and a tendency to minimize lesbian violence considerably impacted participants' responses. Specifically, they found that participants were significantly more likely to rate the heterosexual scenario as more violent than the lesbian scenario and to charge the male batterer with assault. Although these results cannot be generalized to all training programs or the field at large, they do reflect a lack of training regarding lesbian battering and a bias among mental health providers in which heterosexual domestic violence is frequently viewed as more serious than lesbian domestic violence.

Violence in lesbian relationships defies traditional heterosexist[1] ways of defining and understanding battering and demands that we take an individualized, multidimensional approach to partner abuse (Coleman, 1994). To treat batterers successfully, we must develop an understanding of the *particular idiom of being* (Bollas, 1992) that each client possesses, while holding, on a meta level, an understanding of domestic violence that is informed by sociopolitical factors, social learning theory, family dynamics, psychoneurobiology, and psychopathology (Coleman, 1994). Although all of these areas need to be considered to effectively understand and treat domestic violence, this chapter focuses on the role of intrapsychic factors in lesbian battering. In particular, critical elements in the treatment of lesbian battering are considered via an integration of the theoretical constructs of personality development with attachment theory, state and affect regulation, shame, pathological vindictiveness, and variables specific to lesbian domestic violence. Finally, two case examples and treatment considerations are discussed.[2]

CHARACTERISTICS OF LESBIAN BATTERERS

Over the last decade, same-sex domestic violence has begun to be recognized as a serious health concern within the lesbian community. Nevertheless, lesbian battering continues to be significantly under-researched. In contrast to the hundreds of studies examining heterosexual domestic violence, a recent review of the literature (Burke & Follingstad, 1999) identified only 19 empirical/quasi-empirical studies examining violence in same-sex relationships: 15 on lesbian battering, 3 on gay male and lesbian battering, and 1 solely on gay males. The available literature suggests that the frequency of lesbian battering is comparable with that of heterosexual and gay male battering (Burke & Follingstad, 1999; Coleman, 1991, 1994; Waldner-Haugrud, Gratch, & Magruder, 1997). Researchers have found rates of physical violence in lesbian relationships ranging from 7% (Bryant & Demian, 1994) to 48% (Gardner, 1989). This wide range is due to several factors: differences in methodologies, which makes comparisons problematic; difficulty obtaining a representative sample; differing definitions of abuse; and a lack of differentiation between perpetrators and victims.

In general, there appear to be more similarities than differences between heterosexual battering and lesbian battering (see also Leisring, Dowd, & Rosenbaum, 2002). Researchers have found that lesbian battering is a significant problem, with rates of verbal abuse typically exceeding those of sexual and physical abuse (Burke & Follingstad, 1999; Coleman, 1991; Renzetti, 1988; Lie et al., 1991)). Dutton (1995b) compared abuse victimization rates for women who had been in both heterosexual and lesbian relationships, based on data from Lie et al. (1991). Reports of physical, sexual and verbal abuse were all higher for lesbian relationships than for heterosexual, with verbal abuse being the most frequent (64.5% in lesbian relationships). Similarly, milder forms of physical violence (e.g., pushing, slapping, punching) have been found to exceed rates of severe violence (e.g., striking with an object, use of a weapon) (Burke & Follingstad, 1999; Coleman, 1991; Renzetti, 1988; Waldner-Haugrud et al., 1997). The general dynamics of lesbian battering are also comparable to those of heterosexual battering in which there is a cycle of violence (Walker, 1979) and an increase in the frequency and severity of abuse over time (Elliott, 1996; Renzetti, 1988, 1992).

Although no empirical studies have specifically examined the personality dynamics of lesbian batterers, clinical and anecdotal reports suggest that abusive lesbians have personality traits similar to heterosexual male batterers (Coleman, 1994; Elliott, 1996; Renzetti, 1988, 1992). Empirical studies examining the personality characteristics of heterosexual male batterers demonstrate variability in both typology and level of batterer pathology (Gondolf, 1999; Hamberger & Hastings, 1986, 1991; Tweed & Dutton, 1998). However, there are several consistent themes that further inform our understanding of domestic violence. Typically, batterers have faulty appraisal systems and dysfunctional thought patterns that lead to and exacerbate aggressive, violent behaviors (Saunders, 2000; Sonkin, 1995). In terms of specific personality disorders, several studies have identified male batterers as having narcissistic (Barnett & Hamberger, 1992; Gondolf, 1999; Hamberger & Hastings 1986, 1991), borderline (Dutton, 1998; Dutton, van Ginkel & Landolt, 1996; Hamberger & Hastings, 1986, 1991; Tweed & Dutton, 1998), and antisocial (Gondolf, 1999; Hamberger & Hastings, 1986;

Tweed & Dutton, 1998) personality traits. Researchers have also demonstrated a relationship between battering and avoidant, dependent, depressive, compulsive, and anxious personality traits (Gondolf, 1999; Hamberger & Hastings, 1986, 1991; Tweed & Dutton, 1998).

Dutton and his colleagues (1996, 1998) have examined the relationship between borderline personality organization, insecure attachment, posttraumatic stress disorder (PTSD), and the perpetration of violence. Dutton (1998) divided batterers into three groups: overcontrolled batterers, impulsive/undercontrolled batterers, and instrumental/undercontrolled batterers. Most of Dutton's research has focused on the impulsive/undercontrolled batterer, which he argues is the type most consistent with both borderline personality organization and the cyclical nature of domestic violence in intimate relationships. Dutton (1995, 1998) proposed that impulsive batterers have fearful attachment styles, which he reframes as "angry attachment." He found that these men have personality profiles that include jealousy, chronic anger, and PTSD symptoms such as poor sleep patterns, dissociation, depression, and anxiety. My clinical experience indicates that much of Dutton's findings can be generalized to female batterers.

According to the available literature, lesbian batterers frequently feel powerless, have low self-esteem, tend to abuse alcohol and drugs, and are generally overly dependent and jealous (Leeder, 1988; Lobel, 1986; Schilit & Lie, 1990). Leeder (1988) noted that many lesbian batterers fear abandonment, have poor communication skills, tend to be self-absorbed, and are unable to empathically relate to their partners. Consistent with Leeder's descriptions, Renzetti (1988, 1992) found correlations between lesbian batterers' use of violence and levels of dependency, jealousy, and substance abuse.

In a summary of their clinical work with more than 30 lesbian batterers, Margolies and Leeder (1995) reported that all of the women described their violence as an altered state of consciousness and their rage as akin to an adrenaline rush. The researchers found that every batterer had experienced violence in her family of origin: Almost all of them had witnessed abuse of their mothers, approximately 70% had been sexually abused, and 65% had been physically or verbally abused. Typically, the women were appealing and charming; however, they all evidenced low self-esteem, had difficulty expressing their feelings, and utilized splitting as a defense. Margolies and Leeder noted that the batterers were extremely dependent on their lovers for attention and emotional support–which led to the women feeling controlled by their lovers' ability to affect their feelings and sense of self. At times, this perceived vulnerability culminated in a "childlike dependent rage" (p. 145). In some instances, when a woman felt bad about herself or distanced from her lover, battering became a means of re-engaging and establishing intense contact. The authors observed that

> the batterers' underlying feeling was a chronic fear of abandonment and loss. Avoiding those feelings became the organizing principle of their lives. Most violent incidents took place during threatened separations. . . . Violence in these situations was an attempt to maintain connection to the lover, to hold her both physically and psychically. The batterer was lashing out to protect her fragile self from fragmentation and to avoid abandonment. (p. 145)

They also found that batterers had high levels of competitiveness with their lovers, and competed with others for their lovers' attention.

In my clinical experience, and as reflected in the literature, there is not one specific batterer profile but a constellation of personality dynamics that ranges from a specific personality disorder to a combination of traits reflecting the mosaic of that person's distinctive being. As suggested elsewhere (Coleman, 1994), many lesbian batterers evidence personality characteristics that are similar to male batterers and consistent with borderline, narcissistic, or antisocial personality disorders. Batterers may exhibit more than one disorder or present with a mix of personality traits, such as depressive, dependent, passive-aggressive, or compulsive traits. Lesbian batterers with antisocial personality disorder comprise a distinct subgroup; these women typically engage in criminal behaviors as well as intra- and extrafamilial violence. Moreover, they generally do not seek treatment voluntarily. In contrast to batterers with antisocial personality disorder, those with borderline and narcissistic personality organization share a number of characteristics and are often more amenable to treatment. Hence this chapter focuses on the relationship between borderline and narcissistic character pathology and lesbian battering.

PERSONALITY DISORDERS

Borderline and narcissistic personality disorders are both believed to be rooted in early developmental failures resulting from maternal/caretaker misattunement and insecure attachment (Freed, 1984; Schore, 1994). Although there are dynamic and structural differences, these two disorders frequently overlap; many individuals with borderline personality disorder have narcissistic traits, and many individuals with narcissistic personality disorder also have borderline traits. In addition, difficulties in regulating shame, fear of abandonment, and rage are common in both borderline and narcissistic disorders.

Because their capacity for self-soothing is severely compromised, individuals with borderline or narcissistic traits are prone to erupt with rage when faced with unmanageable affects such as anxiety, fear, or shame (Wastell, 1992; Wolf, 1988). At such times, the paranoid-schizoid position conceptualized by Klein (1946/1996) predominates and the individual experiences acute persecutory anxiety. In conjunction with this acute state, the individual falls into (so to speak) a self-preservative mode and is unable to access emotions, behaviors, and cognitions associated with prosocial behavior (C. Lillas, personal communication, October 5, 1999; Wang, 1997). Thus, instead of being able to access thoughts and feelings associated with attachment, empathy, compassion, and trust, the batterer "experiences the anger and fear of self preservation . . . in this state, violence can be inflicted upon others without remorse or conflict" (Wang, 1997, p. 166).

In both borderline and narcissistic disorders, rage and violence become a defense against fragmentation; however, the triggers underlying fragmentation vary based on personality structure. Prior to discussing the relationship between lesbian battering and each of these personality organizations, an overview of attachment theory, affect regulation, shame, and pathological vengeance is provided as a framework for considering aspects of development salient to lesbian batterers.

OVERVIEW OF ATTACHMENT
AND STATE/AFFECT REGULATION

In recent years, several authors have begun to examine the role of attachment theory (Bowlby, 1973, 1988) in several areas that have significant implications for batterer treatment, such as attachment and psychopathology (Dutton, 1998; Fonagy et al., 1996; Pistole, 1995; Sable, 1997; Schore, 1994; Sonkin & Dutton, 2002), attachment and affect regulation (Mikulincer, Orbach, & Iavnieli, 1998; Schore, 1994, 1997; Silverman, 1998), attachment style and assaultiveness (Bowlby, 1984; Dutton, 1998; Dutton et al., 1996; Wallace & Nosko, 1993), attachment and stress (van der Kolk, 1996; Wang, 1997), and attachment and shame (Nathanson, 1987; Schore, 1994; Wallace & Nosko, 1993).

During infancy, we build working models of the world and our self in relation to others. A key component of these models is our representation of attachment figures–who they are, where they can be found, and how likely they are to respond to us in times of need (Bowlby, 1973, 1988). This schema also includes a sense of one's value and acceptability in relation to the attachment figure. A "secure base" (Bowlby, 1973, 1988) develops when an individual experiences the presence of an available and responsive caretaker during times of distress. The consistent presence of such a caretaker (usually the mother) creates confidence in the availability of others and in the self as worthy and valuable. The infant/child's working model of attachment is a set of conscious and unconscious " . . . rules for the organization of information relevant to attachment and for obtaining or limiting access to that information, that is, to information regarding attachment-related experiences, feelings, and ideations" (Main, Kaplan, & Cassidy, 1985, p. 92). According to Main et al., these rules are revealed in the ways an infant organizes thought and language. As summarized by Schore (1997), during "preverbal development, the infant constructs internal working models of the attachment relationship with his caregivers, and these representations, permanently imprinted into maturing brain circuitries, determine the individual's characteristic approach to affect modulation for the rest of the lifespan" (p. 40). In other words, through interaction with her caretaker(s), the infant/child develops affective-cognitive sets that determine how she organizes experience, manages emotions, and relates to others.

Although the mother is generally considered to be the primary attachment figure, the internalized primary object is "a derivative of many experiences with actual others, some occasioned by environmental stresses . . . [and] some determined by character disorders of the mother and the father that are condensed into distressed experiences" (Bollas, 2000, p. 7). It is important to keep in mind that constitutional factors and innate vulnerabilities can significantly impact an infant's capacity for and quality of attachment. For instance, an infant who is constitutionally unable to tolerate delays in gratification will experience her mother as overly frustrating and withholding (Bollas, 2000), thus negatively impacting her internal model of attachment.

Attachment Typologies

Researchers examining infant and child reactions to separations from parents have identified four distinct typologies of attachment (one that is secure and three that are insecure): secure, insecure-avoidant (dismissive), insecure-ambivalent (preoccupied), and insecure-disorganized/disoriented (Ainsworth, Blehar, Waters, & Wall, 1978; Main & Goldwyn, 1991, as cited in Fonagy et al., 1996; Main et al., 1985). Upon reunion after a period of brief separation, secure infants will seek comfort, proximity, and contact with the parent(s) and then return to play. Mothers of secure infants have been found to be responsive to their infants' emotional signals and to permit access when their child seeks proximity (Ainsworth et al., 1978; Main et al., 1985; Schore, 1994). In contrast, "the mother of an insecurely attached infant does not instigate interactive repair nor does she initiate distress-relief sequences. As a result, the infant remains stuck fast in stressful unregulated disorganizing states of unmodulated negative affect" (Schore, 1994, p. 402). Schore argues that remaining in such a state negatively impacts orbitofrontal brain development, leading to deficits in emotionality, affect regulation, and cognitive representational processes. Individuals with such deficits are unable to adaptively modulate their internal states and behavioral responses in stressful situations. In conjunction with other factors, such deficits predispose one to use violence as a means of self-regulation.

Insecure-avoidant infants actively avoid and ignore their parents, often moving away from the parent in what appears to be a defense against rejection (Main et al., 1985; Schore, 1994). Although they may experience a subjective sense of anger, these infants do not openly express anger or distress (Schore, 1994). Mothers of insecure-avoidant infants are emotionally detached, insensitive to their infants' signals, and consistently reject their children's attempts at contact and proximity (Main et al., 1985). In contrast to insecure-avoidant infants, the researchers found that insecure-ambivalent infants demonstrated anger and resistance combined with a desire for contact and proximity. However, attempts to comfort them were unsuccessful; they continued to express distress and were typically unable to be soothed. The infants' ambivalent behavior was in response to mothers' insensitivity to their emotional signals and inconsistency in mothers' physical and emotional availability (Main et al., 1985; Schore, 1994). This attachment style is frequently seen in the push-pull dynamics of batterers with borderline personality organization.

Main et al. (1985) reported that insecure-disorganized/disoriented infants demonstrate "dazed" behavior on reunion with the parent and appear depressed, confused, or disorganized; they seek comfort and security and then become strongly avoidant. These infants also display contradictory behavior patterns, such as approaching their parent with their heads averted or gazing away while in contact with the parent. When interviewed, the parents of these infants evidenced repeated positive-negative oscillations in viewpoint, a refusal to remain on the topic, and irrationality. In their follow-up study of attachment style at 6 years of age, Main et al. (1985) found that upon reunion, these children "seemed to attempt to control the parent, either through directly punitive behavior or through anxious, overly bright 'caregiving' behavior (inappropriate role reversal)" (p. 83). I suspect that these behavioral patterns may later be seen in the charming, caretaking behaviors of many batterers.

Lachmann and Beebe (1997) proposed that an individual's organization of experience and social relatedness is based on the concurrent influences of self and mutual regulation. In mutual regulation, "both partners actively contribute to the regulation of the exchange, although not necessarily in equal measure or in like manner" (p. 93). Self-regulation refers to a capacity to modulate one's states of arousal and predictably organize one's behavior. Through the mutual regulation process involved in healthy, secure attachments, individuals develop self-regulatory functions that enable them to self-soothe under situations of stress (Silverman, 1998). This achievement lays the groundwork for adult relationships and is essential for integrating early emotional experiences, organizing a coherent sense of self and other, and communicating effectively with others. Thus, under conditions of stress, an infant, child, or adult who has developed a secure base is able to utilize effective coping mechanisms to regulate her/his affective experience (Mikulincer et al., 1998; Silverman, 1998) and manage the situation without becoming overwhelmed and dysfunctional.

Psychoneurobiological Correlates

When healthy, secure attachment has not developed, the individual is unable to tolerate dysregulating experiences to such a degree that she/he cannot effectively self-regulate and maladaptive defenses predominate. From a psychoneurobiological perspective, stressful experiences lead to physiological attempts at coping and reestablishing homeostasis; these attempts result in responses that range from hypoaroused (inhibited) to hyperaroused (excitatory/expansive) states (Lillas, 2000). Lillas contends that "chronically excited or inhibited states are the neurophysiological underpinnings of the defensive strategies" (p. 21) identified by Karen Horney: moving against, moving toward, and moving away (Horney, 1950, as cited in Lillas, 2000, p. 21). When Bowlby (1973) observed that children and adolescents who experience repeated separations, threats of separation, and other rejections display both anxious and angry behavior, he was observing behavior consistent with a defensive moving against, hyperaroused physiological state. Under conditions of either hyper- or hypoarousal, an individual is unable to access abilities that are available when she/he is in an "alert processing" mode. As described by Lillas (2000), alert processing (AP) is

> . . . the state of calm, conscious attention. One's sensory, emotional, relational, attentional, and cognitive capacities are at their peak during this AP state, which allows a person to experience a full range of affects while still being engaged relationally. . . . I see this state as the physiological underpinning of the observing ego and the psychoanalytic process of free association. Both the analyst and the analysand must be in the AP state if optimal mutual emotional engagement is to occur. (p. 21)

In my clinical experience, batterers have developed entrenched defensive physiological reactions/states that greatly impair their capacity for alert processing.

Shame

Schore (1994) has explicated the role of anxious attachments, affect dysregulation, and shame in the development of both borderline and narcissistic personality disorder. Individuals with either of these disorders are unable to access the symbolic representations necessary for self-soothing because "due to a preponderance of shame-imprinted interactive representations of the self-in-interaction-with-a-misattuned-other, their ability to autoregulate affect is fundamentally impaired. Both of these primitive emotional disorders are particularly ineffective in regulating shame" (p. 429). Since shame is a fundamental component of all insecure attachment, it is inextricably linked to the need to split off and repress intolerable and unmanageable experiences between self and (m)other. As articulated by Schore, "unregulated, and therefore 'bypassed' and unconscious, shame is a potent motive force that underlies repression. Early forming, nonverbal defenses are erected and maintained to specifically exclude this negative affect from consciousness" (p. 473). As described by Morrison (1999), "shame is that feeling about ourselves of failure, worthlessness, defect, filth, weakness, that makes us feel isolated, different, unlovable . . . that experience that causes one to 'want to disappear into the earth' " (p. 92). Although a healthy level of shame plays an important role in socialization, excessive or inadequate shame can become pathological (Hibbard, 1994; Schore, 1994). In normal levels of shame, libidinally determined, inhibitory, and self-esteem attenuating components predominate; in pathological shame, in contrast, aggressive, persecutory, and humiliating components predominate (Hibbard, 1994). Pathological shame significantly disrupts an individual's ability to develop a cohesive, stable sense of self and is a central component of rage and violence (Balcom, 1991; Dutton, 1995; Hockenberry, 1995; Wallace & Nosko, 1993).

Although controversy exists regarding the age at which the capacity to experience shame emerges, there is evidence to suggest that the earliest triggers for shame are in the misattunements of the attachment relationship (Broucek, 1997; Schore, 1994). The disrupted flow between caretaker/mother and baby results in an early experience of shame due to an experience of failure "to initiate, maintain, or extend a desired emotional engagement with a caretaker" (Broucek, 1997, p. 44). Thus, insecure infants experience an inordinate amount of shame in their attachment relationships. Goldberg (1991) noted that infants who are easily overstimulated may have a heightened sensitivity to experiencing shame. Shame has been correlated with experiences of trauma such as physical and emotional abuse, neglect, and abandonment (Dutton, van Ginkel, & Starzomski, 1995; Hockenberry, 1995; van der Kolk, 1996). As noted by van der Kolk (1996),

> . . . shame is critical to understanding the lack of self-regulation in trauma victims and the capacity of abused persons to become abusers . . . Denial of one's own feelings of shame, as well as those of other people, opens the door for further abuse. Being sensitive to the shame in others is an essential protection against abusing one's fellow human beings, and it requires being in touch with one's own sense of shame. Similarly, not being in touch with one's own shame leaves one vulnerable to further abuse from others. The resulting disorganized patterns of engagement are commonly seen in traumatized people who suffer from borderline personality disorder, who need to be helped to understand how this perpetuates their getting hurt and their hurting others. (p. 15)

Shaming experiences are a painful assault against the self and typically lead to states of "shame-rage" or "humiliated fury" (Lewis, 1987).

Such rage is "a protective, retaliatory attack aimed at wiping out the offending 'other'" (Morrison, 1999, p. 93). Often in love relationships, early shame states are either consciously or unconsciously triggered, resulting in shame-rage and defensive maneuvers that are abusive. Another defense against shame is contempt–which, when combined with rage, creates a formula for likely battering. In contempt, the individual projects her experience of shame onto her partner, who is then devalued and denigrated (Morrison, 1999). Although shame develops out of interactions with others and often occurs in front of others, once shaming experiences have been internalized, shame can be internally induced without the presence of an external other (Morrison, 1999). Many batterers experience feeling shame that is provoked internally–and often unconsciously. Frequently, this shaming internal object is projected onto the batterer's partner, who is then experienced as inducing the shame.

In a study examining the effects of shame, guilt, and abuse on 140 court-referred and self-referred male perpetrators of violence, Dutton et al. (1995) found that shaming experiences in conjunction with parental abusiveness were necessary to account for an individual's later assaultiveness. In other words, when shaming experiences were absent, parental abusiveness had no significant correlation with adult assaultiveness, and when parental abusiveness was absent, shaming experiences were no longer significantly correlated with adult abusiveness. The researchers also found a significant correlation between recollections of shaming experiences and borderline personality organization. (Measures of narcissistic personality organization were not included in the study.) Dutton and his colleagues proposed that although shame and guilt may foster an abuse-prone personality, the modeling of abusive behavior is a necessary second step for becoming an abuser.

Shame is a particularly salient issue for lesbians. During development and throughout life, lesbians must battle misogyny, homophobia, and heterosexism. Kaufman and Raphael (1996) assert that homophobia (an irrational fear of, hatred for, or aversion to anyone lesbian/gay or to aspects of lesbian/gay lifestyle) results from the magnified effects of shame, disgust, dissmell[3], and contempt. In lesbian battering, conscious or unconscious internalized homophobia can contribute to a batterer's negative affect states and "bad" internal objects that increase her vulnerability to shame, shame-rage, disgust, contempt, and dissmell.

In conjunction with homophobia, heterosexism is an ever-present form of cultural abuse that leads to shame and a devalued sense of self, similar to the effects of sexual and physical abuse (Neisen, 1993). Girls who will eventually identify as lesbian (or bisexual) typically grow up feeling different and experience great shame about this dissimilarity. In general, neither heterosexual parents nor society mirror the developing lesbian's homosexuality, which is an integral component of her self-experience. Core experiences of sexual orientation/identity that are not mirrored and accepted (either consciously or unconsciously) by one's primary caretakers result in significant experiences of mis-attunement which must be split-off and sequestered in one's internal world. In addition to experiencing a lack of mirroring, many lesbians are also actively devalued, humiliated, or rejected (either directly or indirectly) by both family members and others in society. Thus, experiencing homophobia and heterosexism, along with their internalized components, adds another dimension to shame and the perpetration of violence. These shame states are often projected onto one's lover, who is then attacked and denigrated.

For example, lesbian batterers who are extremely uncomfortable and ashamed of their lesbian identity often keep their sexual orientation a secret and go to great lengths (criticism, degradation, and/or threats) to control their partner's appearance. One batterer who felt threatened by what her partner wore (she feared that her lover looked "unfeminine" and would be identified as lesbian, thus implicating herself as lesbian) would berate her and devalue her choice in clothes, wrinkling her face in disgust and dissmell. In addition, the batterer would contemptuously distance herself, threatening her partner with rejection and loss of the relationship, if she didn't dress in accordance with her desires.

Pathological Vindictiveness

In their description of the effects of homophobia and heterosexism, Kaufman and Raphael (1996) noted that humiliation breeds vindictiveness, and powerlessness magnifies it. In addition to insecure attachments, poor affect regulation, and shame-rage, I have found that batterers frequently manifest pathological vindictiveness. "Normal" vindictiveness and a desire for revenge are common human reactions to injury and injustice. However, for the pathologically vindictive person vengeance is a central organizing principle and it has an addictive quality (Daniels, 1969; Feiner, 1995; Steiner, 1996). Such pathological vindictiveness can contribute to and enhance the addictive quality of battering and the cycle of violence.

Similar to shame, pathological vindictiveness is rooted in early experiences of humiliation, frustration, deprivation, powerlessness, rejection, and dismissal (Daniels, 1969; Feiner, 1995; Steiner, 1996). One way of conceptualizing vindictiveness is that it develops as a result of the splitting that occurs in an attempt to preserve the good object. As described by Steiner (1996),

> when the self, the good object, or the relationship between them is injured, it is the good object that seems to demand revenge and the patient feels it is his duty to respond as a means of restoring and preserving the lost idealised relationship . . . Revenge is the antithesis of forgiveness and the patient insists that the object cannot be let off the hook until it has been forced to confess and atone for the injury done. (p. 434)

Searles (1965) emphasized the role of vindictive fantasies as a defense against the grief and separation anxiety that results from ruptures in the attachment relationship. These fantasies serve the psychological function of maintaining the self-other bond. Although pathological vindictiveness may evolve initially out of a child's repeated aggressive attempts at getting back the lost object–"to force the parent to love him again" (Daniels, 1969, p. 193)–it

> . . . ultimately become[s] an end in itself, nonetheless retaining, in some psychic realm out of awareness, its original aim–reunion with the evanescent loved one. And, in extreme cases, reunion is purchased at the price of the ultimate merger: the death of the rejecting loved one and the death of the vengeful, rejected suitor. (p. 183)

I propose that such pathological vindictiveness underlies the stalking behavior of batterers and is a central dynamic for batterers who murder their partners. Batterers with significant narcissistic traits are particularly prone to such vindictiveness. As articulated by Schulte, Hall, and Crosby (1994), "self-righteous rage requires revenge, or punishment of the offender, in order that humiliation is repaired and a sense of self, although infantile and grandiose, can be reinstated" (p. 611).

PERSONALITY ORGANIZATION AND BATTERING

Batterers with Borderline Personality Organization

Although there continues to be controversy about whether borderline personality disorder is a distinct diagnostic entity or a personality organization that lies between psychosis and neurosis, there are a number of characteristics common to individuals with borderline personality organization. In general, such individuals vacillate between a fear of engulfment when close with another and fear of catastrophic abandonment when they experience separateness. Other common features include: poor boundaries, lack of a clear sense of self, poor impulse control, lack of frustration tolerance, poor reality testing under stress, need for immediate gratification, lack of an ability to self-soothe, fragile self-cohesion, deficits in superego functioning, affect regulation difficulties, an absence of empathy, dramatic shifts between idealization and devaluation, and lack of a capacity to form stable self and object representations (Goldstein, 1990; Grotstein, 1987; Sable, 1997). These individuals undergo state transitions that can be instantaneous and traumatic–"phenomenologically it [such a shift] is experienced as a precipitous entrance into a shame-associated chaotic state" (Schore, 1994, p. 421). In quoting Lansky, Schore notes that individuals with a borderline disorder are remarkably compromised in their capacity to regulate shame: "most of the defensive operations of borderline patients are reactions to their shameful self-consciousness among others. Borderline patients are exquisitely humiliation prone. They have a pronounced tendency to experience others as deliberately inflicting shame on them" (Lansky, 1992, p. 37 as cited in Schore, 1994, p. 416).

Sable (1997) suggests that borderline pathology may develop out of caregiving that is anxious and intrusive or conversely distant and dismissing, or a combination of the two. Object-relations theorists have conceptualized borderline personality disorder as developing in response to severe difficulties during the process of separation-individuation (Goldstein, 1990; Mahler, Pine, & Bergman, 1975). Based on current knowledge about infant maturation, Brown (1990) proposed a revision of Klein's (1946/1996) concept of the depressive position, in which it would begin around 14 to 16 months and be renamed the "depressive position proper" (p. 507). He suggested that there is a "transitional position" between the paranoid-schizoid position and the "depressive position proper" that coincides with Mahler's differentiation and practicing subphases of the separation-individuation process (p. 507). According to Brown borderline personality organization arises from difficulties in the transitional position that leave individuals "stuck at a maturational point at which they feel neither confused with the object nor do they feel themselves fully distinct from the object" (p. 508). Manic defenses predominate in this position and "the more manic defenses figure into the overall configuration of a borderline's defensive structure, the more likely is that individual to appear narcissistically organized in terms of attitudes of triumph and contempt towards the object" (p. 508). This type of personality structure is frequently seen in individuals who batter.

Self-cohesion is extremely fragile in batterers who have a borderline personality organization, and they lack effective affect-regulation. As a result, seemingly minor disruptions or psychic injuries in relation to their partner can lead to fragmentation (Coleman, 1994). For these women, rage and violence become ways of defending against such fragmentation. Other borderline-level defenses frequently used by batterers include splitting, projection, omnipotent control, idealization, and devaluation.

Both fear of abandonment and fear of engulfment are central issues for batterers with borderline personality organization. Although they tend to seek merger with their partner in an attempt to avoid either real or perceived abandonment, merger leads to a loss of self and fear of engulfment (Coleman, 1994). In addition, closeness intensifies their feelings of need and their fear of abandonment, resulting in periodic episodes of withdrawal (Goldstein, 1990). Individuals with borderline personality disorder are caught in a constant state of tension between closeness and distance–this is the adult version of the insecure-ambivalent infant, and possibly the insecure-disorganized infant. Krestan and Bepko (1980) have suggested that in an attempt to create distance and avoid the stimulation of abandonment fear, lesbians may resort to the use of verbal or physical fights.

Wolf (1988) conceptualized individuals with borderline personality disorder as "merger hungry personalities" who attempt to fuse with their partner in lieu of maintaining their own self-structure (p. 74). Batterers with borderline pathology are prone to becoming enraged by a partner's attempts at separation and independence. They often resort to violence to control the partner and assure her continued function as a selfobject in an attempt to avoid fragmentation and abandonment depression. In addition, manipulative, self-destructive behaviors, such as threats of suicide, may be used as control mechanisms. I have conceptualized these dynamics in relation to the cycle of violence (Walker, 1979) as follows.

The beginning of the relationship is typically marked by the batterer's idealization of the love object and pressure for increased closeness/ merger. A threat to the batterer's self-cohesion, either related to fear of abandonment or fear of engulfment, stimulates the internal representation of the bad object and the resultant intolerable affect states. In an attempt to protect and maintain the good internal object, the batterer projects the bad object representation onto the battered partner and then attacks her. This enraged state is reconstituting for the batterer and shifts her feelings of vulnerability into an experience of strength and power. Following the abuse, there is a return to merger with the good object–which provides the batterer with the needed selfobject function and leads to restabilization of the self (Coleman, 1994).

In general, during the honeymoon phase the batterer is apologetic, remorseful, and makes promises of change. At the same time, she typically blames her lover for her (the batterer's) abusive behavior. Some batterers feel remorse and regret; however, rather than being motivated by genuine guilt and desire for reparation that is characteristic of the depressive position, they are primarily motivated by shame and a desire for reunion with the good object. Wallace and Nosko (1993) noted that guilt "requires an ability to enter into and empathize with the other as an individual to whom harm has been done" (p. 49). Although batterers may have moments of such guilt, concern for the other cannot be sustained.

The following case example highlights the dynamics of attachment style, affect regulation, shame, and pathological vindictiveness in the use of violence as a core defensive strategy specific to borderline personality organization.

Clinical Example–A

Presenting problem and family history. Karen, a 34-year old African-American lesbian, came to me for psychoanalytic psychotherapy at the urging of her friends. She had been obsessing about–and threatening to kill–her ex-lover. Although most of Karen's abusiveness occurred in the context of intimate relationships, she had engaged in criminal behavior up until her mid-20s. Furthermore, she had an ongoing history of assaulting friends and acquaintances when she felt abandoned or disrespected by them. When I went to greet Karen in the waiting room for our initial consultation, I was met with hostile glares and a swaggering, tough persona. The first several sessions were quite tense, as Karen vacillated between expressing a desire for me to help her with her homicidal ideation and proclamations about how the "bitch deserved to die" and there was no point in trying to stop her. Such fluctuations, combined with frequent testing of me, our relationship, and the treatment frame, characterized the first two years of her treatment.

Karen owned a gun and had demanded it back, just prior to beginning treatment, from the friend who had been "holding" it for her. After gaining some confidence in me and our work together, Karen agreed to have another friend hold her gun. I strongly recommended that Karen also participate in a batterers treatment group; however, she refused. In response, I told her that I was not certain that individual treatment alone would be effective, but that we could start at twice a week and then reevaluate. She agreed, and we began a treatment plan that included psychodynamic exploration combined with didactic work on violence and anger management.

Karen had grown up in a middle-class African-American family with two older step-brothers and two younger biological siblings. Her parents had divorced when Karen was a teenager, and she had not seen her father in many years. It soon became clear to her that the way her family appeared to the external world was very different from what happened within the family. At home, Karen witnessed a great deal of domestic violence and was also the victim of her father's violent rages. During the early phases of treatment, Karen would angrily vent her hatred of her father. She described numerous incidents in which he had severely battered her mother, chased and beat up her brothers, whipped her, and severely abused the family pets. Her father's verbal abuse was virtually constant, and he frequently shamed Karen and her brothers. For at least the first 2 years of treatment, Karen's descriptions of these incidents were devoid of any affect other than anger; she was completely cut off from any experience of terror, pain, or shame.

Karen's relationship with her mother was much more ambivalent, ranging from rageful eruptions at her mother to idealization and seeking her support. Her anger toward her mother stemmed primarily from experiences of abandonment. For example, Karen's mother frequently chose her father over protecting the children, bought special gifts for the other children but not for Karen, and minimized Karen's physical and emotional pain. There had also been numerous ways in which her mother was, and continued to be, overly intrusive and controlling. In addition, her mother suffered from an undiagnosed and untreated mental illness that resulted in periodic psychotic episodes, which were extremely dysregulating for Karen.

Attachment style. In terms of Karen's attachment style, she demonstrated traits consistent with both insecure-ambivalent infants and insecure-disorganized/disoriented infants. Her experiences of being shamed and abused by her father were central to her use of violence as a means of self-regulation, whereas her early attachment relationship with her mother, as well as later experiences of abandonment and shaming by her mother, were dominant in her underlying depression and propensity for fragmentation. Karen's identification with the aggressor, her father, was a primary means of escaping intolerable affects related to shame and abandonment, as well as a means of feeling power and control. This dynamic was often demonstrated in manic, omnipotent "highs," during which Karen would contemptuously devalue and taunt women whom she felt had "wronged" her. Underlying Karen's omnipotent aggression was a great deal of shame. On many occasions, she stated that backing down from an altercation made her feel like a "wimp . . . I hate myself for acting afraid . . . I've gotta show them I'm not gonna take that crap!"

Relationship history. Karen's relationship history was replete with conflict and disappointments. In virtually every relationship her verbal abusiveness had quickly escalated into physical assaultiveness. Although Karen's violence during her early 20s was often linked with drinking alcohol, her abusiveness continued after she joined Alcoholics Anonymous and stopped drinking. Prior to coming to treatment, Karen's homicidal ideation developed after a relationship had ended and she had experienced feeling "completely abandoned" by her former lover, Annabelle. In addition to being hurt and angry about the breakup, Karen felt that she had been replaced by Annabelle's new friends. Karen's vindictive fantasies served as (1) a defense against loss of the relationship; (2) a defense against the loss of Annabelle as a selfobject; and (3) enabled her to maintain self-cohesion by warding off unbearable experiences of powerlessness and humiliation.

Initial treatment phase. Initially, Karen would become enraged and defiant when I suggested exploring the feelings underlying her rage. Gradually, I realized that her reaction was partly due to the fact that she lacked an ability to identify and express her feelings. Consequently, my attempts at helping her recognize underlying issues were experienced as an invitation to be shamed and humiliated. In addition, exploring these issues meant having to own and integrate her split-off and projected bad objects and bad object experiences, such as powerlessness, shame, contempt, disgust, devaluation, pain, and terror. Karen also became enraged whenever I referred to her homicidal ideation as her "fantasy" about killing Annabelle. There was no difference for her between fantasy and reality, no capacity for symbolic representation or play. Similarly, there was no potential space in the treatment to allow for an "as if" experience in the transference. Thus, addressing this lack of transitional space (Winnicott, 1971) became an underlying goal of the treatment.

As Karen's homicidal ideation began to resolve, she became extremely depressed and suicidal. At this point, some psychotic symptoms emerged, primarily hearing voices and paranoid ideation. She agreed to a medication consultation and was compliant with the recommendation that she take both an antidepressant (which regulates both serotonin and norepinephrine) and an antipsychotic. This combination of medication proved to be very effective for Karen.

When working with batterers, I have found it extremely helpful to integrate psychoanalytic understanding with cognitive-behavioral interventions designed to improve state and affect regulation as well as interventions that address cognitive distortions and modify behavioral patterns. My work with Karen now increased to three times a week, with one session devoted entirely to addressing her violence, using Sonkin and Durphy's (1982/1989) handbook, *Learning to Live Without Violence* (which we adapted for gender). I also included exercises from a variety of other sources and created a relaxation tape for her to use at home. In addition, we did relaxation exercises at times while in session, which helped Karen improve her state and affect regulation and provided an experience of mutual regulation. She was then able to make use of these experiences to help her self-regulate under conditions of stress. In sum, the didactic work combined readings on violence and stress, with the use of time-outs, assertiveness training, anger intervention worksheets, identification sheets (e.g., identifying the use of threats, intimidation, emotional abuse), and the Iceberg Exercise (described in the section on Treatment Considerations).

The integration of these didactic exercises with psychoanalytic psychotherapy provided a structured holding environment, which enabled us to explore Karen's family and relationship dynamics, as well as issues related to homophobia, heterosexism, and racism. Although much of Karen's violence was rooted in her family's dysfunction and abuse, she also struggled with shame around her sexual orientation and ethnicity. During both elementary and junior high school, Karen was made fun of for being different. She described herself as having been the "typical tomboy," stated that she had always been male-identified, and considered herself to be a "butch" lesbian. She didn't dress like or socialize with the other little girls in the neighborhood. In addition, Karen was often the target of racial jokes. As a result, she struggled a great deal with her identity and typically preferred spending time with, and was attracted to, women from other racial/ethnic groups. However, as she began to integrate various aspects of herself and her racial background, Karen found herself more attracted to other African-American women.

Helping Karen to access and address her early trauma on an affective level and then cognitively link these experiences with her assaultiveness was a critical component of the treatment. Making this connection was extremely hard for Karen because getting in touch with early experiences of pain and longing felt inordinately shameful to her. In addition to addressing the defensive function of her violence and analyzing the ways in which it came up between us (i.e., verbal threats of violence), we repeatedly discussed Karen's experience of her rage and violence as a "high." There was an addictive quality to her abusiveness that was self-reinforcing, making it a difficult cycle to break. Gradually, she was able to recall, with appropriate affect, incidents of being abused by her brothers and father, as well as desperately wanting her mother to intervene–to no avail. Such experiences were replayed many times in the transference, where I was placed in a position of protecting her, and others, from the abusive aspects of herself. Other traumatic memories included times that she was blamed for getting injured when she was abused and then humiliated for crying. For example, when her father broke her hand, she was shamed and blamed for crying and making a "big deal" out of the incident.

The mutual and self-regulatory aspects of our work were an essential foundation of the therapeutic process. Almost from the beginning, Karen started to ask questions about my life and my relationship. My typical response to personal questions is to ask patients to reflect on such questions and for us to use them as a window into their internal world. However, Karen could not tolerate such a stance–she became anxious, demanding, pouty, and threatening. I realized that I needed to shift my analytic stance considerably in order to provide a relational experience in which she could use me as an idealized selfobject. Responding to her questions directly and openly was very effective and over time Karen began to tolerate more reflection and exploration.

Karen also began to develop a capacity for fantasy and play in the treatment relationship, which enabled us to make more direct use of the transference. For instance, at one point, she began tenaciously to test the boundaries of our relationship, requesting that we go for walks instead of staying in the office and demanding that I take her on trips. She became very frustrated by my refusals to give in to such arrangements and at times was even threatening. Slowly I began to engage her in imagining what such experiences might be like. Gradually, Karen was able to start to express these desires in the form of fantasy and then to elaborate on the fantasy. For example, she envisioned us taking a walk where, along the way, I would buy her ice cream; or she would be my baby and my partner and I would set limits on her tantrums and raise her lovingly.

Separations. Much of our work on transference-countertransference dynamics centered on separations. In general, tolerating the breaks between sessions and vacations was extremely difficult for Karen, and during the first few years my vacations precipitated states of fragmentation. These time periods were, for her, fraught with regulatory problems and provided fertile ground for violent explosions in my absence. On one occasion, she landed in jail for assaulting a woman who had ended their brief dating relationship. I conceptualized this behavior as largely a result of Karen's acting out the transference due to her inability to tolerate and manage her feelings of rejection, rage, and disappointment in relation to my absence. Her splitting left her unable to link any of her feelings of rage at this woman with her feelings toward me in relation to the break; she needed to protect me (mother) as the good object and could not tolerate having any ambivalent feelings toward me. Furthermore, for Karen to acknowledge that our separations had an impact on her provoked her shaming, condemning Internal Saboteur (Fairbairn, 1952). Over the years, we did a great deal of work on detoxifying the shame surrounding her affective experience of terror and rage in response to separations. We were then able to anticipate vacations and develop ways that Karen could access her good internalized object-representation of me during separations, while also feeling upset and angry at me for going away. We created a safety plan that helped her to recognize any escalating potential for violence and identify appropriate steps to get support. This measure improved her frustration tolerance and impulse control, and reminded her of our connection.

Karen also began to tolerate linking her feelings of rage and abandonment regarding our separations with her childhood and her mother. Gradually, we were able to "tease out" how conditions of perceived or actual abandonment stimulated her Internal Saboteur, provoking both internal attacks on herself and externalized attacks on others. This process helped Karen to increase her capacity for affect regulation and impulse control, enabling her to make use of her higher cortical functioning and thinking abilities rather than automatically triggering the implicit/procedural memory circuits (Siegel, 1999) linked to her early attachment experiences.

As in the course of any treatment, there were numerous incidents of disruption and repair. One key enactment[4] occurred at the end of a session when, all of a sudden (so it seemed at the time), Karen refused to leave my office. She began taunting me with "What are ya gonna do if I don't leave?" and "You can't make me leave . . . there is nothing you can do." She also threatened to destroy my office and to return and burn down the building if I tried to have her removed forcibly. In response to her bullying behavior and threats, I found myself experiencing a range of emotions. Initially, I was quite anxious, fearful about my safety, and worried about what she might do once I did get her to leave my office. I was also worried about my next appointment and uncertain about the best way to handle the situation. For several minutes it seemed as if I could do nothing right. I felt powerless, ineffective, and afraid. Gradually, I also began to get quite angry and had to take a few minutes to calm down and reflect on what was happening.

Thankfully, I was able to reengage some of my reflective capabilities and recognize that underneath Karen's threatening and abusive behavior was fragmentation due to an inability to regulate her intolerable affects and bad internal objects, which were being stimulated as a result of the ending of the session (and my impending vacation). Finally, I was able to articulate that she must be feeling very anxious, frustrated, and angry about the ending of our session and the fact that I had another appointment. I wondered aloud if perhaps she felt unimportant and imagined that I did not truly care for her. In response Karen stormed out, leaving behind a hail of verbal threats. Remarkably, she called a short time later and left a message on my machine, apologizing and assuring me that she did not mean the things she had said. This was significant change. We were able to process this enactment in several subsequent sessions, using it to better understand the dynamics embedded in her early experiences and how these played out between us, as well as with others.

Indications of progress. Frequently, when overwhelmed by her dependency needs and the pain and terror of separation, Karen utilized splitting and projective identification–inducing terror, shame, confusion, and powerlessness in the other. When we discussed the aforementioned rupture, Karen was able to take in my acknowledgment of having failed her by missing the subtle signs of her distress. She was then able to hear and acknowledge the ramifications of her temper tantrum in terms of my experience. Karen expressed feeling bad about her hurtful behavior and worried that she could or would do something to ruin our relationship. I had always been very clear with Karen that although I valued her and our relationship, I could not work under conditions of threat or abuse. I considered her expression of worry and remorse, in conjunction with the shifts that occurred afterward, as indicative of movement toward the depressive position. This movement contrasted clearly with her previous style of relating, which was almost exclusively from the paranoid-schizoid position, in which she exhibited no true empathy or concern for others.

Play was another important aspect of self and mutual regulation in the treatment. Karen had a good sense of humor and, through play, we were able to address many issues that would otherwise have been too shame-laden for her to acknowledge. For example, sharing some of my own feelings when angry or anxious created a space wherein I could joke with her about how she protected herself with her "gunslinger" persona. At times, I would playfully imitate her glares or her tough posturing to give her a flavor of how she presented herself. In response Karen would laugh in acknowledgment and express feeling glad that I had seen through her defenses. In combination with the Iceberg (Volcano) Exercise (described in Treatment Considerations), this way of playing created a safe space for her that allowed us to talk about the protective nature of her defenses and the affects underlying them.

Another salient segment of the treatment occurred when Karen began to express mixed feelings about a new supervisor at work. She felt attracted to this woman and had developed a "crush" on her. However, she also felt unappreciated and mistreated by her supervisor. She began to have vengeful fantasies of "getting back" at her by physically and sexually assaulting her. I told Karen that I sensed there was something very important for us to understand about these vengeful fantasies. Although she could not yet tolerate considering the meaning of her feelings in regard to the transference, she could examine their relevance to her childhood. I suggested that her feelings of powerlessness and her desire to make her supervisor feel vulnerable and helpless were rooted in earlier experiences of being treated unfairly and feeling vulnerable and powerless as a result. In response Karen began to recall times she had been mistreated and abused by her father and brothers.

In contrast to previous recollections of these memories, this time Karen was able to access the feelings associated with those incidents. For example, in session Karen reexperienced sitting at the dinner table as a young girl and having two of her brothers kick her so hard and so many times that she had bruises up and down her shins. In spite of crying and pleading with her parents to stop them, she was told to "shut up and stop whining" and was sent to her room without dinner. Having this flashback in session with me enabled Karen to have a new object experience in which both her feelings and the injustice of the situation were mirrored and validated. However, shortly thereafter she was flooded by her shaming and condemning internal objects for being "a stupid, weak baby." Furthermore, Karen felt humiliated that she had shown me this weak and vulnerable part of herself. We were then able to discuss this characteristic pattern in which her Internal Saboteur (Fairbarin, 1952) attacked and humiliated her for her vulnerabilities and attachment needs. These dynamics needed to be addressed and relived between us many times before new patterns of object-relating were firmly established, enabling Karen to self-regulate without utilizing her defensive, abusive behaviors.

Batterers with Narcissistic Personality Organization

As with borderline personality organization, the specifics regarding the etiology and diagnosis of narcissistic personality organization remain controversial. Some theorists conceptualize pathological narcissism as a character organization that is diagnosed in conjunction with, but separate from, one's level of functioning (Kernberg, 1984; McWilliams, 1994). From this point of view, one must assess whether an individual with narcissistic character disorder (or any other character disorder) is fundamentally psychotic, borderline, or neurotic in terms of personality structure. Other theorists consider individuals with narcissistic character organization to fall between the borderline and neurotic levels of psychopathology (Goldstein, 1990). According to this perspective, these individuals are considered to have better ego functioning than those with borderline personality organization; however, they exhibit very fragile self-esteem, are prone to shame-rage reactions when narcissistically injured, and frequently utilize primitive defenses, such as splitting, devaluation, idealization, omnipotence, and projection. Other characteristics central to narcissistic character organization include feelings of emptiness or incompleteness, shame and fears of being shamed, feelings of inferiority, a constant need for admiration and affirmation, grandiose self-importance, lack of empathy, interpersonal exploitation, a need for power, fantasies of success or beauty, a sense of entitlement, feelings of envy, and arrogant or haughty behaviors (McWilliams, 1994; Rosen, 1991). Although not all batterers have a narcissistic personality disorder, many of these traits are seen in individuals who batter.

Some authors hypothesize that narcissistic personality structure, in which self and object representations are fused, results either from a fixation during the symbiotic phase of development or as a result of regression to symbiosis due to unsuccessful negotiation of separation-individuation during the rapprochement phase (Freed, 1984; Masterson, 1981). During the symbiotic phase of development, the infant perceives herself/himself as magically controlling the environment in a narcissistic, omnipotent state of oneness with the mother (Mahler et al., 1975). Serious traumas or disappointments during this period interfere with the infant's ability to develop healthy, adaptive narcissism. The child is unable to tolerate the real world and the needs of others and remains defensively linked with the omnipotent object, stuck in a state of infantile narcissism and grandiosity (Masterson, 1981). Schore (1994) contends that the narcissistic individual's ability to access positive affect states, reflected in her/his grandiosity, indicates that she/he has successfully negotiated the symbiotic stage and the early practicing period. He argues that it is "late practicing shame transactions that are central events in narcissistic pathogenesis" (p. 423).

Vulnerable versus Grandiose Narcissism

Shame has generally been considered to be the core of narcissistic pathology. However, there is some evidence that persons with narcissistic character structure can be divided into two phenomenologies that differ in their relationship to shame: a narcissistically vulnerable type and a grandiose, egotistical, and entitled narcissistic type. The vulnerable type is consistent with Hockenberry's (1995) symbiotic narcissist and Broucek's (1982, 1997) dissociative type. Hockenberry (1995) observes that

> fundamental to both styles is a need to maintain an illusion of personal omnipotence and control, in regard to both self-perception as blameless and perfect and to the treatment of others as self-objects. Both types share a propensity for viewing themselves as tragic victims in a hostile, unappreciative world. (p. 307)

Individuals with symbiotic or vulnerable narcissism rely on merger with others to regulate self-esteem and maintain their sense of self (Hockenberry, 1995). Because they tend to split off their grandiose aspects, these individuals often present as vulnerable, self-depreciating, and shame-prone. However, their underlying omnipotence, grandiosity, and rage is demonstrated via control of others, veiled arrogance, projection of anger, and passive-aggressive behaviors (Hockenberry, 1995).

In general, individuals with grandiose narcissism tend to be more limited in their ability to experience and express shame and pride, and they rely more on projection as a means of regulating their anger/aggression (Heiserman & Cook, 1998; Hibbard, 1992; Schore, 1994). Schore (1994) has suggested that individuals with vulnerable/symbiotic narcissism are prone to overt shame experiences and manifest low self-esteem and sensitivity to rejection, whereas those with grandiose narcissism are unable to regulate shameful affect because it is "bypassed" and defended against through grandiosity, entitlement, and contempt of others. However, Hibbard (1992) found that when he statistically eliminated denial of shame, grandiose narcissism continued to be negatively correlated with shame. Thus it is unclear how much those with grandiose narcissism actually experience conscious or unconscious shame. This conceptualization suggests that in the treatment of batterers who present with grandiose narcissism, the practitioner must determine whether there are deficits resulting in a lack of shame or whether the individual is utilizing primitive defenses to defend against shame.

Studies comparing gender with high and low levels of narcissism have found that women are more prone to shame regardless of level of narcissism (Heiserman & Cook, 1998; Hibbard, 1992). In contrast, men with high levels of narcissism have been found to exhibit significantly less shame. Whereas men with a narcissistic character disorder may tend to rely on selfobjects to mirror their grandiosity, women who have a narcissistic disorder may be more likely to obtain and maintain their self-regard, self-worth, and validation through identification or merger with idealized others (Heiserman & Cook, 1998; Hockenberry, 1995). Thus, in contrast to heterosexual male batterers, lesbian batterers with a narcissistic character structure may be more likely to rely on merger with their partners or attuned mirroring of their experiences as a means of sustaining their sense of self.

Schore (1994) proposed that individuals with grandiose narcissism evidence insecure-resistant (ambivalent) attachment patterns, whereas insecure-avoidant attachment is predominant for those with vulnerable narcissism. Narcissistic dysregulation occurs due to "the failure to evolve a practicing affect regulatory system which can neutralize grandiosity, regulate practicing, excitement, or modulate narcissistic distress" (p. 427). Because they do not have the ability to tolerate and recover from narcissistic wounds, these individuals are predisposed to feelings of shame and reactions of narcissistic rage.

In Kohut's (1972) view, narcissistic rage erupts when there is a loss of control over the mirroring selfobject or the idealized, omnipotent selfobject is unavailable. The intensity of narcissistic rage is much greater than that of normal aggression–the individual will resort to any means to right a wrong, undo a hurt, or obtain revenge (Kohut, 1972). Hockenberry (1995) observes that

> latent hatred for internalized objects (for example, due to a frustrating or shaming mother) characteristically leads the person on a search for other objects in which his own mistreated self can be projected and can be similarly attacked, depreciated, or humiliated. Unconsciously, there is an identification with both the suffering, shamed self and with the hated, internalized persecutory objects (identification with the aggressor). However, to avoid painful feelings of unconscious shame, the shamed and vulnerable self is typically dissociated and projected onto the partner. . . . In this way the partner becomes the target of the grandiose narcissist's attempts to triumph over internal shame through "revenge" and victimization. (p. 309)

Consider a batterer with narcissistic personality structure who experiences feeling wounded because her lover has a difference of opinion or takes a phone call at what feels like an inopportune time. This rupture in the merger with her selfobject and/or the lack of mirroring attention is experienced as a selfobject failure that threatens the batterer's grandiose, omnipotent (but fragile) self-cohesion. On an unconscious level there is a reactivation of the original trauma, in response to which she experiences overwhelming feelings of shame, powerlessness, and worthlessness. Rage and violence then become a way to regulate these feelings and return to a state of omnipotence and grandiosity by exerting power and control over her partner. From an object-relations point of view, the bad self-states are split off and projected onto the partner, who is then devalued, shamed, and attacked as a means of restoring the omnipotent, grandiose, good self and object representations.

Lesbian Specific Factors

There are issues specific to the lesbian community that may heighten the difficulties inherent in narcissistic character organization. In addition to the increased potential for merger in lesbian relationships (more on this topic in the treatment section), the mirroring and idealizing functions of the selfobject may be intensified by virtue of the fact that it is a same-sex relationship. As discussed earlier, shame is a particularly salient issue for lesbians, and the experience of both external and internalized prejudices can easily activate shame states in narcissistically vulnerable batterers. Feelings of envy and jealousy may also be exacerbated in lesbian relationships because, in contrast to male-female relationships, where a woman's female friendships do not typically imply the possibility for romantic interest, in the lesbian community friends are not implicitly distinct from potential lovers (Coleman, 1994). This "gray area" can become very threatening for individuals who are prone to jealousy and lack a stable and separate sense of self and other. The following description of Marilyn and Joan illustrates many of these issues. Although most clinicians who offer treatment for domestic violence consider couple therapy ineffective, at the least, and damaging or dangerous, at the worst, the example of Marilyn and Joan is offered to demonstrate the ways in which psychoanalytically informed couple therapy can be effective and beneficial, in some cases.

Clinical Example–B

Presenting problem. Marilyn, a 38-year-old Caucasian woman, called for couple therapy at the urging of her partner, Joan (32, also Caucasian), because they were having "relationship problems." In the initial session, Marilyn stated that she was not interested in therapy and had only come at Joan's insistence. Nonetheless, she dominated a large part of the session with her complaints about the past 3 years of their 5-year relationship, during which, she contended, Joan had been emotionally insensitive and often physically cold and uninterested in sex. Joan was very clear that she was not certain she wanted to continue the relationship, stating that although she still loved Marilyn, she was not sure she wanted to live with her. My attempts to clarify the nature of their difficulties were met with bickering between the two of them. It was not until the second session that it became clear that Joan was threatening to end the relationship if Marilyn did not stop having "tantrums." Exploration revealed that 3 weeks prior, they had had a fight in which Marilyn punched Joan in the stomach, shoved her against a wall, and threatened to "beat her up" if she continued to "flirt and act like a slut" every time they went to a party. Marilyn stated that she was aware that her behavior could be "over the top" but proclaimed that it was a justified response to Joan's disrespectful and insensitive treatment of her. Contrary to many stereotypical assumptions about lesbian batterers, both Marilyn and Joan were quite feminine, and Marilyn was significantly smaller than Joan.

In considering the options for treatment, I realized that providing couple therapy might run the risk of creating an environment in which Joan would feel the need to censure herself or where she might be endangered in the aftermath of a volatile session. On the other hand, it was clear from Marilyn's presentation that she was not open to pursuing individual therapy or joining a batterers group. In addition, they both reported that this recent incident of violence was the most severe; previously, occasional shoves and verbal abuse had been the norm. Given these considerations, I decided to conduct three to four more assessment sessions with them, with a focus on safety. During this time, I also worked to engage them–and Marilyn, in particular–in becoming curious about the dynamics underlying their relationship problems. While mirroring Marilyn's feelings of hurt and betrayal, based on how she experienced Joan's actions, I was also very clear and firm about the abusiveness of her behavior and its negative ramifications. I reviewed the rationale and procedures for time-out and worked with them on recognizing the cues indicating a need for such a break. They both agreed to utilize this technique, and in each session we reviewed their use of it, as well as the times they could have used it but did not.

Initial treatment phase. Although initially resistant to exploring her behavior, by the end of our fourth joint session, Marilyn began to develop an interest in why she interpreted Joan's conversations with other women as flirtatious behavior. She also started to demonstrate mild curiosity about the factors underlying her "over the top" reactions. In addition, she agreed to abstain from physical violence. Based on my assessment, their cooperativeness, and the nature of previous battering incidents, I felt that there was no immediate danger of severe abuse. Moreover, Joan seemed to be using the sessions to verbalize feelings and perceptions she could not express otherwise, and Marilyn was starting to use me as a selfobject, which enabled her to tolerate Joan's feelings and complaints. We were able to examine the ways in which Marilyn's behaviors tended to push Joan away and lead to passive-aggressive responses on Joan's part–which, in turn, led to Marilyn feeling increasingly bewildered, frustrated, and hurt.

Given that the couple therapy seemed to be helpful, I recommended that we continue working in this format and reassess as needed. They agreed and the next several months proved to be constructive in many ways. Marilyn and Joan reacted well to my introduction of the Iceberg Exercise, which was quite effective in helping them to identify the feelings underlying their reactions during arguments. In regard to Marilyn's rages, the Iceberg Exercise facilitated her recognition of the shameful and intolerable feelings underlying her abusive behavior. In addition, our frequent use of the exercise enabled her to separate her feelings from the negative self-talk that fueled her violent reactions. For example, we were able to identify how going to a party was, in fact, a very stressful event for Marilyn. Underneath her grandiosity and charming facade, Marilyn frequently felt insecure and uncertain of her "popularity" with others. When Joan socialized with other women at parties, Marilyn became afraid that their friends would question the "strength" of their relationship. She also felt untrusting of their friends and expected that several of them would try to "seduce Joan if given half a chance." Such fears reflected her early insecure attachments and the dysfunction within her family of origin. In addition, Marilyn's beliefs were fueled by her internalized homophobia, including negative stereotypes about lesbians and lesbian relationships.

We discussed their notions about the lesbian community, their struggles in coming to terms with their sexual orientation, and the impact of homophobia and heterosexism on themselves and their relationship. We also explored how they replayed familial patterns in their relationship as well as in our treatment relationship. Other important areas of discussion included experiences of shame and shaming behaviors in their relationship, their past relationship history, and their current support network within both the heterosexual and lesbian communities. In addition, I provided education on the cycle of violence and battering behaviors.

There were many times during the treatment that maintaining my neutrality and focus was difficult. I had to monitor my countertransference constantly and try not to collude with the ways in which Marilyn would minimize and justify her abusiveness. I also had to carefully monitor my connection with Joan and remain cognizant of the potential to join with her in shaming or condemning Marilyn.

Rupture and repair. In one session, Marilyn became angry and upset with Joan because Joan would not "honor and respect" her feelings by agreeing not to spend time with a friend whom Marilyn found particularly threatening. In response, Joan became frustrated and expressed feeling hopeless about Marilyn ever "getting over her jealous and childish behaviors." Marilyn reacted by increasingly devaluing and attacking Joan. The more controlled and devalued Joan felt, the more rigid and belittling she became toward Marilyn. I commented on this pattern and mirrored the frustration and hurt they were each feeling in response to the other.

In reaction to my responding to *both* of them, Marilyn began to attack me with accusations of not understanding her and not protecting their relationship (from this perceived threat). She stated that I must not be a very experienced and knowledgeable therapist after all, adding, "What the hell are we paying you for?" As I reflected on my countertransference, I was immediately aware of a wish to attack back in a shaming, rageful retort. I was also aware of feeling confused and thrown off guard by her attack. Rather than responding out of identification with the shaming bad object that had been engendered in me, I said to Marilyn, "I think that my acknowledgment of Joan's pain and frustration felt as though I were disregarding your pain and dismissing how threatened you feel." Marilyn responded with an angry "yes." I added, "Perhaps it also feels scary for me to consider Joan's position and feelings alongside yours. In your early experiences, only one person could *win* or have *power*, and you assume that you are going to be the one who will lose and will then be left alone." Marilyn softened slightly and replied, "Yeah, that's just like what would happen in my family . . . I feel dissed." I noted that in feeling "dissed," she seemed to experience both hurt and shame, which then led to her desire to shame the person she had felt hurt by–as had just happened between her and Joan and then between her and me. Marilyn agreed. After a pause, she returned to how unreasonable and uncaring Joan was in her desire to remain in contact with this particular friend. However, as a result of the rupture and subsequent repair, Marilyn was able to experience me as a new object, which allowed us to address this conflict in a more constructive manner. In addition, the continued occurrence of such experiences enabled the two of them to have more frequent moments of empathic connection, gradually expanded the space available for exploration, and furthered the development of their observing egos.

Adding group therapy. After almost a year, I suggested that they consider doing individual work on some of the issues we had identified. Joan stated that she did not feel a need for individual or group therapy. Although Marilyn did not like the idea of participating in individual or group therapy if Joan did not, she acknowledged that group therapy would probably be helpful. She agreed to explore group treatment while continuing with the couple therapy. This was a big step toward differentiation for both of them. It was hard for Marilyn to tolerate feeling like the "sick one"; however, she was now able to use me as a selfobject, which seemed to provide her with the ego strength necessary for the pursuit of group treatment.

TREATMENT CONSIDERATIONS

Basic Requirements

When working with lesbian batterers, it is essential that the analyst/therapist be knowledgeable about lesbian issues and practice lesbian/gay affirmative treatment. From such a perspective, homosexuality and a lesbian lifestyle are healthy and normal cultural variations. As stated by Istar (1996), to provide effective treatment for lesbian batterers, clinicians "must recognize the various systems that are interconnected, including the family of origin, the family of choice, the extended friendship network, and the lesbian community context that has birthed and nurtured an environment in which lesbian couples can create families" (p. 96). The analyst/therapist must also be knowledgeable about lesbian identity development and the impact of homophobia and heterosexism on lesbians. When working with lesbians of color, the impact of racism and the ways in which racism can compound experiences of homophobia and heterosexism should be considered. Yet another important area for examination is the assessment of drug and alcohol abuse.[5]

Gender-Related Dynamics of Merger

Although a continuum of merger-differentiation is thought to exist in all relationships, with many cultural variations in what are considered to be healthy levels of closeness and distance, rigidified rather than fluid states of merger can create conflict. Such rigidity is also a common by-product of the cycle of violence. Because lesbian relationships consist of two women, there are specific gender-related dynamics regarding merger that must be taken into consideration. For example, in contrast to boys, a girl's preoedipal experience of being mothered by a woman leads to " . . . a relational complexity in feminine self-definition and personality which is not characteristic of masculine self-definition or personality . . . Girls come to experience themselves as less separate than boys, [and] as having more permeable ego boundaries" (Chodorow, 1978, p. 93). Accordingly, women typically have a greater capacity for identification with others (Burch, 1986). Although this capacity can intensify intimate relating between women, both psychically and physically, it also increases the possibility of unhealthy levels of intrapsychic merger (Elise, 1986; O'Conner & Ryan, 1993). A propensity toward rigid states of merger may be further exacerbated by the lesbian community, which tends to become a closed system because of its small size and minority status (Coleman, 1994). Thus, when working with lesbians, analyst/therapists must be cognizant of the complexities regarding normative versus pathological states of merger in their intimate relationships.

Lesbian-Specific Aspects

As previously mentioned, internalized homophobia, heterosexism, and misogyny can lead to feelings of shame, powerlessness, and self-hatred, which may then be projected onto the battered partner. Through projection, the batterer is able to rid herself of unbearable affect and intolerable shame states. This defense is readily identifiable in the batterer's devaluation, contempt, and shaming of the battered partner. Treatment providers should also be aware of forms of emotional abuse specific to lesbian battering, which include (1) revealing or threatening to reveal the partner's sexual orientation (for example, to family, at work, or in conjunction with a custody battle); (2) homophobic insults; and (3) threats of heterosexist responses by helping professionals (e.g., intimidating one's partner to stop her from calling the police or others by telling her that they will not believe her or will not help her because she is a "dyke").

Often lesbians present for domestic violence treatment as a couple, and only after an initial assessment does it become clear that there is abuse in the relationship (as in the case of Marilyn and Joan, example B). Frequently, clinicians feel a great deal of internal and external pressure, due to safety concerns and the politics of domestic violence treatment, to recommend separate services and refuse to provide couple therapy. However, sometimes such a rigid stance can backfire and result in clients discontinuing treatment or seeking therapy from someone lacking knowledge about lesbian battering (Istar, 1996; Margolies & Leeder, 1995). Although couple therapy can be dangerous in some situations of domestic violence, it can also be a viable and effective treatment modality (Balcom, 1991). In considering couple therapy as a treatment option, it is essential that the clinician do a careful assessment of the violence and the risks of providing couple therapy. Balcom suggested that in addition to a "no violence" contract, couples in which shaming behaviors are prominent should also agree to a "no shaming" contract. Although it is likely that these contracts will be broken, to some degree, over the course of treatment, such agreements can foster an increased effort toward impulse control.

Although identifying the batterer in a lesbian relationship is often clear, sometimes determining the nature of the abuse and who is battering whom can be difficult. In contrast to heterosexual relationships, there is frequently minimal difference in strength or size between partners. Even where size differences exist, the batterer may be the smaller of the two women; and, due to their experience of feeling victimized, batterers may present as though they are the battered partner. A further complication is that battered lesbians may use violence in self-defense, sometimes even initiating violence in anticipation of abuse. I have done assessments where initially the battered partner described herself as the abuser because she had used violence in self-defense and, as is common in the cycle of violence, she had internalized the batterer's blaming accusations. In treatment it is essential that women who batter are helped to understand their partners' self-defensive use of violence, and it is imperative that they begin to recognize how their early experiences of trauma and maladaptive defenses can result in their *experience* of themselves as victimized by their partners.

Determining which partner is the batterer will generally become clear after a careful process of assessing the cycle of violence, including dynamics of power, control, and fear. As noted by Istar (1996), often "witnessing the partners' interactions will enable the therapist to have the clearest picture of the relationship" (p. 104). Margolies and Leeder (1995) have observed that batterers will often report feeling high, due to the adrenaline-type rush of their rage, whereas the battered partner will be aware of feeling only fear or the sympathetic arousal of a fight-or-flight response. The addictive quality of rage and the enhanced feeling of power that accompanies it must also be addressed when working with batterers. Similarly, pathological vindictiveness has an addictive quality that must be confronted and addressed in order for the early underlying experiences to be worked through.

Treatment Modalities

In terms of treatment modalities, group therapy can be extremely useful. The group creates an environment of support and confrontation wherein batterers can learn new cognitive and behavioral strategies for managing their abusive impulses. Not only is the isolation common in battering eliminated, but new norms for recognizing and expressing emotions are established (Margolies & Leeder, 1995). However, for patients (non-court ordered) who refuse to attend group therapy (as in the case of Karen), many of the exercises used in group treatment can be adapted for individual work. In addition to time-outs and power and control logs, one of the most useful exercises I have used is the Iceberg Exercise. In actual practice I often refer to this as the Volcano Exercise,[6] since the image of a volcano more accurately captures the explosive rage of batterers. The Iceberg Exercise is used to help patients identify the emotions underlying their anger (Fogelman, 1996). The visible tip of the iceberg is the expressed or "visible" anger. Beneath the surface are the underlying and hidden feelings. The diagram of an iceberg is drawn, with anger and its synonyms written in the tip (e.g., rage). A line is drawn to separate the visible emotions in the tip of the iceberg from those "hidden" underneath the water line. The patient is then encouraged to identify those feelings underlying her/his anger, such as hurt, fear, powerlessness, helplessness, confusion, vulnerability, shame, etc. These are then written under the waterline. Phrases that capture these feelings–such as "I felt like a fool" or "I felt she deserved it . . . she shouldn't have said that"–are placed to the side of the iceberg under the heading of "thoughts." Thus, patients are helped to separate their thoughts from their feelings. This step also helps them learn to identify and exert more control over the negative self-talk that frequently escalates batterers' aggression.

Need for Individual Treatment

Although group therapy is an important treatment modality, it is typically not sufficient to create significant changes in personality. In many situations women will stop their physical violence but continue to be controlling and emotionally abusive. In some cases, analytic couple therapy can also be effective. However, in general the effectiveness of couple therapy is increased when combined with either individual or group therapy. In my opinion, the optimal treatment is group therapy combined with long-term psychoanalytic psychotherapy or psychoanalysis.[7] Moreover, individual treatment can most closely approximate early attachment relationships and allow a reworking of developmental failures. As expressed by Bromberg (2001),

> In a growth-facilitating treatment, there is an increased ability to surrender the safety afforded by dissociation and a simultaneous increase in the capacity to bear and process internal conflict. A patient becomes more able, mentally, to play with and creatively struggle with experience that before could only be enacted in the interpersonal field. (p. 389)

Through the secure base provided by the analyst/therapist's consistent presence and relatedness, analytic treatment creates an opportunity for the batterer to construct new working models of attachment. As described by Schore (1997), in treatment the "non-verbal transference-countertransference interactions that take place at preconscious-unconscious levels represent right hemisphere to right hemisphere communications of fast-acting, automatic, regulated, and unregulated emotional states between patient and therapist" (p. 43). He proposed that these nonverbal interactions can create changes in the orbitofrontal cortex, which mediates empathy and the ability to reflect on the emotional states of self and others. In other words, analyzing the patient's split-off, unmetabolized aspects of experience, which are enacted in the transference-countertransference, can create structural change. Of central importance is the identification and confrontation of the individual's defenses against shame and the shame states underlying her/his abusive behavior.

Specific Aspects of Treatment

Reworking Shame

Typically, batterers are only aware of their rage, and much of the therapeutic work entails helping them to recognize their underlying shame and their tendency to project disavowed aspects of themselves onto their partners. As suggested by Schore (1997), for patients with borderline and narcissistic disorders "visual and auditory cues that were perceived during early self-disorganizing episodes of shame-humiliation" are particularly salient and tend to be reactivated in the transference (p. 46). In my experience, the most powerful reworking of early shame experiences occurs in those instances of misattunement and shame in the treatment relationship. By bringing these implicit memories (Siegel, 1999) into conscious awareness through the repeated experiences of misattunement and dysregulation in long-term treatment, there is an opportunity for the repair and regulation of states that were previously intolerable and disorganizing. Similarly, in cases of pathological vindictiveness, the treatment relationship furnishes an opportunity for the expression of hurt and vengeful rage toward the analyst/therapist–though, "with no vindication, but with the in-built [*sic*] guarantee of no analytic counterattack" (Feiner, 1995, p. 391).

Fostering State Regulation

Batterers are particularly prone to feeling shamed, and interpretations regarding their vulnerabilities and the dynamics underlying their abusiveness are likely to provoke shame and shame-rage reactions. Because state regulation underlies affect regulation, a focus on state regulation is often an essential first step in addressing dysregulation and maladaptive defenses (Lillas, 2000). As argued by Lillas, there are times in treatment when one must shift from an interpretive stance to methods that enhance regulatory functioning. By tracking a patient's physiological state shifts (i.e., muscle tension, gaze, tone of voice), one can monitor the patient's level of arousal and, when appropriate, shift from exploration and interpretation to active facilitation of calm, alert processing (Lillas, 2000). This mutual regulation, when repeated, promotes the development of self-regulation and an observing ego, making it possible for patients to identify when they are experiencing shame and tolerate the investigation of shameful affects. In addition, the individual's ability to reflect on the ways in which she/he rationalizes, minimizes, and blames others for her/his abusive behavior increases. The analyst/therapist's ability, "initially at a nonverbal level, to detect, recognize, monitor, and self-regulate the countertransferential stressful alterations in [the patient's] bodily state that are evoked by the patient's transferential communication" (Schore, 1997, p. 49) is an essential component of such treatment.

Creating a Holding Environment

When treating batterers with borderline personality organization, "attunement and responsiveness offer a holding environment (Winnicott, 1965) that is especially important with the fluctuating rage, anxiety, and panic of borderlines" (Sable, 1997, p. 176). Attuned and responsive holding is also a key element in the treatment of batterers with narcissistic personality organization, as they are extremely sensitive and prone to narcissistic wounding and rage reactions. Such adaptiveness on the part of the analyst/therapist allows for mutual influence and the development of a positive reciprocal regulatory system that enhances the patient's self-regulatory system (Silverman, 1998), leading to the internalization of a good object relationship. Furthermore, these experiences enhance the patient's capacity for affective relating, thus enabling her/him to "experience, endure, and regulate affect within a self structure that contains as few disassociated elements as possible" (Ellman & Monk, 1997, p. 85).

Reenacting Encapsulated Traumas

Because early attachment relationships serve as a prototype for intimate adult relationships and are reenacted in the therapeutic dyad, transference-countertransference enactments provide access to early encapsulated traumas and allow for the examination of maladaptive patterns and defenses. As illustrated in my work with Karen (clinical example A), such enactments can be used to (1) understand the terror and rage that accompany separations; (2) make connections between current patterns and the unconscious sequelae of developmental failures; and (3) recognize the alienating effects of tantrums and abusive behavior. In addition to analyzing the affects and behaviors accompanying separations, for batterers with a borderline disorder it is also important to address their ambivalence around connections and the push-pull dance that often ensues. Although the batterer longs for closeness and security within the treatment and within her/his relationship, this longing often leads to unbearable fear and anxiety. In response she/he may pull away and shut down or become critical, hostile, and demeaning. This pattern must be actively confronted and interpreted, illuminating its cycle in both the patient's external relationships and in the treatment relationship.

In order to provide a confrontive, yet nonretaliatory and empathic treatment environment, the analyst/therapist must constantly monitor countertransference issues. This monitoring includes examining and addressing her/his own (1) shame, rage, and capacity for violence; (2) fear of violence and the potential to minimize, deny, or avoid addressing the batterer's abusive behaviors; and (3) internalized homophobia and heterosexism, becoming conscious of the ways in which biases may impinge on the treatment.

CONCLUSION

By integrating personality theory with attachment theory, relevant aspects of state and affect regulation, shame states, and pathological vindictiveness, I have attempted to identify and illuminate variables critical to understanding and treating lesbian batterers. Treating batterers can be both highly rewarding and extraordinarily challenging. The difficulties presented by batterers are extremely complex, and effective treatment requires that the analyst/therapist be intimately familiar with her/his own dynamic issues around violence, attachment, and shame. Working with lesbian batterers also necessitates that the analyst/therapist be knowledgeable about lesbians and the lesbian community, as well as cognizant of her/his own homophobia and heterosexism.

Goals of batterer treatment include (1) improving state and affect regulation; (2) reintegrating unconscious, disavaowed affects and experiences; (3) reducing the use of primitive defenses such as splitting and projective identification; (4) decreasing pathological shame and vindictiveness; (5) developing impulse control and an observing ego; and (6) increasing capacity for empathy. In conjunction with progress in these areas, the batterer is able to move from part-object relating to experiencing others as separate, whole objects. A key component of this developmental movement is the analyst/therapist's ability to resonate empathically with the batterer's affective states and consistently reflect and synthesize her/his experiences, thereby providing the experiential basis that facilitates the patient's readiness for interpretations and enables her/him to tolerate her/his own emotional experiences (Ellman & Monk, 1997, p. 86). In the intimate exchange between patient and analyst/therapist, previously intolerable, encapsulated experiences can be grieved, metabolized, and integrated. Through this transformative process, psychic space and energy become available for new growth–out of and alongside the mourned ruins of the old (Smith, 1999)–providing the basis for nonabusive, even healthy, relationships.

NOTES

1. The ideological denial, denigration, and stigmatization of any non-heterosexual form of identity, relationship, behavior, or community (Herek, 1993, p. 89).

2. Although I refer to various diagnostic categories as a framework for some of the personality dynamics involved in the perpetration of violence, in no way do I mean to imply that an individual's essence can be reduced to a diagnostic label, or that treatment should be exclusively based on that label. Nor am I suggesting that all individuals who suffer from personality disorders are batterers, or that all batterers have personality disorders. Furthermore, in no way am I suggesting that lesbians have higher levels of pathology than other individuals.

3. Dissmell is the innate, human smell response to bad odors that originated as a protective response to poisonous, noxious substances. This response has since evolved into an affect that communicates feelings of dislike and rejection. It is characterized by a raised upper lip and facial retraction from something experienced as foul (Kaufman & Raphael, 1996, pp. 22-23).

4. The analysis of enactments distinguishes psychoanalytic treatment from other forms of therapy. As described by Maroda (1999), "enactment is an affectively driven repetition of converging emotional scenarios from the patient's and the analyst's lives. It is not merely an affectively-driven set of behaviors, it is necessarily a repetition of past events that have been buried in the unconscious due to associated unmanageable or unwanted emotion" (p. 124). The analyst's awareness and examination of her/his countertransference, such that it can be used in the service of treatment rather than dominating treatment, is essential to the constructive use of enactments.

5. Often, particularly in smaller cities, there are few social outlets available for lesbians, and bars become a common arena for socialization. Such socializing, in conjunction with the pressures of being a minority in society, has contributed to high rates of alcoholism in the lesbian community.

6. This name was suggested by Karen.

7. Unfortunately, lack of available resources (i.e., funding, personnel, time) currently makes providing such intensive services untenable in many situations.

REFERENCES

Ainsworth, M. D. S., Blehar, M. C., Waters, E., & Wall, S. (1978). *Patterns of attachment: A psychological study of the strange situation.* Hillsdale, NJ: Erlbaum.

Balcom, D. (1991). Shame and violence: Considerations in couples' treatment. *Journal of Independent Social Work, 5*(3-4), 165-181.

Barnett, O. W., & Hamberger, L. K. (1992). The assessment of maritally violent men on the California Psychological Inventory. *Violence and Victims, 7,* 15-28.

Bollas, C. (1992). *Being a character: Psychoanalysis and self experience.* New York: Hill and Wang.

Bollas, C. (2000). *Hysteria.* New York: Routledge Press.

Bowlby, J. (1973). *Attachment and loss: Vol. 2 Separation: Anxiety and anger.* New York: Basic Books.

Bowlby, J. (1984). Violence in the family as a disorder of the attachment and caregiving systems. *The American Journal of Psychoanalysis, 44*(1), 9-26.

Bowlby, J. (1988). *A secure base: Parent-child attachment and healthy human development.* New York: Basic Books.

Bromberg, P. M. (2001). The gorilla did it: Some thoughts on dissociation, the real and the really real. *Psychoanalytic Dialogues, 11*(3), 385-404.

Broucek, F. J. (1982). Shame and its relationship to early narcissistic developments. *International Journal of Psycho-Analysis, 63,* 369-378.

Broucek, F. J. (1997). Shame: Early developmental issues. In M. Lansky & A. P. Morrison (Eds.), *The widening scope of shame* (pp. 41-62). Hillsdale, NJ: Analytic Press.

Brown, L. J. (1990). Borderline personality organization and the transition to the depressive position. *Journal of the American Academy of Psychoanalysis, 18*(3), 505-511.

Bryant, A. S., & Demian, R. (1994). Relationship characteristics of American gay and lesbian couples: Findings from a national survey. *Journal of Gay and Lesbian Social Services, 1,* 101-117.

Burch, B. (1986). Psychotherapy and the dynamics of merger in lesbian couples. In T. S. Stein & C. J. Cohen (Eds.), *Contemporary perspectives on psychotherapy with lesbians and gay men* (pp. 57-71). New York: Plenum Medical Book.

Burke, L. K., & Follingstad, E. R. (1999). Violence in lesbian and gay relationships: Theory, prevalence, and correlational factors. *Clinical Psychology Review, 5,* 487-512.

Chodorow, N. (1978). *The reproduction of mothering: Psychoanalysis and the sociology of gender.* Berkeley, CA: University of California Press.

Coleman, V. E. (1991). Violence in lesbian couples: A between groups comparison. (Doctoral dissertation, California School of Professional Psychology–Los Angeles, 1990). *Dissertation Abstracts International, 51,* 5634B.

Coleman, V. E. (1994). Lesbian battering: The relationship between personality and the perpetration of violence. *Violence and Victims, 9*(2), 139-152.

Daniels, M. (1969). Pathological vindictiveness and the vindictive character. *Psychoanalytic Review, 56*(2), 169-196.

Dutton, D. G. (1995). *The batterer: A psychological profile.* New York: Basic Books.

Dutton, D. G. (1995b). *The domestic abuse of women.* UBC Press: Vancouver.

Dutton, D. G. (1998). *The abusive personality: Violence and control in intimate relationships.* New York: Guilford Press.

Dutton, D. G., van Ginkel, C., & Landolt, M. A. (1996). Jealousy, intimate abusiveness, and intrusiveness. *Journal of Family Violence, 11*(4), 411-423.

Dutton, D. G., van Ginkel, C, & Starzomski, A. (1995). The role of shame and guilt in the intergenerational transmission of abusiveness. *Violence and Victims, 10*(2), 121-131.

Elise, D. (1986). Lesbian couples: The implications of sex differences in separation and individuation. *Psychotherapy, 23,* 305-310.

Elliott, P. (1996). Shattering illusions: Same-sex domestic violence. In C. M. Renzetti & C. H. Miley (Eds.), *Violence in gay and lesbian domestic partnerships* (pp. 1-8). Binghamton, NY: The Haworth Press, Inc.

Ellman, S., & Monk, C. (1997). The significance of the first few months of life for self-regulation: A reply to Schore. In M. Moskowitz, C. Monk, C. Kaye, & S. Ellman (Eds.), *The neurobiological and developmental basis for psychotherapeutic intervention* (pp. 74-89). Northvale, NJ: Jason Aronson Inc.

Fairbairn, W. R. (1952). *Psychoanalytic studies of the personality.* London: Tavistock/ Routledge Press.

Feiner, A. H. (1995). Laughter among the pear trees: Vengeance, vindictiveness, and vindication. *Contemporary Psychoanalysis, 31*(3), 381-397.

Fogelman, J. (1996). *Stop the violence: An introductory treatment program for gay male batterers.* Unpublished facilitators' Manual.

Fonagy, P., Leigh, T., Steele, M., Kennedy, R., Mattoon, G., & Gerber, A. (1996). The relation of attachment status, psychiatric classification, and response to psychotherapy. *Journal of Consulting and Clinical Psychology, 64*(1), 22-31.

Freed, A. O. (1984). Differentiating between borderline and narcissistic personalities. *Social Casework, 65,* 395-404.

Gardner, R. (1989). Method of conflict resolution and characteristics of abuse and victimization in heterosexual, lesbian, and gay male couples (Doctoral dissertation, University of Georgia, 1988). *Dissertation Abstracts International, 50,* 746B.

Goldberg, C. (1991). *Understanding shame*. Northvale, NJ: Jason Aronson Inc.

Goldstein, E. G. (1990). *Borderline disorders: Clinical models and techniques*. New York: Guilford Press.

Gondolf, E. (1999). MCMI-III results for batterer program participants in four cities: Less "pathological" than expected. *Journal of Family Violence, 14*(1) 1-17.

Grotstein, J. S. (1987). The borderline as a disorder of self-regulation. In J. S. Grotstein, J. Lang, & M. Solomon (Eds.), *The borderline patient: Emerging concepts in diagnosis* (pp. 347-383). London: Analytic Press.

Hamberger, L. K., & Hastings, J. E. (1986). Personality correlates of men who abuse their partners: A cross-validation study. *Journal of Family Violence, 1*, 323-341.

Hamberger, L. K., & Hastings, J. E. (1991). Personality correlates of men who batter and nonviolent men: Some continuities and discontinuities. *Journal of Family Violence, 6*, 131-148.

Hart, B. (1986). Lesbian battering: An examination. In K. Lobel (Ed.), *Naming the violence: Speaking out about lesbian battering* (pp. 173-189). Seattle, WA: Seal Press.

Heiserman, A., & Cook, H. (1998). Narcissism, affect, and gender: An empirical examination of Kernberg's and Kohut's theories of narcissism. *Psychoanalytic Psychology, 15*(1), 74-92.

Herek, G. M. (1993). The context of antigay violence: Notes on cultural and psychological heterosexism. In L. D. Garnets & D. C. Kimmel (Eds.), *Psychological perspectives on lesbian and gay male experiences* (pp. 89-108). New York: Columbia University Press.

Hibbard, S. (1992). Narcissism, shame, masochism, and object relations: An exploratory correlational study. *Psychoanalytic Psychology, 9*(4), 489-508.

Hibbard, S. (1994). An empirical study of the differential roles of libidinous and aggressive shame components in normality and pathology. *Psychoanalytic Psychology, 11*(4), 449-474.

Hockenberry, S. L. (1995). Dyadic violence, shame, and narcissism. *Contemporary Psychoanalysis, 31*(2), 301-325.

Istar, A. (1996). Couple assessment: Identifying and intervening in domestic violence in lesbian relationships. In C. Renzetti & C. H. Miley (Eds.), *Violence in gay and lesbian domestic partnerships* (pp. 93-106). New York: Harrington Park Press.

Kaufman, G., & Raphael, L. (1996). *Coming out of shame*. New York: Doubleday.

Kernberg, O. F. (1984). *Severe personality disorders: Psychotherapeutic strategies*. New Haven: Yale University Press.

Klein, M. (1946/1996). Notes on some schizoid mechanisms. *Journal of Psychotherapy Practice and Research, 5*(2), 164-179. Reprinted from *International Journal of Psycho-Analysis, (1946) 27*, 99-110.

Kohut, H. (1972). Thoughts on narcissism and narcissistic rage. *Psycho-analytic Study of the Child, 27*, 360-400.

Krestan, J., & Bepko, C. (1980). The problem of fusion in the lesbian relationship. *Family Process, 19*, 277-289.

Lachmann, F. M., & Beebe, B. (1997). The contribution of self- and mutual regulation to therapeutic action: A case illustration. In M. Moskowitz, C. Monk, C. Kaye, & S. Ellman (Eds.), *The neurobiological and developmental basis for psychotherapeutic intervention* (pp. 91-122). Northvale, NJ: Jason Aronson Inc.

Leeder, E. (1988). Enmeshed in pain: Counseling the lesbian battering couple. *Women & Therapy*, 7, 81-99.

Leisring, P. A., Dowd, L., & Rosenbaum, A. (2002). Treatment of partner aggressive women. *Journal of Aggression, Maltreatment, & Trauma*, 7(1/2), 257-277.

Lewis, H. B. (1987). Shame and the narcissistic personality. In D. L. Nathanson (Ed.), *The many faces of shame* (pp. 93-132). New York: The Guilford Press.

Lie, G., Schillit, R., Bush, R., Montague, M., & Reyes, L. (1991). Lesbians in currently aggressive relationships: How frequently do they report aggressive past relationships? *Violence & Victims*, 6(2), 121-135.

Lillas, C. (2000). Applying psychoneurobiological principles to psychoanalysis. *Psychologist Psychoanalyst*, 20(3), 21-23.

"Lisa." (1986). Once hitting starts. In K. Lobel (Ed.), *Naming the violence: Speaking out about lesbian battering* (pp. 37-40). Seattle, WA: Seal Press.

Lobel, K. (Ed.). (1986). *Naming the violence: Speaking out about lesbian battering.* Seattle, WA: Seal Press.

Mahler, M., Pine, F., & Bergman, A. (1975). *The psychological birth of the human infant: Symbiosis and individuation.* New York: Basic Books.

Main, M., Kaplan, N., & Cassidy, J. (1985). Security in infancy, childhood, and adulthood: A move to the level of representation. In I. Bretherton, & E. Waters (Eds.), *Growing points of attachment theory and research: Monographs of the society for research in child development*, 50(1-2), serial (209), 66-104.

Margolies, L., & Leeder, E. (1995). Violence at the door: Treatment of lesbian batterers. *Violence Against Women*, 1(2), 139-157.

Maroda, K. J. (1999). *Seduction, surrender and transformation: Emotional engagement in the analytic process.* Hillsdale, NJ: Analytic Press.

Masterson, J. F. (1981). *The narcissistic and borderline disorders.* New York: Brunner/Mazel.

McWilliams, N. (1994). *Psychoanalytic diagnosis: Understanding personality structure in the clinical process.* New York: Guilford Press.

Mikulincer, M., Orbach, I., & Iavnieli, D. (1998). Adult attachment style and affect regulation: Strategic variations in subjective self-other similarity. *Journal of Personality and Social Psychology*, 75(2), 436-448.

Morrison, A. (1999). Shame, on either side of defense. *Contemporary Psychoanalysis*, 35(1), 91-105.

Nathanson, D. L. (1987). A timetable for shame. In D. L. Nathanson (Ed.), *The many faces of shame* (pp. 1-63). New York: Guilford Press.

Neisen, J. H. (1993). Healing from cultural victimization: Recovery from shame due to heterosexism. *Journal of Gay and Lesbian Psychotherapy*, 2(1), 49-63.

O'Conner, N., & Ryan, J. (1993). *Wild desires and mistaken identities: Lesbianism and psychoanalysis.* Camden Town, London: Virago Press.

Pistole, M. C. (1995). Adult attachment style and narcissistic vulnerability. *Psychoanalytic Psychology*, 12(1), 115-126.

Renzetti, C. M. (1988). Violence in lesbian relationships: A preliminary analysis of causal factors. *Journal of Interpersonal Violence*, 3, 381-399.

Renzetti, C. M. (1992). *Violent betrayal: Partner abuse in lesbian relationships.* Newbury Park, CA: Sage Publications.

Rosen, I. (1991). Self-esteem as a factor in social and domestic violence. *British Journal of Psychiatry, 158*, 18-23.

Sable, P. (1997). Attachment, detachment and borderline personality disorder. *Psychotherapy, 34*(2), 171-181.

Saunders, D. G. (2000). Feminist, cognitive, and behavioral group interventions for men who batter: An overview of rationale and methods. In D. B. Wexler (Ed.), *Domestic violence 2000: An integrated skills program for men* (pp. 21-32). New York: W. W. Norton.

Schilit, R., & Lie, G. (1990). Substance use as a correlate of violence in intimate lesbian relationships. *Journal of Homosexuality, 19*, 51-65.

Schore, A. N. (1994). *Affect regulation and the origin of the self: The neurobiology of emotional development*. Hillsdale, NJ: Erlbaum.

Schore, A. N. (1997). Interdisciplinary developmental research as a source of clinical models. In M. Moskowitz, C. Monk, C. Kaye, & S. Ellman (Eds.), *The neurobiological and developmental basis for psychotherapeutic intervention* (pp. 1-72). Northvale, NJ: Jason Aronson, Inc.

Schulte, H. M., Hall, M. J., & Crosby, R. (1994). Violence in patients with narcissistic personality pathology: Observations of a clinical series. *American Journal of Psychotherapy, 48*(4), 610-623.

Searles, H. (1965). The psychodynamics of vengefulness (1956). In H. Searles (Ed.), *Collected papers on schizophrenia and related subjects* (pp. 188-191). New York: International Universities Press.

Siegel, D. J. (1999). *The developing mind: Toward a neurobiology of interpersonal experience*. New York: Guilford Press.

Silverman, D. K. (1998). The tie that binds: Affect regulation, attachment, and psychoanalysis. *Psychoanalytic Psychology, 15*(2), 187-212.

Smith, N. A. (1999). From oedipus to orpha: Revisiting ferenczi and severn's landmark case. *American Journal of Psychoanalysis, 59*(4), 345-366.

Sonkin, D. J. (1995). *The counselor's guide to learning to live without violence*. Volcano, CA: Volcano Press.

Sonkin, D. J., & Durphy, M. (1989). (Rev. Ed.). *Learning to live without violence: A handbook for men*. Volcano, CA: Volcano Press.

Sonkin, D., & Dutton, D. G. (2002). Treating assaultive men from an attachment perspective. *Journal of Aggression, Maltreatment, & Trauma, 7*(1/2), 105-133.

Steiner, J. (1996). Revenge and resentment in the "oedipus situation." *International Journal of Psycho-Analysis, 77*, 433-443.

Tweed, R., & Dutton, D. (1998). A comparison of impulsive and instrumental subgroups of batterers. *Violence and Victims, 13*(3), 217-230.

van der Kolk, B. A. (1996). The complexity of adaptation to trauma: Self-regulation, stimulus discrimination, and characterological development. In B. A. van der Kolk, A. C. McFarlane, & L. Weisaeth (Eds.), *Traumatic stress: The effects of overwhelming experience on mind, body, and society* (pp. 182-213). New York: Guilford Press.

Waldner-Haugrud, L. D., Gratch, L. V., & Magruder, B. (1997). Victimization and perpetration rates of violence in gay and lesbian relationships: Gender issues explored. *Violence and Victims, 12*(2), 173-184.

Walker, L. (1979). *The battered woman*. New York: Harper and Row.

Wallace, B., & Nosko, A. (1993). Working with shame in the group treatment of male batterers. *International Group of Psychotherapy, 43*(1), 45-61.

Wang, S. (1997). Traumatic stress and attachment. *Acta Physiologica Scandinavica, 640*, 164-169.

Wastell, C. A. (1992). Self psychology and the etiology of borderline personality disorder. *Psychotherapy, 29*, 225-233.

Winnicott, D. W. (1971). *Playing and reality.* London: Tavistock.

Wise, A. J., & Bowman, S. L. (1997). Comparison of beginning counselors' responses to lesbian vs. heterosexual partner abuse. *Violence and Victims, 12*(2), 127-135.

Wolf, E. S. (1988). *Treating the self: Elements of clinical self psychology.* New York: Guilford Press.

Beit Noam:
Residential Program for Violent Men

Ophra Keynan
Hannah Rosenberg
Beni Beili
Michal Nir
Shlomit Levin
Ariel Mor
Ibrahim Agabaria
Avi Tefelin

SUMMARY. The initiative of founding the Noam Association, an Israeli association for the prevention of domestic abuse, and Beit Noam, a live-in intervention program for abusive men, was based on the objective of combating the core of the phenomena of intimate violence. The main goals of treating the male batterers are: (1) To allow battered women and their children to remain in their homes and in their natural environment; (2) To treat, re-socialize and teach self-controlling skills and normative behavior to the male batterers; and (3) To stop the pattern of intimate violence from being transferred across generations. This article describes the therapy provided to batterers at Beit Noam, including two case studies, and the results of an assessment report. *[Article copies available for a fee from The Haworth Document Delivery Service: 1-800-HAWORTH. E-mail address: <docdelivery@haworthpress.com> Website: <http://www.HaworthPress.com> © 2003 by The Haworth Press, Inc. All rights reserved.]*

Address correspondence to: Hannah Rosenberg (E-mail: hannahr@netvision.net.il).

[Haworth co-indexing entry note]: "Beit Noam: Residential Program for Violent Men." Keynan, Ophra et al. Co-published simultaneously in *Journal of Aggression, Maltreatment & Trauma* (The Haworth Maltreatment & Trauma Press, an imprint of The Haworth Press, Inc.) Vol. 7, No. 1/2 (#13/14), 2003, pp. 207-236; and: *Intimate Violence: Contemporary Treatment Innovations* (ed: Donald Dutton, and Daniel J. Sonkin) The Haworth Maltreatment & Trauma Press, an imprint of The Haworth Press, Inc., 2003, pp. 207-236. Single or multiple copies of this article are available for a fee from The Haworth Document Delivery Service [1-800-HAWORTH, 9:00 a.m. - 5:00 p.m. (EST). E-mail address: docdelivery@haworthpress.com].

http://www.haworthpress.com/store/product.asp?sku=J146
© 2003 by The Haworth Press, Inc. All rights reserved.
10.1300J146v07n01_09

KEYWORDS. Beit Noam, battered women, residential project, live-in project, group therapy, individual therapy, integrative therapy

BEIT NOAM: BACKGROUND AND RATIONALE

Background

The Noam Association for the Prevention of Domestic Abuse was founded in 1986 in Herzlia, Israel with the aim of initiating, planning, operating, and supervising programs for the prevention of violence in families where one or both partners exert violent physical and/or verbal force towards other family members, including spouses and children. Because women's organizations and government welfare institutions focus on treating battered women, the association decided to concentrate on the perpetrators, whose behavior is the root of the problem. Accordingly, its programs are designed to stop the men's violence so that the women who experience violence in Israel and their children can remain in their homes and natural environment.

In March 1991, the Domestic Violence Act was passed, an act that allows the courts to ban a man who behaves violently toward his spouse and children from his home. This law holds the key to changing the wrongs suffered by women and their children. The period of the violent man's absence from the home can be used for therapy, education, and acquisition of acceptable behavior patterns.

On the basis of this law, the Noam Association for the Prevention of Domestic Abuse introduced the idea of establishing Beit Noam–A New Direction for Violent Men, a program designed as an integrative intervention and educational framework for violent men who are banned by law from their homes and who express a willingness to change their violent behavior patterns. Literally translated, Beit means "home" and Noam means "pleasant"; the name represents the idea to let the male residents be in friendly and accepting surroundings. The establishment of Beit Noam was made possible in 1997, with the cooperation and funding of the Ministry of Labor and Social Affairs and the National Insurance Institute.

Beit Noam was established on the basis of the following basic assumptions:

1. It is important to treat the root of the domestic violence problem, which is the behavior of the violent man.

2. It is important to ban the assailant from his home and offer the victims–his wife and children–a chance to live without terror and fear.
3. It is essential to stop the intergenerational transmission of domestic violence.
4. There is a good chance of eliminating violent behavior among treatable violent men through their residence in an open housing setting that offers an integrated, intensive framework for intervention and education with the support of the law.

Objectives and special features of the program at Beit Noam include:

1. To stop violence and terror toward spouses and children;
2. To cut off the intergenerational cycle of violence transmitted from one generation to the next;
3. To enable the wives and children to remain in their homes.

The Therapeutic Rationale

Treatment at Beit Noam focuses on the fact that abusive behavior is the man's problem. It does not relate to abusive behavior as a symptom of the dynamics of relationships. The man alone is responsible for the effects of his actions. Beit Noam relates to violent men as individuals who have behavioral, cognitive, and emotional problems. The intervention model is, therefore, integrative and intensive. By dealing with the men's difficulties in these three areas, Beit Noam is able to comprehensively contend with the problem. During the course of the program, the male perpetrator undergoes intervention on three levels: the group level, where he experiences a number of different topics; the individual level, where he increases his ability to internalize the learned topics; and the interpersonal level.

Beit Noam's intervention rationale is based on three elements. First, it creates a framework that simulates a home atmosphere. The Beit Noam lifestyle creates a restorative atmosphere that at the same time educates and duplicates normal home life. The residents go to work every morning and return in the evening. Beit Noam enables the men to function in a communal household with a clear division of tasks and to experience relationships as a process. The men are responsible for the maintenance of the center and contribute money to its operation. Second, it creates an integrated intervention model. The intervention process at Beit Noam clearly conveys the following messages to the men:

(1) recognition of gender differences that do not legitimize superiority of either gender; (2) violent behavior is the sole responsibility of the man; (3) violence of any type is forbidden in all circumstances; and (4) each spouse constitutes an independent entity. Finally, Beit Noam focuses attention on the men rather than on their victims. The men participate every evening in diverse intervention workshops, and attend one-on-one intervention sessions.

The Target Population of Beit Noam

Beit Noam is intended for men of any age, socioeconomic status, level of education, and ethnic group who engage in physical, verbal, sexual, and/or psychological violence towards their partner in life, wife, separated wife, or ex-wife. The program does not treat substance abusers or the mentally ill. Men who have been diagnosed for severe personality disorders and criminals who engage in other kinds of crime are allowed to attend on the basis of a comprehensive diagnosis confirming their suitability for the Beit Noam program.

Referrals to Beit Noam

Who Makes Referrals?

Beit Noam is a basic, essential element in the intervention process for abusive men, and serves as part of the community's sequence of therapeutic frameworks. In the first stage, the law enforcement agencies and community therapy frameworks deal with violent men. Depending on need and the degree of danger they pose, men are referred to Beit Noam, which serves as a four-month intensive intervention program. At the end of this period, the men return to intervention follow-up in the community. The achievement and maintenance of Beit Noam's intervention success requires the cooperation of all relevant organizations and agencies in the community; fortunately, such cooperation does exist.

Men are referred to Beit Noam by several sources, including the therapeutic community in the area of the men's residence (e.g., probation officers, welfare workers, centers for the treatment and prevention of domestic violence, and mental health clinics); the district, magistrate and family courts, which are able to bar violent men from their homes for a given period of time; the legal assistance unit that works with the family court; the district attorney's office or the police; various voluntary organizations and national hotlines run by the Ministry of Labor and Social Affairs; the abusive man's extended family; and self-referrals.

The Referral Process

After the referring agencies approach Beit Noam by telephone, they are asked to complete a referral form that includes the history of family violence, a description of the most violent incidents, an estimation of the degree to which the man is dangerous, and an evaluation of the degree to which the man is willing to receive treatment. If the basic details correspond to Beit Noam's criteria for acceptance (i.e., the man must not be addicted to chemical products and cannot be suffering from a mental illness), the man is immediately asked to come for an interview to determine his potential to change. If the man agrees to the terms of residence at Beit Noam, a date is set in accordance with space available.

Upon arrival at Beit Noam, the man undergoes an in-depth interview and signs documents that bind him to observe the rules and regulations of the house. The man also commits himself to pay for the entire period of his stay. The referral and diagnosis process at Beit Noam represent a sort of filter for suitability, ability, and willingness to be part of the intensive homelike framework offered by Beit Noam.

Group Treatment

Beit Noam's primary focus is on group rather than individual intervention because of the emphasis it places on the dynamic that evolves from simulating a home framework, as well as the therapeutic impact of the group. There are a total of six groups that are conducted. One group, the daily group, meets for thirty minutes every evening in order to discuss "here and now" issues, led by the educational coordinator. In addition, five different types of intervention groups are conducted, one every evening, and are obligatory for all residents. The subjects and/or techniques of the groups were chosen for their intervention/educational content based on the special needs of the residents of Beit Noam. The groups include an open group dealing with interpersonal relations among the residents; a cognitive self-control group; a group for the development of self-awareness; a parenting group dealing with child witnesses of violence; and a follow-up support group for the men who completed the four-month residence program. Each of these six groups is described in detail below.

The Daily Group

Every evening, a discussion is held under the leadership of Beit Noam's educational coordinator, or "house supervisor." The discussion opens the intervention evening program at the center. The daily group is mainly a free-flow conversation, lasting thirty minutes. Because the men maintain the house themselves, and for many it is the first time in their lives they have done such work, this often gives rise to conflicts and group tension. The purpose of the daily talk is to provide a setting for sorting out these conflicts and finding alternative ways to resolve them and encouraging dialogue.

This group differs from the intervention groups, which are led by the social workers. Here the emphasis is more educational, and less on intervention. In addition, the group is unique in that it meets daily, reminiscent of the format of a home and a family. Cleaning, dishwashing, and tidying the house are simple, technical activities. For most of the residents, they are new activities, and they are emotionally loaded. For example, in the daily discussion, the men spontaneously bring up their rigid positions about sex roles: "Why should men be cleaning? If they would see me in the neighborhood, they'd call me a woman." In addition to allowing the spontaneous expression of attitudes and opinions, this is also a forum in which the men learn to settle conflicts among themselves, rather than in the violent way familiar to them. For example, one of the men complained to the group that his roommate was inconsiderate, turned the light on late at night, and noisily got ready for bed. He brought this complaint to the group in an accusing voice, in an aggressive, projective tone: "Who are you to bother me? What are you, my wife? You're probably doing this on purpose. I'm warning you . . ." The group members helped the man convey his complaint more calmly. In addition, this man learned from the others' comments how his wife felt when he talked to her in the same way.

Each man at some point brings up a difficulty, claim, or problem, and the other men apply themselves to helping him solve the problem through their own personal examples. In most of the discussions, problems are raised around the upkeep of the house. The men are charged with maintenance and cleaning, and complaints are often raised about some of the residents who avoid this burden and refrain from taking an active part in the housework. The group is responsible for sorting out the difficulties, reflecting their behavior to the evaders and getting them to help the other group members.

For many men in our setting, this is the first opportunity to have someone relate to their behavior. Usually, the behavior patterns that characterized them in their homes also arise here. Men who avoid the cleaning work, men who use verbal violence towards other men while executing tasks, men who use threatening language towards the others, men who tyrannize and dominate the others–all these are expressed in the group, through the daily dialogue.

These group sessions are brief and intensive in frequency because they are held five times per week. The daily continuity is highly significant. The men learn that each of them has a place on both the verbal level, to express himself verbally, and on the group level, to learn to substitute a problematic group role with another.

The contact between the house supervisor and the social worker staff is extremely important. Every evening, after the daily talk with the men, the house supervisor updates the social worker that will lead the group session of the evening on what happened during the daily discussion.

Open Group

The Open Group meets once a week, and is facilitated by a social worker. This group provides the men with an opportunity to learn from the problems and experiences that result from living together at Beit Noam, participating in intervention and learning groups, housekeeping issues, and issues that emerge from sharing close quarters. In essence, the group is a laboratory where the men examine situations that parallel their home lives. The group assumes that Beit Noam is a simulation of family life and the workplace. The group creates a framework that encourages the emotional expression that enhances openness and flexibility in human relations (e.g., a veteran resident complains that a new man is not fulfilling one of the house rules, so the veteran points to the new man's need for compliance).

Cognitive Self-Control Group

The rationale of this group is that violent behavior indicates an absence of self-control, and that self-control is one of the main tools for dealing with violent behavior. This group teaches the men self-control by a cognitive-behavioral method that is geared to achieving behavioral change by changing thinking patterns. In doing so, the men discover that there are several aspects to all situations. They learn the processes of decision making and creating hierarchies of importance. The group is didactic and educational. The men also learn new concepts (e.g., definitions of violence), identify the ingredients of anger, discuss the underlying feelings of anger (e.g., helplessness, guilt, shame), and learn assertive communication (e.g., how to express themselves effectively and how to negotiate while respecting the other).

The Group for Development of Self-Awareness and Insight

A resident at Beit Noam said of the sculpture of a head that he had made, "This is me and my big mouth. With harsh words I insisted on voicing harsh criticism, exerting pressure, and refusing to give in until I got the answer I wanted to hear that would prove I was right. My big mouth that I just had to open every time and with it, to injure and control. Now I understand how violent words can be." Another resident made a clay figure of a tall, broad, muscular man, with a tiny head. The resident, himself a sportsman, picked the figure up so that all the members of the group would look at it. He said, "This is me. This is how I always was. A small head–I didn't think at all, I didn't stop for one moment to think what would happen afterwards, what the consequences of my actions would be. I just used my physical strength. I solved every problem with force. I frightened people and I got what I wanted through violence. This worked for the moment; it made me feel strong. Now I understand that it took a very heavy toll on my relationships, especially with my wife."

These are two examples of things said by men in the self-awareness group in reference to clay sculptures that they made during the session. This group uses projective means to develop the men's self-awareness of their emotions, personal patterns of reaction (emotional and behavioral), attitudes, world view, tendencies, ways of coping with difficulties and problems, different needs within intimate and other relationships, strengths and weaknesses, and all other internal material that does not generally emerge to the level of consciousness. The development of awareness is not a goal in itself, but rather a means to expose the hidden parts, to make them accessible to therapy. The working assumption at Beit Noam is that violent behavior takes place, among other reasons, because of unconscious processes. Transferring these to the conscious level makes it possible to choose another behavior and thus contributes to diminishing the violence. The rationale for using projective means is that they circumvent the individual's defense mechanisms and offer a non-threatening way to deal with the inner self. This constitutes an easier, more pleasant way to expose matters that are embarrassing and threatening to deal with directly. Furthermore, the non-verbal tools also enable free expression among the men who have trouble doing so in words.

No less important is the secondary profit gained through the exposure of the men to new means of expression that provide them with satisfaction and pleasure. They discover abilities and skills that they were not aware they had, thus enriching their world, enhancing their ability to express emotion, and broadening their range of choices. Extensive use is made in the sessions of the plastic arts (paint, plasticine, clay, newspaper cuttings), texts, watching videotapes, music, and games that use photos and drawings. The sessions follow a set structure. At the beginning of every session, the facilitator presents the tasks and means to be used. The first part of the session is devoted to implementation (personal and/or group, depending on the task). The second part is a discussion of the "products." In this part, every participant receives feedback from the others and has an opportunity to talk about his creation or experience.

The facilitator's intervention at this stage is directed toward identifying the themes that emerge and helping incorporate them into a message or an insight that the men can take with them. The facilitator directs the men to observe both the issues that emerge (thus transmitting unconscious material to the conscious) and the patterns of interaction that take place in the process, with constant linkage of all issues that arise to the subject of violence.

Example. In one session, the men were asked to draw their homes. The instructions were deliberately very open, in order to allow the men to relate spontaneously to the significant home for them, in the here and now. Some drew the house where they grew up, some drew the home they had established, and some drew both, emphasizing the comparison between them. Some drew their home as they experienced it in reality, while others drew their fantasy home, the one that they dreamed of. Observing their choices and discussing the reasons for these choices created a new awareness. In studying the drawings, the participants related to their choice of colors, the relationship between inside and outside, the presence or absence of people in the picture, and which members of the family were present and where. The closeness and distance expressed in the painting, the borders of the house (rigid, broken, blurred, or clear), its stability, and anything else that arose from within the picture were considered. Special attention was given to existence or nonexistence of violence in the house: Does violence accompany me all my life or did it begin in the home that I established? Am I capable of removing the violence from the house and building a new home? What enables me to do so?

One resident, Yossi, drew three houses. The first one depicts the house he dreamed of: he is arriving home and his wife and five children await him. The house is warm and there is an aroma of food cooking. When he first got married, he dreamt of such a house. In the second picture, the house is cold. Yossi is standing alone, outside the house. This is the situation he has gotten to: far from his family, alone, not knowing how to create the family he dreamed of. In the third picture, black paint covers the center of the page, so that we see nothing at all of a house. Yossi describes the destruction and his present feelings: Everything is ruined, confused, and chaotic. The future is unknown. Violence has destroyed every good bit.

The members of the group asked Yossi how his future house would look. Yossi turned the page over and returned to the first picture he drew. He stated, "I hope that with the help of therapy I will nevertheless succeed in creating a warm home and that I won't destroy relationships anymore with my violence." For Yossi, who until this point had demonstrated no ability of self-examination, this was a significant achievement. He was able to tell his story through the pictures and see the process he was involved in and the destructive role of violence in his life. Through observing his pictures, he also saw his goal in therapy more clearly.

Parenting Group Dealing with Child Witnesses of Violence

A resident, Avi, recalled an episode of violence against his wife. He grabbed her, pushed her body up against the living room wall, and kicked her in the stomach. As he did so, he threatened her, "I'll tear you apart, you'll regret the day you were born." His five children, ages one through six, sat close together on the living room couch, embraced each other and trembled, praying that the incident would end.

This is one of a countless series of similar incidents, involving one of twelve violent men in a group on child witnesses of violence. This group meets once per week, with the aim of stopping the incidence of children witnessing violence between their parents. Like all the groups we hold, every man must complete its tasks within 16 sessions carried out over four months of the intervention. Most of the men join the group when they are in denial, repression, or consciously detached from emotion regarding the cumulative damage their children suffer by witnessing their violence. Therefore, this group is assigned a difficult task in a short period of time. The denial, repression, and detachment from feelings are the response to the psychological difficulty of recognizing and accepting that they have injured their children, whom they love, and difficulty in acknowledging the wounded and wounding places within them.

The gap between the dream of a perfect family and the actual behavior and reactions of their children often gives rise to emotions such as severe guilt, shame, a sense of failure as parents, and despair. These feelings are significant to the group work and, in our opinion, constitute the transition from behavior without thinking (doing) to the acquisition of new behavior with their children through self-observation (being).

Most of the men in the group were child witnesses of violence themselves and were battered as children; as adults, they reenacted this behavior pattern with their own children. Some of them internalized violent language as effective and essential, and some expressed a desire and an inability to change. The group deals with adult men/fathers, but it was given its name for two reasons: to acknowledge that many of the men were child witnesses of violence themselves and to create the initial suggestion that as fathers they were in turn making their own children witnesses to violence. In this group, it is our intention to address both aspects.

The main goal of the group is integrative emotional and cognitive recognition of the damage caused to their children by witnessing violence and cessation of this cumulative damage. In order to achieve this goal within the given time span of 16 group sessions for each man/father, the Beit Noam staff initially tried different means of intervention that were based on different approaches to group leadership. On the basis of this accumulated knowledge, the leadership of the group is currently based on three approaches:

- The existential approach, which is founded on the principle that choice is in the hands of the man/father and he is able to choose differently.
- The intergenerational approach allows the men to explore the link between their own witnessing of their parents' violence in the past to their children's witnessing of their own violence in the present. This approach helps men to recognize the patterns transmitted intergenerationally and to recognize that they had repeated their parents' behavior toward them.
- The dynamic approach is based on the principle of understanding the sources and motives of behavior, and helps the men understand

how they reached the violent behavior that their children have witnessed.

The group facilitators combine the three different approaches. At times, the combination is for a given period of time, and at others one central approach is used every evening. The combination of these approaches is implemented in practice through a set format, using psychodrama as the medium of exploration. The emphasis is not on role-play, but on reconstruction of the incident at the behavioral and, in particular, the emotional level. We found that the psychodrama method is very effective in circumventing the men's rigid defenses and connecting them emotionally to these difficult and loaded experiences.

Use of psychodrama. In order to enable meaningful intervention, the men have to experience the group as a protective, containing place with clear limits. In every session, the men become child witnesses to violence on the emotional level through the use of psychodrama. According to their choice, a man/father sits in the center. He chooses some of the men to play his family, while the remaining men become witnesses of the violence. The man reconstructs and directs the enactment of a specific violent event that occurred between he and his wife, with his children witnessing.

Every man/father sits on the psychodrama "chair" several times in the course of the 16 sessions that he participates in the group. Sometimes he sits there as a father, a wife, or a child, and sometimes as an observing witness. The dynamic transition between the different roles enables him to increase his level of self-observation, and to lower the level of his denial of the pain his children experienced. In most cases, returning to his primary experiences as a child witness of violence creates a bridge to his children.

For example, one man, whose wife was saved from near death after he hit her on the head with a rolling pin while ordering his children to hold her arms, constantly repeated that he was "father of the year" and beat his wife "only educational blows." In the psychodrama that he directed, the group (both the men who played his wife and children and the others who were witness to his violence) provided an emotional reflection of his deeds, in a supportive yet challenging environment. Such reenactment of the event enabled him to get in touch with the gaps between his behavior outside of the home and his behavior in the family, and enabled him to begin taking responsibility for his violence.

Most of the men focus initially on treating their own pain and unsatisfied needs. At the beginning, they are not able to observe their children and accept them as separate beings, possessing instead their own emotional and developmental needs. For example, in one of his first sessions in the group, Avi, a man who hit and threatened his wife while his five children watched television, claimed that his children were not injured because they were otherwise occupied. After six weeks of intervention, however, Avi sat down in the "empty chair." He chose one of the men as his wife and five others as his children; the remaining five group members became bystanders witnessing the violence. He described the details of the incident in a few minutes (the same event he had described a few sessions earlier from the position of emotional detachment). The five men enacted the incident, with the group facilitator's supervision and guidance. After the enactment, each of the participants shared the feelings he had felt as either an actor or a spectator. Avi heard from all the men in the group what they had felt when he was violent. For the first time, he heard from "his children" (the men) that they felt emotions such as fright, tremendous anxiety, despair, worthlessness, a decline in self-image, and guilt, as though he was violent because of them. In addition, Avi heard from "his children" that when he was violent he looked frightening, dangerous, and out of control, and that there were many noticeable physical signs.

A few weeks after sitting in "the chair," Avi told the group that he now understood for the first time and took responsibility for the damage he caused his children. He was beginning to make the connection between their behavioral expressions (e.g., bedwetting, physical contraction when he approached them, nightmares) and the experience of witnessing his violence. Avi shared this with great pain and expressed a wish that the group would help him learn to provide his children with healthier experiences. The men's newfound connection to their children, through their own childhood experiences, and through authentic reconstruction of their violent behavior in front of their children, along with feedback from the group members, facilitates powerful and emotional self-observation. It also enables them to see their children as separate from them.

The integration in the sessions of men who are at different stages of their intervention also enables and catalyzes the group process. For example, one of the men/fathers who was two months ahead in the group process turned to Avi and shared with him that he had experienced similar feelings of pain and despair after he recognized, in the group, the damage he had caused his children. He was now in a different situation: he spoke with his children, according to their respective ages, about the violent incidents they had witnessed. He heard from them how much they were afraid and hurt. He overcame this difficulty and was now aware that his attitude toward them and ways of coping with them had changed.

About 90% of the men at Beit Noam are child witnesses of their fathers' violence toward their mothers. The fantasy that their own children will not experience the difficulties the men experienced as witnesses to violence is repeatedly shattered by their violence toward their wives. The discrepancy between the dream of the perfect family and their actual behavior gives them feelings of guilt, shame, and a sense of parental failure. Getting in touch with what their children have experienced, through both their experiences as children in psychodrama and through authentic reenactment of their own violent behavior while receiving feedback from group members, enables them powerful self-observation and, later, allows them to see their children as separate from them.

The solidarity and sense of belonging that they feel in the peer group enables most of the men to touch the difficult spots that reflect their injury to what is most precious–their children. The denial is replaced by awareness; this opens the way for behavioral change, which leads to emotional openness with their children, both from a point of identification and from a point of the motivation to repair. In addition, the re-experiencing of their own violence, seen this time through the eyes of their children, enables the men, within in a short period of time, to stop allowing their children to witness violence, to see the children as separate individuals with different needs, and to start to develop a different parenthood based on the personality strengths of each man and father.

Follow-Up Group

The follow-up group is designed for men who have completed the intervention program at Beit Noam. It operates parallel to community intervention. Men come to the group on a voluntary basis, once a week for several months. The group offers a support framework and helps men readjust to their lives outside Beit Noam. The topics discussed at the group are chosen by the men themselves and often relate to fears of separation from Beit Noam and from their families, getting along in the community, as well as the function and technical problems of returning to society. In addition to being supportive, the group also serves as an alternative to loneliness and isolation.

INDIVIDUAL THERAPEUTIC WORK

The following case studies are examples of the intervention work that is done on an individual basis, alongside the group work, at Beit Noam. The setting of the individual counseling is one hour per week, as opposed to ten hours of group work. Indeed, our view is that the group forum is the main "workshop" for the client to share his violent experiences and behaviors and to cope with the challenges of the program. The rationale behind the individual counseling is that it will serve as a facilitating ground for the group sessions: a good positive therapeutic alliance between a patient and therapist will accelerate the patient's competence for the intervention process. These case studies illustrate the process that a client has gone through in the individual counseling, alongside his progress and development in the group.

Case Study 1: Dani

Dani was referred to Beit Noam by his parole officer following a plea bargain in a lawsuit filed against him by his wife. Additional claims had been closed in a plea bargain, including "finding" a full bag of firearms and drugs and keeping it in his home for about a year. As part of the plea bargain, Dani received a seven-month ban from his home, during which he lived in the home of a rabbi who took responsibility for him. Dani's parole officer indicated that that Dani was extremely violent and should be perceived as dangerous. The parole officer, and later Dani himself, felt that Beit Noam was the last intervention option before a long-term prison sentence.

According to the reports received before the meeting with Dani, he was 25 years old, married, and had five children (ages one through six). He had lost custody of the two oldest children, who were transferred to the guardianship of his parents; he had received intensive attention from welfare services regarding raising the other three children. At the same time, he had engaged in intense, severe violence against his wife, who had been defined by welfare services as an "unfit mother" for the two oldest children.

At the first one-on-one session, a boyish looking man entered the room. He wore a skullcap, had a bashful yet provocative smile, and a dazed look in his eyes. Dani's first sentence–"I was born into a cruel life, in which all the evil fell upon me, I don't understand how"–constituted the first step in creating a therapy contract between us. As the focus of the intervention, we agreed upon the transformation of Dani into the protagonist and director of his life, instead of a passive spectator. The aim was for him to gain control over his violent behavior and take responsibility for his life. In retrospect, his first sentence may have served as the key to all Dani's therapeutic activity at Beit Noam.

In the course of the first two months with us, Dani continued to function as he always had: broadcasting verbally and non-verbally that "everything was all right" and continuing to live in a destructive inner world. Dani complied with all the rules of the center in an exemplary manner. He was never late to a session or activity, he did not argue, and he did not have conflicts with anyone. However, neither did he allow verbal and emotional contact with his inner world.

The one-on-one sessions were the first sphere in which he began to bridge the many gaps in his life. The therapeutic material that Dani brought up in the sessions was related to his internalized narrative as a victim–his life was in ruins and he had no idea why. In the one-on-one intervention, Dani managed without difficulty to identify the physical signs that characterized him prior to violent events: trembling legs, grinding teeth, a locked jaw, nervous and clenched eyes, restlessness expressed in endless pacing, perspiring hands, and pressure in his stomach and chest that was accompanied by hot flushes.

The impressive list of signs and the excellent ability to identify them was again dissonant with his feeling that he had no control, that there was no inner dialogue between his body and himself. This impressive cognitive process was cut off from the emotional process. Therefore, I sensed that the work on connecting the different parts of the split world (so that he could take responsibility for his life) should take the form of empathetic connection to the sources that created the primary narrative in his childhood. From there, Dani could begin to build a new narrative in which he would be the protagonist and director of his life.

The facilitator's request that Dani talk about his childhood quickly changed the dynamics in the room, and he took a more significant role in the interpersonal space. Dani brought up extremely harsh childhood experiences–recurrent incidents of violence, severe neglect, and a basic primary experience that the home is dangerous and the world in general is a cruel and cold place. His father relentlessly and blindly whipped Dani and his brothers with a belt. In such situations, his mother would stand by watching, sometimes weeping quietly and sometimes muttering, almost inaudibly, "Stop" or "They deserve it." According to Dani, it was impossible to rely upon her reactions, and she did not protect her children from their father.

At the age of 7, Dani's father tied him to the toilet, whipped him several times with a belt, left him there for many hours, and forbade the other members of the family to approach him. In addition, Dani's parents decided that his aging paternal grandfather needed help, and moved Dani and his brothers to his house to assist him. Dani experienced this parental decision as another form of rejection and abandonment. For two years during his adolescence, Dani and his brothers lived in their grandfather's home, nursing him. They bathed, fed, and cleaned up after him, and they were ordered by their parents not to eat anything, ask for anything, or be anything but their grandfather's caregivers. Therefore, Dani had to go to his parent's home for any personal need (i.e., to use the bathroom, shower, eat).

After two years of caring for his grandfather, Dani returned to his parents' home having decided that he would no longer allow anyone in the world to torture, humiliate, and batter him. The first time that his father took out his belt, Dani hit him and threatened that he would "tear him apart" if his father dared hit him again. On that day, Dani chose to move to a boarding school framework and to closely monitor his father. Instead of attending the boarding school, he would wander throughout the city on his bike, looking for his adulterous father and confronting him every time he found him with a woman other than his mother. (At the time, his mother was hospitalized and his father did not visit her.) In addition, he began developing ties with a peer group with whom he would disappear for several days at a time, engaging in illegal motorcycles trips or vagrancy.

Dani met his wife in his late teens on one of these wanderings. She had run away from an extremely violent home, in which she had been battered and abandoned many times during her adolescence and had moved from one foster family to another. Dani promised, as he often did, "everything would be all right." He saw her as a twin spirit, and fantasized that with her help he could find a place where he would be loved unconditionally, where he would never be abandoned, and where he would be contained and protected from becoming a criminal. In the couple dynamic, it was only a matter of time before the first slap, which occurred when she (then his girlfriend) failed to smile when he came to pick her up for a date.

Dani told these difficult stories with emotional distance, in his monotonous, quiet voice with a slight smile at the corners of this mouth. When I shared with him the pain I felt in the story of his childhood events and the detached way he told the stories, Dani was moved but did not understand what I was making a fuss about. His reaction was one of suspicion, readiness, and detachment: "What is there to get so excited about, why does this interest you?"

However, the emotion that had touched him in individual therapy began to sink in. In the informal activities, Dani began to challenge other men to share their childhood events and stories of violence with him. He began to develop a need to find out whether the others had perhaps experienced such serious childhood events as his own. In my view, unconsciously, Dani began to examine whether it might be possible for things to be different, whether what had been was not necessarily what would be. However, in the group process, Dani continued to convey the message to the other men and the facilitators that "everything was all right." He quickly became popular among the other violent men in the program, and this aroused our concern.

Dani's automatic reaction in therapy was that "I have no chance of changing." In the intervention contract, it was decided that Dani would examine this assumption through even the smallest experiments with change. Subsequent sessions were accompanied by his excitement about every small revelation of change (he dared ask another man for a cigarette, despite his high anxiety about being helped; another man told him he seemed tense and he listened without hitting him). Alongside this excitement, however, his initial perceptions continued to accompany the sessions: "Life is cruel, and all its evil falls on me, and I don't understand how."

Dani introduced metaphor to the sessions: he named his inner world "my closed box." In examining the metaphor, it emerged that he perceived his inner world as locked to him, so that he did not know it or control it. However, boxes also have keys. In addition, Dani called the box "my box," thus transforming himself from the spectator in a play to its protagonist. He was still a beginner protagonist, unsure of himself.

Another significant stage in the intervention began when I asked about the scar on his hand. This question opened a window to another childhood event, when he was hospitalized for surgery after two fractures in his hand failed to heal. At the same time, Dani began to recall associative, disorganized memories. The memories revolved around experiences of sleeping alone in the hospital, anxiety about the surgery, and loneliness. His mother came to visit him only once after the surgery; she sat next to him and cried. This memory was his only experience of maternal concern. In moments of difficulty, the memory of his mother crying in the hospital emerged from his "closed box" and comforted him.

In the group work, Dani continued the former patterns of "everything's okay," without allowing contact with his inner world. The changes that he did allow were preliminary and specific, and did not counterbalance the patterns of the past. As is sometimes customary at Beit Noam, I assigned another man to him who had been in the intervention process two months longer than Dani. This "tutor" was a Moslem Arab, a father of eight small children who had also been severely violent toward his wife. He was to be available for Dani to turn to, to help him gather the courage to ask for help when he felt it was appropriate. Through him, Dani heard for the first time that there are men who hug their children, change their diapers, and express feelings. Through him, Dani experienced hope and began to envision himself several months ahead in the intervention. However, past patterns also dominated this relationship. At the one-on-one sessions, Dani expressed great difficulty in daring to turn to him and ask for help. He expressed this in his perception that if he asked for help, he would see himself as dependent and lacking control, and he would thus become violent. Therefore, as he saw it, his tutor "secretly" helped him.

Dani continued to avoid contact with the professional facilitators in the intervention groups. He answered when asked questions, avoided direct interaction and initiative, and continued to lock "his box." However, in the individual sessions, Dani began to deal with the question of whether he would be desirable and loved without violence, domination, extreme jealousy and his compliance. He said that was the question he had not dared ask in the past; when he did dare to ask, it was hard for him to believe that such a situation was possible.

After six one-on-one sessions, the primary therapeutic relationship was established; at this point, Dani began to request an absence on evenings for "different occasions." He revealed that he had met his wife "by chance" in the city. He said that this was not contrary to the court order, which forbade him to meet her at home. It was clear to me that these things were related. In his inner world, it was not possible that there would be significant relations without rejection, abandonment, and an outburst in the relationship. At the same time, joint sessions at Beit Noam were held with the parole officer and the social worker that worked with the wife. At the first session with them, we discussed our common concern about whether it was possible, in such a short time, to connect the split aspects of Dani's world and generate the desired behavioral change. The wife's social worker shared her impression that, contrary to the court order, Dani was meeting his wife and had entered their apartment. She got this impression from something the wife had said unintentionally.

The next one-on-one session with Dani was different. I confronted him with what the social worker had said. Dani told me that he was meeting his wife, almost daily, even though he was aware that this was in breach of the court order. Dani opened up and shared another aspect of his inner world–a primary, archaic, and suspicious aspect. It included some psychopathic traits, such as his belief that the world was so cruel and cold that it was simply stupid not to act accordingly. In this context, the daily meetings, which until then had not been discovered, increased his feeling of omnipotence and destructiveness.

Dani was amazed when the group facilitator shared my perception that he was not only breaching the court order, but also betraying my basic trust as well as that of the group social workers and the other men at Beit Noam. The surprise came from his inner, primal world, where there was no such thing as relations of trust. Furthermore, Dani told me that although he felt and heard from me that everyone cared about him, inside he did not allow himself to feel such caring, because it endangered him with feelings that were unfamiliar to him and not in his full control.

At this stage in the intervention (after two months), Dani's case was presented to the Beit Noam team and a major question was raised: Should we let Dani stay at our center or stop the intervention? There were many considerations, at several levels. We reexamined Dani's ego strengths to cope with the task of the intervention in our framework in such a brief period. The entire team felt that we could not promote Dani to the desired goal–to make him into a man who controls his violent urges–within the short period available. At the same time, it was clear to us that regardless of any decision we made, the court might not allow continuation of the follow-up intervention after disclosure of the information about his numerous breaches of its order.

In order to promote the professional discussion, we isolated ourselves from the legal process, over which we had no control, and focused on the intervention-related questions only. As a team, we estimated that Dani would have a very difficult time completing the process and we decided to terminate his intervention. However, despite this decision, the director of Beit Noam decided that Dani would remain. This process in the staff was highly significant to the continuation of the intervention. In retrospect, the split that was created between the intervention team and the director regarding Dani's intervention process was no coincidence. Perhaps as a team, we had more intensely witnessed the splitting that

Dani had experienced all his life, whereas the director had distance from this situation.

After reporting the decision to the parole officer and the wife's social worker, the facilitator informed Dani of the decision to continue the intervention. He received outlined specific conditions (any further breach would lead to immediate expulsion from Beit Noam) and told him about the split among the staff (without citing names). Both the conditions and the information that some of the staff was in favor and others against his remaining increased the progress that followed. At the one-on-one sessions during the third month of the intervention, Dani gained better understanding of his automatic behavior, and thereby began to take responsibility for his past violence and for his life, and began to "direct the play." In a concomitant process, Dani began to be present, in the emotional sense, in the intervention groups and to raise subject matter and experiences in the one-on-one sessions. For example, in the consciousness group, which works with nonverbal tools, Dani drew a house in reality (an empty house, broken into and black) opposite a fantasy house (closed, with a wife and children waiting for him on the path, surrounding by flowers and smiling). Both the group facilitator and Dani shared that the picture was related to contents from inside "the closed box."

At the beginning of the third month of the intervention, Dani came to the one-on-one session, sat down, and for the first time, did not start with the sentence "everything's all right." Instead, he began with harsh feelings of despair, helplessness, and a desire to destroy himself and the environment because of these feelings. To this point, Dani had raised such feelings only after a process in the session, and certainly not at his own initiative. Dani easily identified the automatic patterns that in the past–in order to avoid having these hard feelings–he would cut himself off emotionally and react immediately with violence, or physically flee to other women, to horses, or to motorcycles. At the same time, Dani continued to bring up incidents that seemed insignificant in the outside world, but were significant in his inner world, in which he experienced an interaction of acceptance with the group social workers. In one of the incidents, he was late for a skills group session, and the facilitator commented on this. Dani was aware that it was he who had been late and he listened without acting out the inner dialogue that developed within him–a feeling that the social worker was rejecting him and wanted to get rid of him, and the consequent desire to leave everything, destroy our setting, do damage and flee. He would then experience our expulsion of him, and again prove to himself the basic assumption that "the world is a cold, cruel and rejecting place." He was able to make the connection between the work he did in the first months of intervention, and its application now in the group.

The despair that he felt about stopping the past patterns began to be countered by increased familiarity with alternative patterns. In one session, I examined with Dani whether he could interpret the facilitator's comment about his tardiness as an expression of concern and caring. This possibility surprised him; it seemed impossible but appealing. Was it possible that someone would limit him out of concern and love, without violence, rejection, or exploitation? Dani was able to say that this was what happened to him in our setting, but he was still unable to put such "strange and moving" experiences into the "closed box."

The occasions on which Dani dared open the "closed box" in groups became more numerous. For example, in the group on child witnesses of violence Dani directed an enactment of his relationship with his children. The third month and the beginning of the fourth month of the intervention were intensive for him, as he struggled between old patterns and new awareness. These few weeks demanded clear, strong therapeutic limits together with great containment. However, Dani continued to make progress. For example, at the beginning of the fourth month, Dani was the house monitor for one week (responsible for collecting money for shopping, preparing and planning suppers, and keeping to schedule). While his initial, automatic response was that he could not fulfill this job, by the end of the week he experienced joy and pleasure as well as a sense of pride and self-worth because of his success in the task.

His experiences of competence grew in the one-on-one intervention, the groups, and with the peer group. Dani heard from the other men that it was when he dared to allow them to be acquainted with his less "attractive" aspects (i.e., the "closed box") that they felt closer and more genuine with him. Dani developed social relationships with two of the residents. In my view, these two symbolized the connections between the internal splits in his life. The first relationship was with another violent man, and was based on former patterns: social relations through the false parts, including giggling during difficult moments in the group sessions, talking about women with whom they betrayed their wives, and speaking as victims. The relationship with the other man represented the change that Dani was undergoing and included parts of the true self. The relationship was authentic, revealing, and mutually caring. For the first time in his life, Dani developed a relationship based on mutual trust, with a similar/different character. This relationship continues to this day. The two men protect each other from returning to past patterns, holding phone conversations several times a day, despite the physical distance between their places of residence.

In light of the changes that had taken place and the work that still needed to be done, the professional staff decided to extend Dani's therapy in our setting by another month. The decision was based on the belief that in an extra month we could strengthen the points of change, which would serve as a protective wall in the future when facing difficulties and the desire to revert to past patterns. This decision required the approval of the court and, in fact, led to a delay in the court hearing regarding Dani's sentence. The legal threat of possible imprisonment was another therapeutic catalyst.

In the fifth and last month of Dani's intervention, he took full responsibility for his life and made many changes, ultimately becoming the protagonist and director of his own life. In the one-on-one and group meetings, Dani revealed violent events from his past and took full responsibility for them, declaring that "I was a violent man, I behaved violently, I belittled, humiliated, prevented her from having freedom and rights. I chased her and didn't let her live her life, I made a terrible mistake with the arms and the drugs, I had sexual intercourse with her regardless of what she wanted." Dani became emotionally prepared for the possibility that his wife would want to divorce him. Furthermore, he initiated talks with her through her social workers; he opened these talks by saying he wanted to return home after the intervention and after the sentence, but only if she wanted him and not out of her fear of him. Moreover, he physically and emotionally took responsibility for his children, and implemented his visiting rights. In the group, we saw a transition before our very eyes, from a child who was raising five neglected children to a father with difficulties setting limits and getting in touch with his children.

For this first time since he had come to Beit Noam, Dani reacted aggressively to two of the men, whom he felt were belittling and rejecting him. In my view, this incident was actually testimony to progress, because he allowed himself to be authentic with his peer group, and trusted himself to engage in a dialogue with them without violence.

In the inner struggle, the knowledge that the entire staff was aware of his breaches of the court order, and the restrictive conditions of his continued stay at Beit Noam were perceived as healthy limits. In addition, he was developing a sense that the entire staff cared about him and wanted the best for him. These experiences enabled the inner dialogue to choose change. His belief that he could change his fate was expressed in new thinking about a struggle against the threat of the sentence. Dani initiated meetings with the parole office, in which he described the change he had undergone and his desire that the parole officer fight against a prison sentence. In the parting session, after 20 minutes had gone by, Dani, for the first time in the five months he had been at the center, expressed a desire to "skip over" the separation from me and expressed a desire to continue the intervention relationship.

Dani returned home on the basis of a mutual agreement. The court decided not to send him to prison, in light of the changes he had made. Dani returned to one-on-one sessions with his parole officer and came to Beit Noam once a week to attend a supervision and follow-up group. He also began attending a follow-up intervention group in his area of his residence.

Case Study 2: Davian

Davian, a 33-year-old male, had been married for eight years to his twenty-nine-year-old wife. They had two children, ages six and one. Davian lived in a small town and worked as a supervisor in a cleaning company. Prior to coming Beit Noam for an intervention, he had undergone five years of treatment, comprised of both individual counseling and group sessions, for his violent behavior.

At the beginning of his treatment at Beit Noam, Davian claimed that he felt he needed a more intensive treatment framework that would help him overcome feelings of low self-confidence, meaninglessness in his life, and dissatisfaction with his marriage and family life. In his opinion, these feelings were the cause for his inability to control his violent behavior towards his wife. When one of the authors [B.B.] met him, Davian took full responsibility for the physical, verbal, and psychological abuse he perpetrated against his wife. At the time he came to Beit Noam and expressed his wish to enter the program, six months had elapsed since the last violent incident between he and his wife. During that incident, Davian had slapped her. In the months that followed, they lived in separate rooms in the same house. We assumed that, sub-consciously, Davian created situations in which he was bound to be rejected. For example, in one of our sessions, Davian saw me putting on hand cream, told me that they get hand creams for free at his place of work, and asked me if I would like him to bring me some. I thanked him and said that it was nice of him to offer it, but stated that there was no need for that. A week later, Davian left me a hand cream in my room. I addressed it as a therapeutic issue and gently refused his gift.

Socially, Davian assimilated very quickly into the group life and dynamics, acquired a unique position, and was rather active in revealing his intimate thoughts and feelings, both with himself and with the group and myself. On the other hand, Davian experienced unexplained shifts in mood, with the tendency to fall into a state of confusion, self-reproach, and depression that manifested in frequent wishes to commit suicide.

Davian's history included growing up with emotional deprivation, being physically abused as a child, being a child witness to his father's violence towards his mother, and experiencing permanent feelings of mistrust and loneliness. Davian acceded that his pattern of being passive-aggressive was the basis of many of the crises and violent behavior he had experienced with his wife. In other words, Davian did not know how one behaves in an intimate relationship: in situations of intimacy or situations that were about to create intimacy, Davian felt confusion and fear. To deflect these feelings, he created a situation that dispelled the intimacy and created the opposite: rejection of his partner and tension. Rejection and tension for Davian were known dynamics for gaining power and control, psychic terrains in which he felt comfortable.

At that point, my feeling and assessment was that Davian was afraid and unsure of his ability to make a precedent breakthrough to other, less known parts of himself, such as consideration, self-acceptance, satisfaction, and friendship. To put it metaphorically, my assessment was that Davian knew his "darker" terrain inside out, but that he was paralyzed by fears that he might not find anything if he started "turning on the light" in his other parts. This paralyzing fear meant being caught in a cycle that comprised the following phases: experiencing intimacy, feeling confused, seeking control in provocative or aggressive testing, encountering rejection, acting in non-productive (passive-aggression) or destructive (violence) behavior, and feeling morbid. My therapeutic intention was to become for Davian a self-object: to create a therapeutic relationship that would enable Davian to experience a full, safe, and rewarding intimate experience through me. Thus, in our individual sessions, I supported and encouraged Davian's expressions of his good self (parts of himself he could find meaning in and be proud of), while simultaneously holding a mirror up to his failings when they occurred. I believed that if we succeeded in forming a successful self-object relationship, it would assist Davian in gaining confidence in his ability to create and integrate intimate situations, leaving alienation and destruction behind. In addition, the group sessions provided the main arena for testing himself, through topics of control, violent and aggressive behavior, and his interpersonal relationships. There, as well, Davian developed awareness of his tendency to dispel intimacy.

Ten weeks into the program Davian moved from one extreme to the other. From a generally morbid affect, Davian's affect changed to a happy one; for example, he became very flexible about issues in the group's daily life. This clear switch in affect was discussed between us, and Davian was aware of it. Our goal for the last month had been to find the proper middle path that suits Davian's stage, abilities, and personality. I pointed out to Davian that a stage of euphoria is an unrealistic and worrying extreme, and that the result would not be so. Indeed, in the last month, Davian shifted to a more focused and less easygoing position, and I became less directive.

Davian gradually processed his interactions differently, and by capturing the changed narrative, he could normalize his relapses, so their impact was shorter and less alarming. My proof to that was the way in which Davian parted from the staff. This was a clear moment of intimacy, and Davian feared and warned me that he would sabotage his relationships with people around him before leaving. Eventually, however, Davian parted in a very peaceful way. In my view, the positive experience that we had on the emotional interpersonal level widened and deepened the impact of his stay in Beit Noam and increased his ability to pursue constructive patterns of interaction in the future.

ASSESSMENT REPORT OF BEIT NOAM

An assessment of the Beit Noam project was carried out over a period of more than two years by the Mishtanim Corporation (project assessors and organizational consultants) and the National Insurance Institute (Special Projects Section). In the course of the assessment, a variety of open and closed tracking tools were utilized (including interviews, observation, and statistical analysis of questionnaires) and five interim assessment reports were presented. The final report was published by the national insurance institute in September 2000.

These preliminary findings were based on the following data:

- 19 interviews with women whose partners had completed the residency period at Beit Noam at least 6 months prior to the interview;
- 52 questionnaires completed by male residents, 35 of whom were at the beginning of the residency period at Beit Noam and 17 of whom were at the end of their stay. The questionnaires were com-

posed of both closed-ended questions that were submitted to statistical analysis and open-ended questions that were submitted to quantitative, as well as qualitative, analytic mapping; the questionnaires were completed pre and post.

- 16 interviews with professionals involved with re-integrating the Beit Noam graduates into the community. The interviews were personal and related to various patients.

In addition, a quantitative mapping of activity and intensive observations of groups and group activity was performed, and interviews were conducted with the social workers, clients, and senior professionals within the community. Finally, interviews were conducted within the domestic violence treatment centers, and observations were made of the steering committee, the professional committees, and the grassroots connections.

Preliminary Results

Combating Intimacy Violence

The abused women and the professionals who work with the residents within the community and probation services all reported that Beit Noam had been successful in dealing with the physical violence symptoms of battering men. As of the date of the fifth assessment report, the probation office reported no complaints and no reports of physical violence against the women (based on in-depth interviews with complainants and professionals within the community). A detailed analysis follows.

The wives of Beit Noam graduate residents. Wives of battering men involved in the program reported considerable changes in the behavior of the men. In fact, each woman interviewed reported a decrease in violence. The women reported that the men no longer assaulted or threatened them; they also reported that they no longer felt afraid of the men, as they had been in the past. They pointed out that the men now make efforts to control their anger. Nevertheless, there were still patterns of verbal violence and there were occasional reports of physical violence towards a security guard at work. Except for one woman, all the women noted that the communication patterns between the treated battering men and their wives and children had improved: There was an improvement in the way the men expressed themselves, it was possible to talk with the men more, and the men were more open, gentle, and patient.

Better communication was reported in all the families where the man had returned to cohabit with the wife following the intervention (50% of the 19 cases), but of course not in cases where the couple had separated. However, various professional sources indicated that the very ability of the Beit Noam graduates to separate from their wives and end an unsuccessful relationship in a normative and violence-free manner should be considered a professional success.

In addition, the women who were interviewed were asked about treatment services that they might have sought. It was found that, whereas the battering men undergoing integrative intervention at Beit Noam go through meaningful experiences that included processes that brought about change (see below), their wives undergo only partial treatment within the community. According to the women, this fact creates dissonance and difficulties within the relationship.

Thus, based on the reports of 19 of the wives of men who underwent treatment at Beit Noam, the program appears to be effective in the short-term in reducing prevalence of physical violence. However, the long-term effectiveness of the treatment still remains an open question, a question that can only be answered by longitudinal, follow-up studies.

Men who have completed the intervention program at Beit Noam. The men who were part of the assessment and completed the intervention program at Beit Noam reported on the changes that they underwent and the characteristics of intervention that they received. On comparing the pre and post questionnaires, the men who completed the intervention program reported taking more responsibility for their violent behavior.

The men reported that the program at Beit Noam offered advantages over previous treatment methods they have experienced. The intensive integrative intervention method at Beit Noam allowed the men to acquire coping tools and new patterns of behavior, as well as new means of self-expression and enrichment. The men believed that their range of behavior towards their spouses and towards others was enlarged and improved.

The men also reported feeling that they had succeeded in changing things by themselves. They credited the learning, the experience of shared-living with others who are facing similar difficulties, as well as the professional intervention by the Beit Noam staff. At the conclusion of their stay, they were more focused on themselves and saw the need for change in themselves (as opposed to the external focus that was typical of them in the pre-treatment stage).

The men arrived at Beit Noam with the expectation of receiving specific intervention for their violent behavior as well as concrete tools to deal with their spousal relationship. At the conclusion of the intervention program they achieved a deeper, more introspective understanding and an internal relating of the violence, yet they also were now more aware of the inherent difficulties of living with others. The men credited the graduate support groups that take place at Beit Noam. They noted the great need for continuing follow-up intervention. At the same time, we found that the "buddy" system is very important, both during the intervention and at its conclusion.

The Intervention Group Sessions

As mentioned previously, Beit Noam hosts five intervention group sessions every week (one session per evening), as well as a follow-up session for graduates. The type of group session may change depending on the professional and administrative needs. The groups combine into an entire holistic intervention fabric, since each one of the group sessions deals with a different area, using a different intervention model and different therapeutic tools.

We have found that the group sessions are the most important intervention element for the men. Each man expresses himself differently in different group sessions. The intensity of intervention is likewise important. The follow-up session for graduates has special significance as the ability of the men to return to the community to implement and continue to fortify the coping tools he has acquired can be monitored and reinforced. In addition, the buddy system work that takes place within the group session has been beneficial to the participants, as well as the significant integration of daily life at the center with the group session discussion.

The Professional Elements within the Community

Although at first the community professionals were unfamiliar with the project, the Beit Noam steering committee and administration succeeded in creating a fertile dialogue with the various community professionals (both the referring and receiving elements). This dialogue was created through public relations work and exposure of the Beit Noam staff within the community, as well as a series of planning and procedure-building meetings involving a number of partners: The Ministry of Labor and Social Affairs, probation services, the Beit Noam staff, the

Noam Association for the Prevention of Domestic Abuse, and other professionals in the community (e.g., welfare services and the domestic violence treatment centers).

There has been an intensive implementation of the recommendations of the various assessment reports, the work of the steering committee, and the community-integrated committees. According to these recommendations, there is a need to continue to develop organized connection patterns with the community and, in particular, with the social workers and therapists in the communities. This experiment is taking place, especially through the use of the concept of a case manager and by devoting the time to working with the case manager and tracking the work. Tracking the work of the case manager assists over time in ensuring that the perpetrator (the abusive man) arrives more prepared for the intervention program at Beit Noam.

CONCLUSION

Beit Noam represents a program that deals with the care of the abusive behavior of men against their spouse. It is a residential intensive and integrative program in Israel that was started as an experimental pilot program, and after only five years has become known as one of the most important methods of working with and treating batterers in Israel.

Integrating Spirituality
and Domestic Violence Treatment:
Treatment of Aboriginal Men

Robert Kiyoshk

SUMMARY. This article provides a brief reflection on how the Change of Seasons treatment model developed and the reasons for its success with Aboriginal men. Parallels between Aboriginal perspectives, or worldviews, and Ken Wilber's transpersonal psychology, Rupert Sheldrake's fields theory, and Peter Senge's systems thinking are also discussed. Practical rituals and ceremonies that have been successfully integrated into psycho-educational group counselling as practiced in the Change of Seasons model are explained. These musings are included to initiate further dialogue on holistic approaches to counselling and other community initiatives. *[Article copies available for a fee from The Haworth Document Delivery Service: 1-800-HAWORTH. E-mail address: <docdelivery@haworthpress.com> Website: <http://www.HaworthPress.com> © 2003 by The Haworth Press, Inc. All rights reserved.]*

KEYWORDS. Aboriginals, Aboriginal spirituality, group counselling, treatment, spousal abuse, systems thinking

Address correspondence to: Robert Kiyoshk (E-mail: mukwamanitou@telus.net).

[Haworth co-indexing entry note]: "Integrating Spirituality and Domestic Violence Treatment: Treatment of Aboriginal Men." Kiyoshk, Robert. Co-published simultaneously in *Journal of Aggression, Maltreatment & Trauma* (The Haworth Maltreatment & Trauma Press, an imprint of The Haworth Press, Inc.) Vol. 7, No. 1/2 (#13/14), 2003, pp. 237-256; and: *Intimate Violence: Contemporary Treatment Innovations* (ed: Donald Dutton, and Daniel J. Sonkin) The Haworth Maltreatment & Trauma Press, an imprint of The Haworth Press, Inc., 2003, pp. 237-256. Single or multiple copies of this article are available for a fee from The Haworth Document Delivery Service [1-800-HAWORTH, 9:00 a.m. - 5:00 p.m. (EST). E-mail address: docdelivery@haworthpress.com].

http://www.haworthpress.com/store/product.asp?sku=J146
© 2003 by The Haworth Press, Inc. All rights reserved.
10.1300J146v07n01_10

A MODEL FOR WORKING WITH ABORIGINAL[1] CLIENTS

The Change of Seasons model is a 28-session psycho-educational group counselling model that has been used over the past ten years by the Change of Seasons Society in North Vancouver, British Columbia. Spiritual practices are an integral part of the entire program, and every third session is completely focused on such activities. In 1990, when I first set foot in a meeting of the British Columbia Association of Counsellors of Abusive Men (ACAM), very few Aboriginal people were actively involved in the work of counselling assaultive men. At that time I met Bruce Wood, who had been working extensively with a psycho-educational approach. We collaborated on a model for working with Aboriginal men; the result was the Change of Seasons model, a combination of Bruce's model and Aboriginal cultural healing methods. Since then hundreds of Aboriginal men have participated in the counselling groups, and the model has been adapted for working with Aboriginal women and youth by the Warriors Against Violence Society in Vancouver.

We developed a model for working with Aboriginal men because we felt that models in common usage had much to offer but did not accommodate the particular cultural and spiritual needs of Aboriginal men. Our clients have many issues with mainstream approaches and service providers, all of these issues deriving from historical and contemporary relations with the dominant society's structures and values. Our model has been accepted by Aboriginal clients because it fits with their community's spiritual beliefs and worldviews.

As time passed, I began to realize the importance of being able to articulate for other counsellors the underlying processes of development taking place in the group therapy. This understanding is also essential for our own counsellors, in order to for them to become clearly cognizant of the processes in which they were engaging their clients. Although a client may not necessarily be aware of the treatment theories and processes, it is imperative that the counsellor be totally aware. The approaches of Ken Wilber (1996, 1998a, 1998b), Rupert Sheldrake (1988) and Peter Senge (1990, 1994) are used here to draw parallel between some mainstream approaches and Aboriginal perspectives.

HISTORY OF OPPRESSION: COLONIZATION AND ANOMIE[2]

Assaultive men's counselling in the Aboriginal community is a lot different than in mainstream programs. This is because the dynamics and circumstances affecting the aboriginal population are quite different. Domestic violence statistics in Canadian general population figures show high degrees of domestic assault occurring nationally, while Aboriginal figures show astoundingly higher rates of domestic assault and other forms of family violence (Kiyoshk, 2001). Mainstream figures show perhaps one or three in ten women as victims of spousal abuse; Aboriginal figures run as high as eight and nine out of ten, depending upon the study and location.

The 1996 Royal Commission on Aboriginal Peoples did much to emphasize the social and economic conditions that contribute to the serious violence within the Aboriginal population. However, the problem among the Aboriginal population is as serious today as it was when the British Columbia Task Force on Family Violence (1992) submitted its report *Is Anyone Listening?* and the accompanying *Family Violence in Aboriginal Communities* (Frank, 1992). Unfortunately, such studies objectify and quantify abuse without really getting down to the reality of the oppression and its long-term effects on aboriginal people. If one were to conduct substantial research into the effects of historical white-aboriginal relations, the findings might be quite alarming. For example, Dr. Anthony J. Hall, Associate Chair of the Department of Native American Studies at the University of Lethbridge, wrote the following:

> Until well into the 1970s, the Canadian government paid the major Christian churches in Canada to conspire actively in the coercive silencing of these Aboriginal languages and preventing Indian children from honouring the Great Spirit in the way of their ancestors.
>
> The history of these Indian residential schools, which existed in the United States but were forced on Indian Country with a singular intensity in Canada, illustrate the very clear existence of government laws, policies and institutions that generated outcomes which clearly lie within the United Nations Convention on Genocide, which was first ratified in 1948 but was not adopted by the USA until 40 years later. Article 2(e) of the Convention defines genocide to include "forcibly transferring children of the group to another group." That is precisely what the Indian residential schools did, the receiving group being the Christian churches that ran these organizations.
>
> Moreover, given the high rate of physical and sexual abuse which took place in these institutions, and the fact that the whole

purpose of these Christian institutions was to teach Indian children to despise and renounce their own Aboriginal heritages of language and religion, they easily meet definition 2(b). That provision refers to "causing serious bodily or mental harm to members of the group." Section 2(c) is also applicable. It defines genocide as "deliberately inflicting on the group conditions of life calculated to bring about physical destruction in whole or in part." (Hall, 1999, p. 5)

Needless to say, the survivors of this legacy have been traumatized, and it is little wonder that their presenting symptoms are often those of Post-traumatic Stress Disorder as listed in the *Diagnostic and Statistical Manual of Mental Disorders* (DSM-IV-R; American Psychiatric Association, 2000). Many Aboriginal men receiving counselling today are survivors of this Residential School Syndrome, or suffer the residual effects of having parents who were survivors or casualties.

CULTURAL AWARENESS AND THERAPY

What makes a good spousal abuse counsellor in the Aboriginal community? Sharing the same cultural background and beliefs is a good starting point. What approaches work best? Circumspect, eclectic and egalitarian are desirable characteristics of an effective approach. Many approaches have been effective in working with Aboriginal men, leading one to conclude that it may well be the therapist who is responsible for the results more so than the particular approach used. In any case, understanding the etiology of an Aboriginal client plays the more significant role. The question of cultural relevance has been posed many times in Aboriginal and cross-cultural settings. Cultural background plays a large part in a client's etiology, and therefore must be considered in the approach to therapy. Aboriginal men can be placed at any number of spots along a continuum to determine where they are in terms of awareness of, or acceptance/non-acceptance of their culture of origin, and to what degree they have been acculturated or assimilated (see Table 1). In forming an etiology and understanding the role of anomie in counselling Aboriginal men, it is important to understand the personal situation of the client in respect to these possibilities, and to remember that perhaps the client does have a drastically different set of experiences that influence their perspectives and circumstances today. In addition, shifts in worldview[3] can occur for a client; change

TABLE 1. Continuum of Cultural Acceptance

Aboriginal:	Has had extensive exposure to aboriginal life and is grounded in aboriginal value systems and beliefs.
Bicultural:	Identity has been nurtured in family and through childhood; functions comfortably as bi-cultural individual (acculturated).
Assimilated:	Aboriginal heritage is peripheral to daily life, and lives primarily in mainstream society.
Between Worlds:	Caught between the expectations, values and demands of two worlds; unable to find a point of balance.

(e.g., from assimilated to Aboriginal) or movement (e.g., from Between-Words to Bicultural to Aboriginal) can occur back and forth between categories depending upon situations.

MODELS OF TREATMENT: CIRCLES OF UNDERSTANDING

Native American Worldview and Systems Thinking

A system is a collection of parts that interact with each other to function as a whole. The worldview of Native North Americans is holistic. Systems thinking is also holistic. The two are identical in every respect except terminology. Systems thinking is actually an ancient way of thinking and perceiving the world. Systems thinking has been the underpinning of Native American consciousness and worldview since the earliest times. In *The Fifth Discipline*, Senge (1994) uses the term "nature's templates" in reference to the universal applications and presence of systems principles. Systems thinking considers all factors, forces and players influencing any given circumstance.

A contemporary term and symbol used by Native Americans to describe their philosophies is the Medicine Wheel (see Figure 1). It is a recently developed symbolic tool for explaining the various dimensions of human processes and their relationships to each other. It is widely used in the education of Native Americans who have been deprived of, or lost touch with, their heritage. It is also widely used in the cross-cultural education of those wanting to grasp an understanding of Aboriginal clients. In the Medicine Wheel philosophy, the basis of all thinking and acting lies in the unceasing effort to bring the four worlds,

FIGURE 1. Medicine Wheel

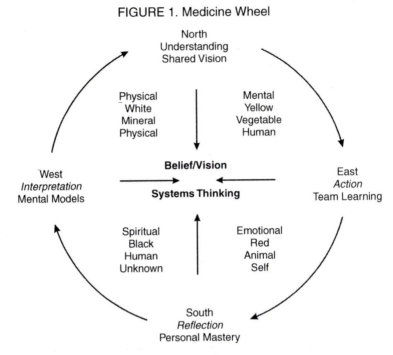

(Integration of Senge, 1990, 1994, and Bopp & Bopp, 1982)

Belief and vision occur at the center with the four components of knowledge–action, reflection, interpretation and understanding. These components are transposed with Senge's team learning, personal mastery, mental models and shared vision, with **systems thinking** as the central factor. This holistic framework is useful to those working in program and community development. Application to program development is discussed at the end of this article.

in whichever dimension they are being expressed, into perfect balance within the developing individual, his or her community, and all of Creation (Bopp & Bopp, 1982a).

Holistic thinking has been the underpinning of Native American consciousness and worldview since the earliest times. Well-known quotes attributed to Chief Seattle focus on the interconnectedness of all things. On the west coast of British Columbia, the Nuu-Chah-Nulth people have an expression "hishuk-ish-ts'awalk," which translated into English means "everything is one." The Dakota expression "mitakuye oyasin," which begins and ends many prayers, translates to "all my relations" in reference to all of Creation, i.e., all beings, past, present and future. A similar notion expressed by Ken Wilber (1998a) is one of "non-duality," meaning not dichotomized or fragmented, but inclusive of body and spirit, and even more so, one with the universe. Basically, these terms are all in reference to a way of acknowledging, not perceiving, reality. Wilber (1996) believes: "If we string these orienting generalizations together, we will arrive at some astonishing and often profound conclusions, conclusions that, extraordinary as they might be, nonetheless embody nothing more than our already agreed upon knowledge. These beads of knowledge are already accepted: It is only necessary to string them together into a necklace" (p. 18).

Wilber's Integral Philosophy

To understand the whole, it is necessary to understand the parts. To understand the parts it is necessary to understand the whole. Such is the circle of understanding. We move part to whole and back again, and in that dance of comprehension, in that amazing circle of understanding, we come alive to meaning, to value, and to vision: the very circle of understanding guides our way, weaving together the pieces, healing the fractures, mending the torn and tortured fragments, lighting the way ahead–this extraordinary movement from part to whole and back again, with healing the hallmark of each and every step, and grace the tender reward. (Wilber, 1998a, p. 1)

A genuinely holistic approach to viewing life is that espoused by Ken Wilber (1998a) in *The Eye of Spirit: An Integral Vision for a World Gone Slightly Mad*. Integral means integrative, inclusive, comprehensive, and balanced. Wilber applies this approach to various fields of human knowledge and endeavours, including the integration of science and spirituality. Jack Crittendon summarizes the approach:

Truths from such fields as physics and biology; the ecosciences; chaos theory and systems sciences; medicine; neurophysiology; biochemistry; art, poetry, and aesthetics in general; developmental psychology and a spectrum of psychotherapeutic endeavors, from Freud to Jung to Piaget; the Great Chain theorists from Plato and Plotinus in the West to Shankara and Nagarjuna in the East; the modernists from Descartes and Locke to Kant; the Idealists from Schelling to Hegel; the postmodernists from Foucalt and Derrida to Taylor and Habermas: the major hermeneutic tradition, Dilthey to Heidegger to Gadamer: the social, systems theorists from Comte and Marx to Parsons and Luhmann; the contemplative and mystical schools of the great meditative traditions, East and West, in the world's major religious traditions (cited in Wilber, 1998a, viii-xi).

Figure 2 provides an illustration of the various dimensions of Wilber's approach. The approach initially examines the evolution of consciousness, applies and compares this to the discipline of transpersonal psychology, and eventually explores the application of these theories to a host of other beliefs and disciplines.

It is my assertion that Aboriginal worldviews are indeed within the category of what Wilber calls the "perennial philosophies."[4] Perennial philosophies pay particular attention to "spirit,"[5] which is often missing from mainstream counselling approaches. Basically in his "four-quadrants" he has created his own 'medicine wheel' to explain human consciousness. Spousal abuse counselling in aboriginal communities can benefit from an approach that demands a comprehensive holistic theoretical base that underpins the work. The pragmatic work, where theory becomes practice, can then be articulated from such a perspective.

Wilber's approach covers all the major capacities of the "human bodymind" (i.e., physical, emotional, mental, social, cultural, spiritual; see Figure 2). In his research on worldviews, he attempted to find a single and basic "holarchy"[6] that he felt was common across cultures. Of the perennial philosophies worldwide, he distilled four factors that were in common to all. These factors discovered are actually very simple, yet inclusive or holistic. They are the *inside* and *outside* of a holon,[7] in both its *individual* and *collective* forms, and are referred to as the "Four Corners of the Kosmos" (Wilber, 1996, 1998a, 1998b). Aboriginal worldview and symbolism are remarkably similar as evident in the various Medicine Wheel configurations and perspectives. The directions of the medicine wheel are in fact meant to position oneself in the universe, relative to everything else, hence the expression "all my relations," which includes all of Creation, and all creatures, beings and spirits of the past, present and future. Wilber's theory is shown here in the same quadrant-circle configuration as the Medicine Wheel.

Aboriginal perspectives and Wilber's transpersonal psychology emphasize holism, change, and process. Both contend that material reality and spiritual reality are functionally inseparable, and that human beings exist in connection to all other aspects of Creation. Humans are in a process of becoming, and that as humans we transcend the limitations of materiality by virtue of our ability to direct the process of our own be-

FIGURE 2. Wilber's Integral Theory Transposed to the Medicine Wheel

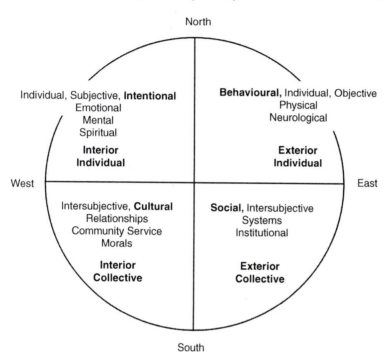

The system is that of a whole person in all his/her dimensions, and is the basis for the study of consciousness and transpersonal psychology (adapted from Wilber, 1996, 1997, 1998a).

coming. Aboriginal worldview is encapsulated in this statement: "The essence of human actualization is the process of coming to know and to love the ultimate unknowns underlying the ordering of the universe. This infinite process is expressed by individuals and by human collectives" (Bopp & Bopp, 1982a, pp. 8).

Role of Ritual and Ceremony in Therapy

Ritual is a significant part of counselling in the aboriginal community. As a counsellor training coordinator I received interesting feedback from our trainees. Trainees were placed in group counselling situations in mainstream agencies and were asked to comment on their experiences. Invariably what they said was missing was a formal opening ritual, such as a "smudge," a ritual cleansing used to begin most aboriginal counselling circles. Also absent was a symbolic object that embodied spiritual significance and a commitment to honesty, such as an eagle feather. Ritual can be trivialized by those not in touch with the spiritual aspect of existence; however, for cultures with a strong spiritual basis ritual is essential. It is not something that is mystical or impractical, but necessary to establish the tone and energy for the activity to follow.

When rituals and ceremonies are practiced, memory-energies are aroused, come alive, or awaken, as does the possibility for their repetition and replication in both physical and energetic form. In many indigenous cultures it is believed that spiritual energies can be influenced through ritual. The understanding is of oneness within spiritual-material construction, and that each cannot and does not occur without the other in human experience. Indeed the purpose of spiritual ritual is to access, to express, to recreate and experience spiritual energies or fields.

Rupert Sheldrake (1988) refers to the phenomenon that makes the revival of these memories possible as *morphic resonance*. In his theory, a field is a non-material region of influence; however, it can have a physical influence. He defines a morphic field as "A field within and around a morphic unit which organizes its characteristic structure and pattern of activity. Morphic fields underlie the form and behaviour of holons or morphic units at all levels of complexity. *The term morphic field includes morphogenetic, behavioural, social, cultural, and mental fields*" (p. 371). He further states "Fields interrelate and interconnect matter and energy within their realm of influence. Fields are not a form of matter, rather, matter is energy bound within fields" (p. 367). Some examples of fields in physics are gravitational and electro-magnetic fields, and the matter fields of quantum physics.

Central to the concept of morphic resonance is the transmission of forms and behaviours through repetition in time, in a pattern known as "formative causation," which theorizes that organisms or morphic units at all levels of complexity are organized by these fields. Sheldrake (1988) states, "Morphic fields are shaped and stabilized by morphic resonance from previous similar morphic units, which were under the influence of fields of the same kind. They consequently contain a kind of cumulative memory and tend to become increasingly habitual" (p. 371). It is explanations such as these that make an integral connection possible between spirituality and physical realities.

It is manifestations of these energies and forms Sheldrake is referring to that are awakened when organizations achieve 'synergy.' Lloyd

Haraala, an Ojibway elder (personal communication, April 1999) explains that the Eagle Sundance pledge meeting is highly ritualized because "we are trying to get a rhythm going here." It is these same energies that are awakened when a ceremonial participant has a spiritual experience. 'Knowing' in ritual is inherent in custom, tradition and in the continual invoking of energies, as well as in the doing. Certainly some of the great achievements experienced in human systems through true dialogue and principle-centered cooperation are no less spiritual experiences than those occurring in ceremonies. It is for these reasons that sweat lodge ceremonies, pipe ceremonies, and smudges are employed frequently and effectively in the format of the Change of Seasons and other First Nations men's spousal abuse counselling programs.

Group Facilitator as Therapist and Guide

The changes a group participant is guided through are part of a quest to achieve a higher level of consciousness. Thus, at the outset it is essential that the counsellor is aware of this: that their role is more than that of didactic educator. Transpersonal psychology can help determine where the damage has been done to a person and to a soul, and it can therefore be helpful in identifying the work that needs to be done to achieve a higher consciousness. Basically, it can identify what work needs to be done to transcend the damage that has occurred. The work needs to be able to move the person through the stages of consciousness not accessible because of the trauma experienced. A crucial part of this journey is to provide access to the stage where spirit is not only acknowledged, but where it can be experienced. Higher forms of consciousness manifest in "issues in social action of mercy and compassion on behalf of all sentient beings"(Wilber, 1998b, p. 8). Likewise, it is the objective of counselling, and the rituals that augment it, to raise the consciousness of clients to a point where they are cognizant of the imbalance in their relationships. This awareness of *conscience* that evolves through heightened experiences of ceremony and ritual provide peak experiences in which participants get a glimpse and taste of what is possible.

Many men perhaps do not relate well to the concept of spirituality that is so often referred to in Aboriginal cultures and traditions. This extraordinary and elusive part of our beings is so closely intertwined with the emotional, psychological and physical aspects that at first it is viewed as something fundamentally different and separate, but it is not. It is a common thread that binds all the other aspects. It is the ever-present element that allows us to appreciate the beauty of a sunrise. It is the sentiment that brings sadness to us when the sun is setting, or when we lose a close friend, relative or child. It may be that part of us that hurts when we abuse those we love, telling us that something is wrong and out of balance. It is the mystery that makes our children grow and develop as persons, the energy that makes us perform physical feats beyond our expectations, and the creativity that connects us to others through the spoken word, song, or artistic achievement. Without it there is no real life. Certainly *indigenous* peoples do not have a monopoly on this thing. It is something that can enrich the lives of all people.

MY PERSONAL CIRCLE OF UNDERSTANDING: THE CHANGE OF SEASONS

When I set out on this journey I had no great aspirations that my work would eventually touch the lives of hundreds of Aboriginal men. I had seen what spiritual involvement could do for others, but at the time was driven by the pragmatic notion that Aboriginal family violence could be addressed in more effective ways than those most widely used at the time. Those approaches were incarceration and disease model alcohol and drug programs. For a long time I was suggesting to others that our Aboriginal cultural and spiritual heritage could change lives for the better. The more I espoused this, the stronger the reality became for myself. The journey I was suggesting for others became a journey of my own, and many of my closest colleagues set out on similar paths.

It is not assumed that clients will immediately experience the higher levels of consciousness attainable through consistent and focused spiritual practice. The role of the therapist therefore is merely to assist clients in taking the first steps on this journey. In retrospect, I feel it is also important as counsellors to map our own development towards spirit, towards peace. What teachers, techniques and rituals helped us on our path? This knowledge can be useful to others. Counsellors must also rise to the challenge of confronting violence in our communities by returning to the spiritual ways of our ancestors. As leaders and guides for others we must develop those qualities and virtues in ourselves that promote the creation of healthy Aboriginal families and communities.

Rituals and Ceremonies in Change of Seasons Model

Ceremonies and rituals that effectively augment group counselling are the focus of this section. I will briefly touch upon those that are most common. These are the smudge, the talking circle, and the sweatlodge purification ceremony. Brief mention is made of the pipe ceremony.

In the manual *A Change of Seasons: A Training Manual for Counsellors Working with Aboriginal Men Who Abuse their Partners/Spouses* (Wood & Kiyoshk, 1998), the cultural content is integral to the program. Every third session is a cultural activity that augments the psycho-educational group format. However every session includes cultural and spiritual ritual and symbolism.

All the rituals mentioned are performed within a circle, either standing or sitting. The men's groups, which are the focus of this chapter, incorporate elements of the smudge as well as the talking circle; therefore, those topics will be covered first.

The Smudge Ceremony

A smudge ceremony is conducted at the beginning of each group session. A smudge is a means of cleansing oneself and one's surroundings of negative energies and thoughts. The primary element necessary for this ritual is an herb for burning as an offering. In most common use are sage, sweetgrass, cedar and juniper. The herb is lighted with a wooden match so as to smolder in a container such as a seashell, a flat or hollow rock, or similar vessel. Participants stand in a circle, and the person leading the ceremony will fan the smoldering herb with an eagle feather or fan. As he passes from person to person, each person wafts the smoke over themselves with their hands in a motion similar to washing themselves. As each person does this, the leader holds the feather or fan over their heads. Each person is involved in a silent prayer or meditation at this time; as prayer is a private, it is impolite for others in the circle to be staring at one another. Sometimes participants smudge their personal effects such as medicine pouches or jewelry. The herbs used are held to be sacred by those performing and/or participating in the ritual, and are considered to be gifts from the Creator. Each of these herbs has a special significance to the tribes in the territory to which they are indigenous. These gifts are from the plant world, and are given so curing and healing of the mind, body and spirit may occur when respectfully used. The smoke signifies that one's prayers are being sent to the Creator. This ritual is performed prior to any event of significance to ensure success and productivity. It can be performed in private, particularly to greet a new day, or whenever it is needed. In the case of a men's group, it is done to create a positive atmosphere and to ensure that one's words are forthcoming and truthful.

Talking Circle

This ritual is used in the personal sharing segment of each session. A talking circle is simply a gathering of people who have something of importance to talk about. Sometimes it is referred to as a sharing circle. When people come together in this way, respectful conduct is imperative and a given. The leader of the circle is generally a person held in high regard by those assembled. Hopefully this will be the case in an abusive men's group. In a talking circle, everything said is held to be strictly confidential. The leader usually describes the process and protocol of the circle. An object of some spiritual significance, sometimes called a "power object," is held by the speaker; for example, an object such as an eagle feather or a rock can be used. Customarily in a talking circle, people share whatever is on their mind and they are allowed to continue uninterrupted for whatever time they require. Others do not get up and leave or talk amongst themselves while sharing is occurring. When finished, the speaker utters words of closure and passes the power object to the person on their left. This person will then share, or pass the object with acknowledgment by offering words such as "all my relations" or "thank you" in their native tongue. Opting out however, is not always an option in a men's group.

The key difference in a men's group, however, is that after sharing a man will place the sacred object in the center of the circle and he then will be given feedback and/or confronted on what he has shared. Also, he will be required to stick to the topic at hand, usually concerning his abusive behaviour. In these instances, the sacred object of the culture is used to facilitate truthful sharing, and cannot be used to avoid feedback and confrontation. Generally, both types of sharing are preceded by a smudge.

The Sweatlodge Ceremony

The sweatlodge ceremony, a rite of purification, is probably the most common of all Native North American ceremonies. It is used for physical, mental and spiritual cleansing. It is usually done in preparation to any major undertaking, such as Sundancing or Fasting.

The lodge itself is circular in layout, with a dome-like shape. The lodge is usually no more than four feet high and varies in width from one culture/society to another. The direction in which the door of the lodge faces also varies across cultures, usually predicated by the season or society. The number of saplings, and the type of wood used to construct the frame is also determined by the society and purpose of the ceremony. There are many variations, but willow is most common. The frame was traditionally covered with hides, but today tarps and blankets are used. The lodge is completely dark within to allow the Spirits to visit when summoning prayers and offerings are made.

A fire is built at a specified distance from the lodge. This distance is stipulated by the society. In this *sacred fire*, rocks are heated until they are red hot. These rocks are referred to as *Grandfathers* in the native tongue. The number of rocks varies according to the purpose of the ceremony. Participants usually smudge and/or offer tobacco in the sacred fire before entering the lodge. The rocks, once heated, are brought into the lodge and placed in a pit in the center. All movement within the lodge is in a clockwise direction, as well as movement outside the lodge. Once all participants have taken their place, prayers are offered verbally and/or through songs, and herbs are sprinkled upon the red hot Grandfathers. Water then is splashed upon the rocks causing steam and intense heat within the lodge. The ceremony generally consists of four rounds, but I have been in ceremonies that have involved two and three rounds. A round is a time of praying, singing and chanting, and is dedicated to a specific purpose. At the end of the round, the door flap is opened for a breath of fresh air. On some occasions a sacred pipe is used in the ceremony.

What is shared during the sweatlodge ceremony is viewed as sacred and therefore is not for discussion outside of the lodge, except perhaps when consulting with an Elder or spiritual leader. Within the lodge, a participant can remove the masks that are worn in daily life, and is open to receive healing from the spiritual energies. The sweatlodge is viewed as a womb, and participants are renewed through ritual. This is an ideal place for releasing tension, shame and guilt, and an appropriate place to make or reaffirm commitments to positive change. This ritual is introduced with a didactic overview of the ceremony to prepare those who are not familiar with the practice. It is effectively used after particularly difficult sessions, such as sessions involving discussion of the most violent incident or the family of origin, or when the woman has shared her story.

The Pipe Ceremony

The smoking of the sacred pipe is viewed as a prerequisite to all events of significance by all Nations that have the pipe as part of their traditions. Perhaps the strongest message that First Nations can offer the mainstream society is embodied in this ritual. The pipe bowl and stem are viewed as being female and male respectively, and joining of the two is essential for the successful and natural completion of any task. It is symbolic of male and female forces working together for the betterment of humanity. Out of the joining of these two separate entities comes the potential for the creation of something that is more than the sum of the parts. In this ceremony lies the potential for the creation of humanity, for the creation of Life. Likewise, effective First Nations approaches to dealing with family violence are cooperative in nature rather than adversarial. This differs from the time-proven ineffectiveness of approaches that employ methods such as jail therapy and shame-basing. The pipe carrier offers prayers to the Creator, by offering the pipe to the six directions of the universe. The smoke from the tobacco takes one's prayers to the far-reaching corners of the universe, to the *Great Mystery*.

This brief description of some of the ceremonies included in the program for aboriginal men was written to provide information about cultural tools that may complement existing programs. Numerous other ceremonies exist, such as ceremonial dancing, fasting, and cold water purification baths in mountain streams and pools. However, a culturally appropriate program consists of more than merely beginning sessions with a smudge or a prayer. A minimum of paper work is given out on cultural teachings. Concepts can be explained in charts and diagrams in black and white, but the real learning and *transformation* comes from involvement. The real long-term goal of this type of treatment is for the men to practice these things daily throughout their lives.

SYSTEMS THINKING IN COMMUNITY AND PROGRAM DEVELOPMENT

A system is a collection of parts that interact with each other to function as a whole. We may associate the word "system" with everyday terms such as social system, nervous system, legal system, or information system. For many years, scientists believed the best way to learn about something was to take it apart and find out what it was made of. This approach has been somewhat useful in physics, biology and chemistry. However, when this approach is taken to its extreme it is known as "reductionism," meaning that something is nothing but the sum of its parts. In the 1920s, a group of scientists who realized the shortcomings of this approach began a serious study of the *patterns* of interactions taking place between the parts, in fact looking at the *organization* of things. An interesting discovery was that no matter how different the ingredients of different systems looked, they were put together according to the same *general rules of organization.* This new field of study provided a linking together of numerous fields of knowledge, showing what they had in common. It became known as *"general systems theory"* (Kauffman, 1980). This knowledge underpins today's technological and human systems, and provides important direction for managing massive growth and change.

System thinking is a solid foundation for effective Aboriginal program and community development initiatives. The work of Peter Senge and the MIT-grounded systems thinking applied to organizational development gained widespread recognition as a result of the book *The Fifth Discipline: The Art and Practice of the Learning Organization* (Senge, 1990). This book presents the basic criteria necessary for the creation and maintenance of a *learning organization.* These "disciplines" are: *personal mastery, mental models, building shared vision,* and *team learning.* The fifth discipline, *systems thinking*, integrates the other four into a coherent body of theory and practice. These disciplines working in synergistic fashion create a place where people are continually discovering how they create their reality, and how they can change it. In such an organization, a shift in thinking occurs that is conducive to heightened experiences of creativity, and learning takes on a meaning well beyond its conventional usage (Senge, 1990). The five disciplines advanced by Senge are briefly summarized here.

Personal Mastery is learning to expand our personal capacity to create the results we most desire, and creating an organizational environment that encourages all its members to develop themselves toward the goals and purposes they choose. Personal mastery means developing both people skills as well as skilled knowledge and managerial competency.

Mental Models is reflecting upon, continually clarifying, and improving our internal pictures of the world, and seeing how they shape our actions and decisions.

Shared Vision is building a sense of commitment in a group, by developing shared images of the future we seek to create, and the principles and guiding practices by which we hope to get there.

Team Learning is transforming conversational and collective thinking skills in terms of open dialogue, so that groups of people can reliably develop intelligence and ability greater than the sum of the individual members' talents.

Systems Thinking is a way of thinking about and a language for describing and understanding, the forces and interrelationships that shape the behaviour of systems. This discipline helps us to change systems more effectively, and to act more in tune with the larger processes of the natural and economic world (Senge, Kleiner, Roberts, Ross, & Smith, 1994).

Culturally Appropriate Initiatives

Community and program development work requires that we know the history and dynamics of the local area. Aboriginal communities are a collective of the individual experiences of its members. As they are also systems, systems thinking approaches are suitable and applicable to them.

Historically, the systems perspectives integral to Aboriginal peoples' existence were of a pragmatic nature. The following quote from Vine Deloria (1995) demonstrates their practical application:

> Indians came to understand that all things were related, and while many tribes understood this knowledge in terms of religious rituals, it was also a methodology/guideline which instructed them in making their observations of the behavior of other forms of life. Attuned to their environment, Indians could find food, locate trails, protect themselves from inclement weather, and anticipate coming events by their understanding of how entities related to each other. (p. 57)

This notion of practical, relational interdependence needs to be revisited in our Aboriginal communities. An excellent resource for the practical applications of systems theory for building community is *The Fifth Discipline Fieldbook: Strategies and Tools for Building a Learning Organization* (Senge et al., 1994).

CONCLUSION

The First Peoples of North America have held out against the ravages of colonization for several centuries. The survival of the indigenous peoples in these demanding circumstances can be largely attributed to their adaptability to ever changing environments. Having made it this far through repeated cycles of crisis and renewal, the current challenge is to live within the structures of modern day society and contribute to positive change. The challenge is not only to survive, but also to thrive in a complex world of government and politics, business and economics, education and technology, while restoring and maintaining customary values and traditions. The key to survival has been a worldview that does not separate spirituality from everyday life. This characteristic is also what ensures success in counselling assaultive men.

NOTES

1. Aboriginal: Terms often used in reference to Native North Americans are *indigenous, Native,* and/or *Aboriginal.* In Canada a widely used term is *First Nations.* For clarity and to appeal to an international audience *Aboriginal* is used here most frequently. Other synonymous terms will be used only in the context of quotes or titles.

2. Anomie: a loss of identity resulting in a sense of alienation and confusion.

3. Worldview: 1. Cosmology, study of the order of the universe. 2. a perception of the world in which one lives (Corrigan, 1995). The term *worldview* will be used here to describe cultural perspectives, or ways of perceiving reality.

4. Perennial philosophy: "the worldview that has been embraced by the vast majority of the world's greatest spiritual teachers, philosophers, thinkers, and even scientists. It's called 'perennial' or 'universal' because it shows up in virtually all cultures across the globe and across the ages" (Wilber, 1998b, p. 7), and, "that absolute Truth which is timeless, formless, and spaceless, radically whole and complete, outside of which nothing exists–a Truth that can be known, but which can never be adequately or fully captured in any form, doctrine, system, philosophy, proposition, thought or idea . . ." (Wilber, 1998a, p. 60).

5. Spirit: "the upper reaches of consciousness itself . . . a Spirit that shines forth in every I and every we and every it, a Spirit that sings as the rain and dances as the wind, a Spirit of which every conversation is the sincerest worship, a Spirit that speaks with your tongue and looks out from your eyes, that touches with these hands and cries out with this voice–and a Spirit that has always whispered lovingly in our ears: Never forget the Good, and never forget the True, and never forget the Beautiful" (Wilber, 1998a, pp. 35-36).

6. Holarchy: in systems theory, all complex hierarchies are composed of holons, or increasing orders of wholeness, hence holarchy is the word for a *growth* or *actualization hierarchy.*

7. Holon: a whole that is a part of other wholes, e.g. a whole atom is part of a whole molecule; a whole molecule is part of a whole cell, and so forth.

REFERENCES

American Psychiatric Association. (2000). *Diagnostic and statistical manual of mental disorders* (4th ed., text rev.). Washington, DC: Author.

Bopp, M., & Bopp, J. (1982a). *Overview: The four worlds development project.* Alberta: University of Lethbridge.

Bopp, M., & Bopp, J. (1982b). *The sacred tree*. Lethbridge: Four Worlds.

British Columbia Task Force on Family Violence. (1992). *Is anyone listening?* Victoria, B.C.: Ministry of Women's Equality.

Corrigan, S. (1995). *Readings in aboriginal studies: World View* (Vol. 3). Brandon: Bearpaw, Brandon University.

Deloria, V. (1995). *Red earth: White lies*. New York: Scribner.

Frank, S. (1992). *Family violence in Aboriginal communities*. Victoria, B.C.: Ministry of Women's equality.

Hall, A. J. (1999). *Ethnic cleansing and genocide in North America and Kosovo*. Unpublished manuscript.

Kauffman, D. (1980). *Systems one: An introduction to systems thinking*. Minneapolis: Future Systems.

Kiyoshk, R. (2001). *Family violence in Aboriginal communities. A review*. Ottawa: The Aboriginal Nurses Association of Canada and Royal Canadian Mounted Police.

Royal Commission on Aboriginal Peoples. (1996). *Royal Commission on Aboriginal Peoples–Final report*. Ottawa: Ministry of Supply & Services.

Senge, P. (1990). *The fifth discipline: The art & practice of the learning organization*. New York: Currency Doubleday.

Senge, P., Kleiner, A., Roberts, C., Ross, R.B., & Smith, B.J. (1994). *The fifth discipline fieldbook: Strategies and tools for building a learning organization*. New York: Currency Doubleday.

Sheldrake, R. (1988). *The presence of the past: Morphic resonance and the habits of nature*. New York: Random House.

Wilber, K. (1996). *A brief history of everything*. Boston: Shambhala.

Wilber, K. (1998a). *The eye of spirit: An integral vision for a world gone slightly mad*. Boston: Shambhala.

Wilber, K. (1998b). *The essential Ken Wilber*. Boston: Shambhala.

Wood, B., & Kiyoshk, R. (1998). *A change of seasons: A training manual for counsellors working with aboriginal men who abuse their partners/spouses* (Rev. ed.). North Vancouver: Change of Seasons Society.

Treatment of Partner Aggressive Women

Penny A. Leisring
Lynn Dowd
Alan Rosenbaum

SUMMARY. The examination of partner aggression perpetrated by women has been a controversial but important development in domestic violence research. Previous studies have suggested that women's use of aggression in romantic relationships may place women at increased risk of being assaulted by their partners. Furthermore, children who witness the aggression may be at increased risk for mental health and behavioral problems. This article describes what we know about the characteristics of partner aggressive women, and how this information might inform our understanding of their behavior and the design of treatment programs to assist them. The group treatment program for partner aggressive woman at the University of Massachusetts Medical School is described in detail. Recommendations about necessary components of treatment for aggressive women and a description of how treatment for female perpetrators should differ from treatment for male batterers are provided. Suggestions are made for future research to evaluate current programs and to further develop and refine effective treatments. *[Article copies available for a fee from The Haworth Document Delivery Service: 1-800-HAWORTH. E-mail address: <docdelivery@haworthpress.com> Website: <http://www.HaworthPress.com> © 2003 by The Haworth Press, Inc. All rights reserved.]*

Address correspondence to: Penny A. Leisring, PhD, Quinnipiac University, Department of Psychology, 275 Mount Carmel Avenue, Hamden, CT 06518-1940 (E-mail: penny.leisring@quinnipiac.edu).

[Haworth co-indexing entry note]: "Treatment of Partner Aggressive Women." Leisring, Penny A., Lynn Dowd, and Alan Rosenbaum. Co-published simultaneously in *Journal of Aggression, Maltreatment & Trauma* (The Haworth Maltreatment & Trauma Press, an imprint of The Haworth Press, Inc.) Vol. 7, No. 1/2 (#13/14), 2003, pp. 257-277; and: *Intimate Violence: Contemporary Treatment Innovations* (ed: Donald Dutton, and Daniel J. Sonkin) The Haworth Maltreatment & Trauma Press, an imprint of The Haworth Press, Inc., 2003, pp. 257-277. Single or multiple copies of this article are available for a fee from The Haworth Document Delivery Service [1-800-HAWORTH, 9:00 a.m. - 5:00 p.m. (EST). E-mail address: docdelivery@haworthpress.com].

http://www.haworthpress.com/store/product.asp?sku=J146
© 2003 by The Haworth Press, Inc. All rights reserved.
10.1300J146v07n01_11

KEYWORDS. Domestic violence, treatment, aggression, female perpetrators, family violence

Most research conducted on partner aggression has examined male to female violence, due to findings from crime surveys demonstrating that most perpetrators of partner aggression are male (Kurz, 1993). However, national surveys asking respondents about family problems have found that approximately equal numbers of men and women assault their partners (Straus & Gelles, 1990). While much research has been conducted about male-perpetrated aggression, far less has been conducted on women's violence toward male partners. With the exception of work by Hamberger and Potente (1994), Nichols and Dutton (2001) and Dowd (2001), little information is available to guide those engaging in the treatment of partner aggressive women. This article will provide a brief summary of the controversy surrounding women's aggression, an overview of the characteristics of partner aggressive women, and a description of the similarities and differences between group treatment formats for partner aggressive men and women. In addition, suggestions for further research will be offered.

THE CONTROVERSY SURROUNDING WOMEN'S AGGRESSION

Female perpetration of relationship aggression has been a controversial topic (Saunders, 1986; Straus, 1993). For various reasons it has been suggested that aggression by women should not be examined. One reason to avoid addressing women's aggression is the fact that male to female partner aggression is considered to be more serious and damaging than female to male aggression. This is in part due to the difference in the severity of consequences resulting from aggression perpetrated by men and women. Cascardi, Langhinrichsen, and Vivian (1992) found that wives were more likely than husbands to be negatively affected by marital aggression, and wives were more likely than husbands to have clinical levels of depressive symptomatology. Injuries resulting from male to female aggression occur more frequently and tend to be more severe than injuries resulting from female to male aggression (Cascardi et al., 1992; Vivian & Langhinrichsen-Rohling, 1994). In addition, Stets and Straus (1990) found that female victims of partner aggression were more likely than male victims to require medical treatment as a result of partner aggression.

The feminist perspective on domestic violence has been extremely influential in the field and brought the issue of domestic violence to public attention in the 1970s (Dobash & Dobash, 1979). This perspective views partner violence as a "tactic of entitlement that is deeply gendered, rather than as a conflict tactic that is personal and gender neutral" (Yllo, 1993, p. 57). Male privileges of power and control over women, which are reinforced by societal factors, are thought to be at the heart of domestic violence. This perspective has greatly influenced the structure of treatment for male batterers and the "Power and Control" wheel developed by Pence and Paymar (1993) is one of the most commonly discussed and emphasized topics in treatment for male perpetrators of domestic violence (Rosenbaum & Leisring, 2001). The wheel was designed with input by over 200 battered women in Duluth, Minnesota (Pence & Paymar, 1993). It details the many tactics that men use in addition to physical violence to control their partners, including behaviors such as economic abuse, male privilege, coercion, intimidation, emotional abuse, isolation, using children, and minimizing abuse (Pence & Paymar, 1993). Violence is thought to take place within the context of inequality between men and women (Kurz, 1993) and thus, the feminist view has encouraged a focus on male rather than female perpetrators.

Addressing women's aggression has also been discouraged due to fear that attending to women's aggression may be invoked as an excuse for male perpetrated aggression and result in victim-blaming (Kurz, 1993). Because many partner aggressive women are also victimized by their partners (Hamberger & Potente, 1994; Stets & Straus, 1990), female aggression is often viewed as self-defensive or retaliatory, and not as the mirror image of male aggression. Understanding the dynamics and consequences of women's use of aggression, as we will argue, might have implications for the safety and well being of women and children that are too significant to ignore out of fear that this information might be misinterpreted or misused. Helping women to take responsibility for their own behavior and to choose non-violent ways of solving conflict does not place the responsibility for all relationship aggression on them.

According to family violence surveys, approximately 12% of women and men assault their romantic partners per year (Straus & Gelles, 1990). Severe assaults against partners are perpetrated by 4.8% of women and 3.4% of men each year (Straus & Gelles, 1990). Women's violence has been explained as occurring in self-defense (Saunders, 1986). Women who have been arrested for partner aggression have been described as being primarily battered women who are fighting back in self-defense, in retaliation for prior abuse by their partners, or to protect themselves from imminent violence by their partners (Hamberger, 1997; Hamberger & Potente, 1994). This may be the case for some, and perhaps for a significant portion of the population. However, women have been found to initiate aggression in relationships as often as men (Straus & Gelles, 1990) and women have been found to be the sole aggressor within the past year in 25.5% of violent couples (Straus, 1993). Men were the sole aggressor in 25.9% of cases, and both partners were violent in 48.6% of the cases (Straus, 1993). Thus, the degree to which women are aggressing against their partners in self-defense is unclear.

Although there are realistic concerns about attending to, or addressing, female to male aggression, women are being arrested and sent to diversion programs for treatment. Without sufficient research examining women's aggression, clinicians working with partner aggressive women cannot look to the literature for effective interventions. Programs designed for aggressive men may not be well suited for aggressive women. At the University of Massachusetts Medical School (UMass), the treatment program for male batterers has been substantially modified to fit the needs of aggressive women presenting for treatment.

THE IMPORTANCE OF ADDRESSING WOMEN'S AGGRESSION

Family violence researchers have pointed out that relationship aggression affects all family members in destructive ways (Straus & Gelles, 1990). Aggression perpetrated by women, as well as by men, negatively affects child witnesses (Jaffe, Wolfe, & Wilson, 1990; Straus, Gelles, & Steinmetz, 1980). Children exposed to violence in their family of origin are more likely than other children to develop psychopathology including depression, anxiety, conduct problems, and aggressive behavior (Cummings & Davies, 1994; Jouriles, Murphy, & O'Leary, 1989). Rosenbaum and O'Leary (1981) found that 45% of male batterers witnessed partner aggression in their families of origin while growing up. Witnessing aggression in one's family of origin is one of the most consistent predictors of male-perpetrated partner aggression (Feldman, 1997). Prevention of aggression by men *and women* may reduce the rates of child psychopathology and the intergenerational transmission of domestic violence.

In addition, successfully treating aggressive women may ultimately prevent aggression perpetrated against women. Feld and Straus (1989) found that women's mild aggression toward their spouses predicted future severe violence perpetrated by their husbands against them. Murphy and O'Leary (1989) found that even psychological aggression perpetrated by women predicted future physical violence by their husbands. Furthermore, women's use of psychological aggression has been shown to predict future physical aggression by husbands who have not previously been physically aggressive (Murphy & O'Leary, 1989). Thus, not only are women who engage in psychological aggression at risk of engaging in future physical aggression themselves but they are at risk of being physically victimized by their partners even if their partners have not previously been physically violent. Slapping their husbands or putting their husbands down verbally may be placing women in danger of being assaulted by their partners in the future. Women's actions do not justify men's violence and women should not be blamed for the actions of men. Men must be held accountable for their perpetration of domestic violence. Similarly, women should also be held accountable for their use of verbal and physical aggression.

CHARACTERISTICS OF WOMEN
WHO ASSAULT THEIR PARTNERS

Unfortunately little research has been done to shed light on the nature of this population, and much of the information available is embedded in the literature in a way that is fragmented and difficult to access directly. As is the case with male batterers, domestically violent women are likely a diverse group, ranging from those who engage in infrequent and mild aggression which has been called "ordinary marital violence" (Straus, 1990, p. 405) and "common couple violence" (Johnson, 1995), to women who use or threaten to use weapons and who inflict serious injury on their partners. To date, only a few small samples of domestically violent women have been described in the literature. Issues of context, and motivation in particular, have not been fully explored across groups of domestically violent women. There are problems in making assumptions and generalizations across potentially dissimilar groups of domestically violent women, such as representative community samples and clinical samples (Kwong, Bartholomew, & Dutton, 1999; Straus, 1993; Straus, 1999).

While the focus of this paper is primarily on heterosexual women who assault male partners, there exists a substantial literature on partner assault in lesbian couples. The prevalence of violence in lesbian couples is thought to equal, or exceed, that in heterosexual couples, ranging among studies from 30% to 75% (Waldner-Haugrud, Gratch, & Magruder, 1997). Partner aggressive lesbians have been described as unable to relate empathetically to their partners, fearful of abandonment, dependent, jealous, and as having poor communication skills (Leeder, 1988; Renzetti, 1988).

A picture of heterosexual women who are treated for partner aggression is beginning to emerge, based on several court-mandated samples that have been described in the past few years (Abel, 1999; Hamberger, 1997; Leisring, Dowd, & Rosenbaum, 1999). The Abel (1999) and Hamberger (1997) samples were composed of women who were arrested specifically for domestic violence, while the women in the Leisring et al. (1999) sample were mandated to anger management treatment for a variety of interpersonally aggressive acts, including partner aggression. The women in all three samples reported high rates of childhood victimization of all types, as well as physical victimization in adulthood. Over a third of the Leisring et al. (1999) sample and over half of the Hamberger (1997) sample reported having witnessed parental aggression. Past and current substance abuse was a significant problem for many women across the samples. In the Leisring et al. (1999) sample, nearly two thirds of the women had a history of outpatient mental health treatment, and nearly a third had attempted suicide at least once. It has also been found that approximately 45% of the women in the anger management program at UMass were experiencing clinical levels of posttraumatic stress disorder symptoms at the time of admission into the program (Leisring, Dowd, & Rosenbaum, 2000). Abel (1999) found that women in batterer treatment programs appeared to be more similar to female domestic violence victims than to male batterers in terms of arrest history, victimization history, social service utilization, and trauma symptomology. In summary, women mandated to treatment for partner aggression are likely to have been previously traumatized and are at high risk for substance abuse, Posttraumatic Stress Disorder (PTSD), and other mental health problems.

In addition to the above areas of investigation, a growing literature on adult attachment has begun to focus on marital violence in recent years. A number of studies have explored attachment styles and their correlates in domestically violent men (e.g., Dutton, Saunders, Starzomski, & Bartholomew, 1994; Sonkin & Dutton, 2003) and their victims (Dutton & Haring, 1999; Kesner & McKenry, 1998). Dutton et al. (1994) found that anxious attachment was associated with abusiveness in men. We are unaware of any parallel findings about attachment style and domestically violent women, although the link between attachment disturbances, trauma, and complex posttraumatic stress disorder has been noted for women hospitalized for trauma-related disorders (Allen, Coyne, & Huntoon, 1998). Based on the above discussion, it is tempting to speculate that a problematic attachment style, formed in an environment of ongoing psychological, physical, and/or sexual injury, and exacerbated in later years by accompanying mental health and substance abuse issues, could be a significant vehicle for the intergenerational transmission of domestic violence for women.

GROUP TREATMENT FOR AGGRESSIVE WOMEN

Lacking treatment models tailored to domestically violent women, a natural strategy was to base treatment for aggressive women on male batterer treatment programs. General guidelines and many treatment modules typically included in treatment programs for men are also relevant to the treatment of aggressive women, and will be reviewed here. However, as Hamberger and Potente (1994) have pointed out, treatment for aggressive women should differ from treatment for aggressive men because aggressive women have unique needs. Six modifications to men's treatment protocols, based on current knowledge of aggressive women and our experiences treating them over the past four years, will be described.

Description of Guidelines for UMass' Men's and Women's Programs

An initial intake evaluation is performed, with special attention to circumstances surrounding the referral incident, previous aggression, and patterns of initiation and interaction in relationships in which aggression has occurred. Treatment is offered through groups, which meet weekly for 90 minutes, for 20 weeks. Group rules include a commitment to keeping information about each other confidential, and abstinence from drugs or alcohol prior to coming to group.

Clinical Experience with Partner Aggressive Women

The first and second authors of this paper have experience leading both men's batterers' groups and women's anger management groups. The observations described in this section are derived not from research, but on experience working with both partner aggressive men and women treated in the domestic violence programs at UMass. The women's groups seem to build more cohesiveness than the men's groups. Women seem on average to be less resistant during initial sessions than men and they are more willing to take responsibility for their actions than men. The majority of the women are parents, and many are motivated to change for the sake of their children. The women typically provide each other with support, encouragement, and information about resources in the community. They require more referrals for treatment of depression, PTSD, substance abuse, and parenting skills in addition to the anger management program. It is not unusual for numerous group members in a given session to discuss pressing issues such as severe depression, suicidal ideation, addictions, and homelessness in addition to difficulties with anger or aggression.

Treatment Components Modeled from Treatment Components for Men

Partner abusive women, as we have stated, are often victims, as well as perpetrators, of domestic aggression. Group leaders must remain aware of this possibility and sensitive to its implications for treatment. Many of these considerations are discussed later as modifications of batterer treatment programs. However, in each of the strategies employed in group, whether borrowed from treatment for male batterers, or unique to the treatment of female perpetrators, safety considerations are always paramount. Nine components typically incorporated in treatment programs for men will be described here in detail (cf. Dutton, 2002; Waltz, 2002). We feel that these components should be incorporated into treatment for aggressive women.

Component 1: Teach women to be responsible for their own actions. Partner aggressive women need to recognize that their partners do not "make" them engage in psychological or physical aggression. Women are taught that engaging in aggressive behavior is a choice that they have made. They are encouraged to recognize that there are usually alternative ways to handle situations and that aggression is not their only choice. This goal is accomplished by brainstorming various ways of handling a conflict. For example, options may include taking time-outs, explaining to their partner why they are angry in a non-threatening and constructive way, ignoring the situation temporarily while using skills to reduce arousal, or calling someone for support and/or guidance.

Component 2: Teach women to recognize anger signs. Women are taught that anger occurs on a continuum. Learning to recognize anger cues, such as the physical sensations in their bodies, the cognitions, and the behavior that they typically engage in at various points along the continuum, is emphasized early in the program. They are encouraged to use these as early warning signs to become aware that their anger is escalating. Once they recognize that their anger is escalating they can stop and think about the various options available for handling their present situation and de-escalating their anger. Women are also taught to identify situations and times when they are most likely to have difficulty with anger management.

Component 3: Teach women how to use time-outs safely. The time-out technique is presented as a method to prevent the dangerous escalation of anger in one or both partners. Women are taught the steps involved in taking a time-out: making the decision to leave, knowing all available exits, engaging in calming activities during the time-out, and calling the partner prior to returning to determine if he is calm enough for her to return. Women are encouraged to talk to their partners about the purpose and elements of time-out at a time when they are both calm. In addition, women are encouraged after each time-out to discuss the original problematic issue with their partner or to set a time in the future to discuss the issue. Discussing the technique ahead of time and eventually discussing difficult issues will increase the likelihood that the partners of the women will agree that time-outs should be used in their relationship. However, despite these efforts some partners may feel threatened or abandoned by their partners' attempts to take time-outs and may attempt to struggle with the women to keep them from taking a time-out. Women are encouraged to evaluate whether they can feel safe in a home with a partner who will not allow them to take time-outs.

Component 4: Teach women about the consequences of their own aggression. A brainstorming exercise is used to help group members identify the consequences, for themselves and others, of their own aggression. Most poignant is the discussion about the effects of aggression on witnessing children. Many women in the program have open cases with child protection agencies because, in Massachusetts, exposing children to inter-parental aggression is considered a form of child neglect. Increases in child behavior problems and psychopathology as a result of witnessing aggression are discussed. Potential consequences of aggression for their partners, such as injuries, fear, and depression are mentioned, but are not emphasized as much as in men's treatment due to the lower frequency of these consequences resulting from women's violence. The women discuss the consequences of their anger and aggression for themselves at length. These often include: relationship strain or loss, guilt, stress, legal charges, financial strain, effects on their job, and effects on their health. Women are also informed about the research findings of Feld and Straus (1989) and Murphy and O'Leary (1989) suggesting that their use of physical and psychological aggression may place them at risk for being physically victimized by their partners in the future.

Component 5: Teach women about the "anger suitcase." The feelings typically underlying anger are identified in a brainstorming exercise. The "anger suitcase" is described as a container for a mixture of important feelings that may be difficult to identify and communicate. Identifying feelings that underlie anger guides us in determining how to handle a situation. Women typically identify any combination of the following underlying feelings: jealous, sad, hurt, powerless, confused, afraid, frustrated, irritated, anxious, insecure, humiliated, trapped, unheard, overwhelmed, betrayed, embarrassed, disrespected, abandoned, stressed, and insulted. Many women describe feeling angry when they engage in psychological or physical aggression. It is hoped that helping them to recognize and label the feelings underlying their anger will aid them in generating appropriate behaviors to reduce their negative feelings. They are encouraged to communicate with others in an effective manner instead of escalating a situation by engaging in psychological or physical aggression.

Component 6: Communication training. Effective communication skills are discussed and demonstrated through role-plays. Women are encouraged to communicate their feelings in non-threatening ways. They are taught to attend to the content of their speech and their tone of voice and they are urged to communicate using "I statements" instead of "you statements." It is suggested that they avoid using words like "never" and "always" and they are encouraged to suggest reasonable compromises to problems. Women are taught to communicate in an assertive, non-aggressive manner to get their needs met. This is similar to communication training in treatment for partner aggressive men but a focus on maintaining the safety of the women in the program is given priority. Previously it has been suggested that teaching abused wives to be more assertive may place them at risk of being victimized by their partners in the future (O'Leary, Curley, Rosenbaum, & Clarke, 1986). Women remaining in abusive relationships are encouraged to continually monitor their safety. If they are concerned that their partners may respond aggressively to assertive communication, they are urged to communicate in ways that will ensure their safety and the safety of their children. Meanwhile, they are supported to make their own decisions about whether they want to remain in relationships in which they feel unsafe.

Component 7: Changing cognitions. Emphasis is placed on the role of thoughts in anger escalation and de-escalation. Women are taught to recognize several types of thinking errors that can lead to increased distress and they are urged to engage in alternative ways of thinking that can reduce distress. The role of extreme thinking, false assumptions, and inappropriate attributions is discussed. Specifically, women are encouraged to avoid the following: labeling themselves and others, mind reading, fortune telling, and exaggerating. They are taught to take responsibility for their own actions but not for the actions of others. These techniques are often used in cognitive therapy for depression (see Beck, 1995, for a thorough description of cognitive techniques).

Component 8: Alcohol and substance abuse. While alcohol and other substance use does not directly *cause* aggression, their use does significantly predict marital aggression in males (Pan, Neidig, & O'Leary, 1994). The differences among substance use, substance abuse, and addiction are discussed by group members. Treatment options for substance abuse are discussed and group members are given handouts with contact information about local substance abuse treatment facilities. Typically each women's anger management group has several members in it who are in recovery from addiction. These members often share their experiences with others, including the relationships between their substance use and aggression in their lives, and their use of 12-step recovery programs. Group members currently abusing substances are strongly encouraged by group leaders and other group members to seek substance abuse counseling in addition to anger management.

Component 9: Stress reduction. Group members often describe themselves as being under significant stress. Straus, Gelles, and Steinmetz (1980) found that over 50% of women with 10 or more life stressors were aggressive toward their husbands. Group members are taught problem-solving skills to help them relieve stress. Cognitive-behavioral skills such as deep-muscle relaxation, deep breathing, and mental imagery are demonstrated during group sessions. In addition, women discuss other appropriate methods for handling stress such as exercising, listening to music, reading, etc. Group members are encouraged to engage in stress-reducing activities on a regular basis.

Modifications of Group Treatment for Men

The treatment program for partner aggressive women at UMass has been evolving since it began in 1996. Since the start of the women's program, it has become evident that several modifications to the men's program were necessary due to women's unique needs. Over the years, this program has been changing in response to our awareness of the relevant issues. The following modifications to men's treatment have been incorporated into the women's treatment program at UMass.

Modification 1: Increased emphasis on the safety of the group members. Safety of the women in treatment programs for aggressive women should be a top priority. Results from the 1975 and 1985 National Family Violence Surveys suggest that two-thirds of women who assault their partners are also victimized by their partners (Stets & Straus, 1990; Straus et al., 1980). By the time women are referred to a treatment program it is expected that some women will have left their partners and some women will have remained in their relationships. Despite the status of the relationship, group leaders need to be aware of the potential danger that these women could be victimized in the future.

Treatment of aggressive women has been described as a means of providing support and treatment to battered women (Hamberger & Arnold, 1990; Hamberger & Potente, 1994). Safety plans are discussed with group members to ensure that women are capable of getting away from an abuser quickly. This may involve keeping money, extra car keys, important documents, or clothes packed and ready for a quick escape from danger. Women should have a clearly articulated plan about where they would go in the case of an emergency and how they would get to their destination. Group members are provided with phone numbers for local women's centers and shelters, and they are given information about the services available to them, including instruction about how to obtain restraining orders.

Because some women are currently in abusive relationships and some are contemplating returning to an abusive relationship, information is provided about the effects of abuse on women and witnessing children. Characteristics of healthy and unhealthy relationships are discussed at length during treatment. Group leaders express concern about the safety of group members in abusive relationships while staying mindful that in order to empower their female clients, the leaders cannot instruct or pressure a woman to leave her relationship. If a woman is not feeling ready to leave a relationship, her group leader may only succeed in alienating her or causing her to drop out of treatment by suggesting that she must leave an abusive partner.

Modification 2: Attention to women's hierarchy of needs. Maslow (1970) put forward the belief that humans need to satisfy their lower-order needs (e.g., food, sleep, money, security) before they will be motivated to work toward higher-order goals such as attaining knowledge, having high self-esteem, and maximizing one's potential. Many women in treatment programs may be dealing with urgent issues that take precedence over learning to control their anger and aggression. While this is also an important issue in treatment for many men, it seems to be a more frequent and pressing issue for aggressive women. Many women referred to treatment are dealing with issues like lack of shelter, food, and employment if they have just left an abusive partner or if their partner has left them due to their own aggression. It is important to raise women's awareness of housing options available in their communities. In addition, women are in need of information and referrals to guide them through the process of applying for welfare, health insurance, legal counseling, financial counseling, and vocational counseling. Once women have consistent shelter and food for themselves and their children, they are better able to address their higher needs and work on taking responsibility for their actions and changing their behavior patterns.

Modification 3: Increased emphasis on Posttraumatic Stress Disorder. Dutton (1995) has emphasized the potential importance of PTSD symptoms in male batterers. While we agree that PTSD and previous trauma need to be addressed in men's treatment, we feel that a greater emphasis on PTSD ought to be incorporated into treatment for women due to the high rate of trauma suffered by aggressive women as indicated above. Trauma symptom checklists such as the PTSD Checklist-Civilian Version (PCL-C; Weathers, Huska, & Keane, 1991) are used to quickly assess the presence and severity of trauma symptoms in group members. PTSD may contribute to women's difficulties in controlling their anger and aggressive impulses, as well as coping with stress in general. Women are educated about the symptoms and treatments for posttraumatic stress disorder. We feel that many of the women in our groups would benefit from learning grounding techniques to cope with flashbacks and dissociation. While such techniques are beyond the scope of our program, many group members are given appropriate referrals for treatment of PTSD.

Modification 4: Increased emphasis on conditions that undermine mood stability. Moffit, Robins, and Caspi (2001) recommend that targeting negative emotionality should be a focus of intervention with female and male perpetrators of domestic violence. Leisring et al. (1999) found that almost two-thirds (63%) of women in the anger management program at UMass reported a history of depressive symptoms and 7.4% reported having a diagnosis of Bipolar Disorder. Approximately one third (32.3%) of women in that sample had made at least one suicide attempt (Leisring et al., 1999). Group members are educated about the symptoms and treatments for mood disorders and given appropriate referrals for treatment. In addition, many women in the anger management program at UMass have described having problems with their mood related to premenstrual syndrome and menopause. Thus, discussions of the symptoms and treatments for PMS and menopause have been incorporated into the treatment program as well. Menstrual diaries are distributed to the group members so that they can track the presence and severity of their symptoms across three months.

Modification 5: More emphasis on parenting behavior. While parenting behavior is a critical topic to be included in treatment for aggressive men, we feel that this issue should be especially emphasized in women's treatment due to the fact that women continue to be more involved in child care than men (Lamb, Pleck, Charnov, & Levine, 1987). Children raised in maritally violent homes are four times more likely to have psychological difficulties than children raised in nonviolent homes (Jouriles et al., 1989). Furthermore, findings from the 1985 National Family Violence Survey indicate that families in which the husband or wife has been aggressive toward their spouse have an increased risk of child abuse (Straus & Smith, 1990). Women who have been abused in childhood by family members may need guidance and information about appropriate parenting behavior.

The parenting module of our program emphasizes the main points often covered in parent training groups (see Barkley, 1997; Barkley, Edwards, & Robin, 1999). Women are taught how to give clear and effective commands and consequences. Consequences should be as immediate as possible and in proportion to the misbehavior. Group members are encouraged to set consequences that they know they can follow through with, and avoid assigning consequences that they will not be able to effectively enforce. Women are urged to avoid the use of corporal punishment because it has been shown to lead to child aggression and delinquency (Straus, 2000) and to child cognitive difficulties (Straus & Paschall, 1999). Furthermore, many of the women in treatment describe having difficulties managing anger, and spanking a child while angry may result in the parent spanking harder than intended. It may be frightening for a child to be hit by an angry parent and children may learn from the parent's example that hitting while angry is acceptable.

Time-outs, grounding, and privilege removal as alternatives to corporal punishment are described in detail. Women are given the names of books on parenting and/or child development such as *Your Defiant Child* (Barkley & Benton, 1998) and *Touchpoints: Your Child's Emotional and Behavioral Development* (Brazelton, 1994). In addition, group leaders are knowledgeable about parenting resources in the community and make referrals for parenting groups and respite care as needed.

Clinicians are mandated in Massachusetts to report suspected cases of child abuse to child protection agencies. At intake and during the first session, group members are informed about this during a discussion of the limits of confidentiality. Group members are promptly notified if/when their actions are reported to child protection agencies by group leaders.

Modification 6: Less emphasis on power and control. Modifications 1-5 described above involve adding components to treatment for partner aggressive women. However, determining how to add treatment modules while being constrained by program length can be difficult. Power and control issues are discussed and emphasized in the great majority of treatment programs for partner-abusive men (Rosenbaum & Leisring, 2001), but we advocate spending less time on these issues in treatment programs for women. Women typically exert power and control in different ways than do men and the consequences of women's behavior are far different. For example, by intimidating and assaulting women, men control women by placing them in fear of their safety. Women may also use aggression to control others. For example, they may verbally assault or slap their partners if their partners come home late from an evening out with friends. The men may decide in the future to return home on time so that they do not have to listen to their partners yelling and to avoid being physically assaulted by them. However, men in violent relationships are less likely than women to fear bodily injury (Tjaden & Thoennes, 2000). In most cases it is likely that men who alter their behavior do so less out of fear of serious bodily injury than their female victim counterparts.

The Power and Control Wheel developed by battered women in Duluth, Minnesota (Pence & Paymar, 1993) is typically discussed and distributed in treatment programs for male batterers. As described earlier in this article, the Power and Control Wheel illustrates tactics that are used by men to establish and maintain control over their partners. Though we acknowledge that some women may "batter" men (Steinmetz & Lucca, 1988) the majority of women being mandated to treatment programs for domestic violence are not considered batterers because their aggressive behavior is not severe and does not result in the victim changing his behavior due to fear of bodily injury. While women should be encouraged during treatment to examine the degree to which they use emotional and physical abuse to obtain power and control in their relationships, overall we believe that less emphasis should be placed on these issues.

FUTURE RESEARCH NEEDED TO INFORM TREATMENT

Further research examining women's aggression is needed and may benefit aggressive women, their partners, and their children. This article offers guidelines to be considered when treating aggressive women. However, it is acknowledged that treatment programs for aggressive women have yet to be evaluated. It is unknown how many women arrested and mandated to attend anger management or batterers treatment go on to assault their partners again after completing treatment.

Considerable research is needed examining the characteristics of partner aggressive women as well as predictors and precursors of aggression perpetrated by women. Such research may highlight additional treatment components that will enhance the effectiveness of intervention programs for women, and inform prevention efforts. Leisring et al. (1999) found that only 53% of court-mandated women who had an intake for the anger management program at UMass actually completed the 20-session program. Research studies comparing the characteristics of women who complete treatment with those of women who drop out of treatment have not been conducted. If predictors of treatment drop-out are identified, adjustments to interventions can be made in an attempt to increase treatment completion.

Previous research has found that partner aggression perpetrated by women results in fewer and less severe injuries than partner aggression perpetrated by males (Vivian & Langhinrichsen-Rohling, 1994). However, women who engage in partner aggression may be placing themselves at risk of future victimization at the hands of their partners (Feld & Straus, 1989). The mechanisms by which this occurs warrant further study. Does women's aggression give men the idea that aggression is acceptable in their relationship as Straus (1993) suggests? Does women's violence cause relationship discord, which in turn leads to aggression perpetrated by men? Marital discord is one of the strongest predictors of men's partner-aggression (Pan et al., 1994). Do men retaliate with aggression because they are trying to use fear and intimidation to stop further assaults by their female partners? These questions remain unanswered.

CONCLUSION

It is hoped that this article will guide clinicians interested in treating partner aggressive women. While treatment for partner aggressive women should incorporate some of the same components of treatment for men, aggressive women also have unique needs that must be addressed. Many of the aggressive women have been victimized by their partners and the safety of women needs to be the top priority of treatment. Women should be aided in developing safety plans to facilitate their ability to leave dangerous situations as quickly as possible. It must be recognized that most partner aggressive women have been victimized in some way either in childhood, adulthood, or both. Symptoms of posttraumatic stress disorder and mood disorders should be assessed and additional treatments recommended when warranted. Helping women discipline their children in a non-aggressive manner should be a major goal of treatment, in addition to reducing partner-violence. Many women in treatment will need help in fulfilling their basic needs of shelter and food. Once women's basic needs are met, it is hoped that they will benefit from cognitive-behavioral anger management skills, and will be less likely to engage in partner aggression in the future. Men, women, and children have the right to live in a non-violent home.

REFERENCES

Abel, E. M. (1999, July). *Who are women in batterer intervention programs: Implications for practice.* Paper presented at the 6th International Family Violence Research Conference, Durham, NH.

Allen, J. G., Coyne, L., & Huntoon, J. (1998). Complex posttraumatic stress disorder in women from a psychometric perspective. *Journal of Personality Assessment, 70*(2), 277-298.

Barkley, R. A. (1997). *Defiant children: A clinician's manual for assessment and parent training* (2nd ed.). New York: Guilford Press.

Barkley, R. A., & Benton, C. M. (1998). *Your defiant child: 8 steps to better behavior.* New York: Guilford Press.

Barkley, R. A., Edwards, G. H., & Robin, A. L. (1999). *Defiant teens: A clinician's manual for assessment and family intervention.* New York: Guilford Press.

Beck, J. S. (1995). *Cognitive therapy: Basics and beyond.* New York: Guilford Press.

Bland, R., & Orn, H. (1986). Family violence and psychiatric disorder. *Canadian Journal of Psychiatry, 31,* 129-137.

Brazelton, T. B. (1994). *Touchpoints: Your child's emotional and behavioral development.* New York: Harper-Collins.

Cascardi, M., Langhinrichsen, J., & Vivian, D. (1992). Marital aggression: Impact, injury, and health correlates for husbands and wives. *Archives of Internal Medicine, 152,* 1178-1184.

Cummings, E. M., & Davies, P. (1994). *Children and marital conflict: The impact of family dispute and resolution.* New York: Guilford Press.

Dobash, R. P., & Dobash, R. E. (1979). *Violence against wives: A case against the patriarchy.* New York: Free Press.

Dowd, L. (2001). Female perpetrators of partner aggression: Relevant issues and treatment. *Journal of Aggression, Maltreatment & Trauma,* 5(2), 73-104.

Dutton, D. G. (1995). Trauma symptoms and PTSD-like profiles in perpetrators of intimate abuse. *Journal of Traumatic Stress, 8*(2), 299-316.

Dutton, D. G. (2002). Treatment of assaultiveness. *Journal of Aggression, Maltreatment, Trauma, 7*(1/2), 7-28.

Dutton, D. G., & Haring, M. (1999). Perpetrator personality effects on post-separation victim reactions in abusive relationships. *Journal of Family Violence, 14*(2), 193-204.

Dutton, D. G., Saunders, K., Starzomski, A., & Bartholomew, K. (1994). Intimacy-anger and insecure attachment as precursors of abuse in intimate relationships. *Journal of Applied Social Psychology, 24*(15), 1367-1386.

Feld, S. L., & Straus, M. A. (1989). Escalation and desistance of wife assault in marriage. *Criminology, 27,* 141-161.

Feldman, C. M. (1997). Childhood precursors of adult interpartner violence. *Clinical Psychology, Science, and Practice, 4*(4), 307-334.

Hamberger, L. K. (1997). Female offenders in domestic violence: A look at actions in context. *Journal of Aggression, Maltreatment, & Trauma, 1*(1), 117-129.

Hamberger, L. K., & Arnold, J. (1990). The impact of mandatory arrest on domestic violence perpetrator counseling services. *Family Violence Bulletin, 6,* 10-12.

Hamberger, L. K., & Potente, T. (1994). Counseling heterosexual women arrested for domestic violence: Implications for theory and practice. *Violence and Victims, 9*(2), 125-137.

Jaffe, P. G., Wolfe, D. A., & Wilson, S. K. (1990). *Children of battered women.* Newbury Park, CA: Sage.

Johnson, M. P. (1995). Patriarchal terrorism and common couple violence: Two forms of violence against women. *Journal of Marriage and the Family, 57*(2), 283-294.

Jouriles, E. N., Murphy, C. M., & O'Leary, K. D. (1989). Interspousal aggression, marital discord, and child problems. *Journal of Consulting and Clinical Psychology, 57,* 453-455.

Kesner, J. E., & McKenry, P. C. (1998). The role of childhood attachment factors in predicting male violence toward female intimates. *Journal of Family Violence, 13*(4), 417-432.

Kurz, D. (1993). Physical assaults by husbands: A major social problem. In R. J. Gelles & D. R. Loseke (Eds.), *Current controversies on family violence* (pp. 88-103). Newbury Park, CA: Sage.

Kwong, M. J., Bartholomew, K., & Dutton, D. G. (1999). Gender differences in patterns of relationship violence in Alberta. *Canadian Journal of Behavioral Science, 31*(3), 150-160.

Lamb, M. E., Pleck, J. H., Charnov, E. L., & Levine, J. A. (1987). A biosocial perspective on paternal behavior and involvement. In J. B. Lancaster, J. Altmann, A. S. Rossi, & L. R. Sherrod (Eds.), *Parenting across the life span: Biosocial dimensions* (pp. 111-142). New York: Aldine De Gruyter.

Leeder, E. (1988). Enmeshed in pain: Counseling the lesbian battering couple. *Women & Therapy, 7*(1), 81-99.

Leisring, P. A., Dowd, L., & Rosenbaum, A. (1999, July). *Characteristics of women mandated to anger management.* Paper presented at the 6th International Family Violence Research Conference, Durham, NH.

Leisring, P. A., Dowd, L., & Rosenbaum, A. (2000). *Trauma histories, PTSD symptoms, and aggression in partner-abusive women.* Paper presented at the 34th Annual Meeting of the Association for the Advancement of Behavior Therapy, New Orleans, LA.

Maker, A. H., Kemmelmeier, M., & Peterson, C. (1998). Long-term psychological consequences in women of witnessing parental physical conflict and experiencing abuse in childhood. *Journal of Interpersonal Violence, 13*(5), 574-589.

Maslow, A. (1970). *Motivation and personality* (2nd ed.). New York: Harper and Row.

Miller, B. A., Downs, W. R., & Testa, M. (1993). Interrelationships between victimization experiences and women's alcohol use. *Journal of Studies on Alcohol, 11*, 109-117.

Moffit, T. E., Robins, R. W., & Caspi, A. (2001). A couples analysis of partner abuse with implications for abuse prevention policy. *Criminology, 1*, 5-36.

Murphy, C. M., & O'Leary, K. D. (1989). Psychological aggression predicts physical aggression in early marriage. *Journal of Consulting and Clinical Psychology, 57*, 579-582.

Najavits, L. M., Weiss, R. D., & Liese, B. S. (1996). Group cognitive-behavioral therapy with women with PTSD and Substance Use Disorder. *Journal of Substance Abuse Treatment, 13*(1), 13-22.

Nichols, T., & Dutton. D. G. (2001). Violence committed by women against intimates. *Journal of Couples Therapy, 10*(1), 41-57.

O'Leary, K. D., Curley, A., Rosenbaum, A., & Clarke, C. (1986). Assertion training for abused wives: A potentially hazardous treatment. *Journal of Marital & Family Therapy, 11*(3), 319-322.

Pan, H. S., Neidig, P. H., & O'Leary, K. D. (1994). Predicting mild and severe husband-to-wife physical aggression. *Journal of Consulting and Clinical Psychology, 62*, 975-981.

Pence, E., & Paymar, M. (1993). *Education groups for men who batter: The Duluth model.* New York: Springer Publishing Company, Inc.

Renzetti, C. (1988). Violence in lesbian relationships: A preliminary analysis of causal factors. *Journal of Interpersonal Violence, 3*(4), 7-27.

Rosenbaum, A., & Leisring, P. A. (2001). Group intervention programs for batterers. *Journal of Aggression, Maltreatment, & Trauma, 5*(2), 57-71.

Rosenbaum, A., & O'Leary, K. D. (1981). Children: The unintended victims of marital violence. *American Journal of Orthopsychiatry, 51*, 692-699.

Saunders, D. G. (1986). When battered women use violence: Husband abuse or self-defense? *Violence and Victims, 1*, 47-60.

Steinmetz, S. K., & Lucca, J. S. (1988). Husband battering. In V. B. Van Hasselt, R. L. Morrison, A. S. Bellack, & M. Hersen, (Eds.), *Handbook of Family Violence* (pp. 233-246). New York: Plenum Press.

Stets, J., & Straus, M. A. (1990). Gender differences in reporting marital violence and its medical and psychological consequences. In M. A. Straus & R. J. Gelles (Eds.), *Physical Violence in American Families: Risk Factors and Adaptations in 8145 American Families* (pp. 151-166). New Brunswick, NJ: Transaction Books.

Straus, M. A. (1990). Ordinary violence, child abuse, and wife beating: What do they have in common? In M. A. Straus & R. E. Gelles (Eds.), *Physical violence in American families: Risk factors and adaptations to violence in 8,145 families* (pp. 403-424). New Brunswick, NJ: Transaction Publishers.

Straus, M. A. (1993). Physical assaults by wives: A major social problem. In R. J. Gelles & D. R. Loseke (Eds.), *Current controversies on family violence* (pp. 67-87). Newbury Park, CA: Sage Publications.

Straus, M. A. (1999). The controversy over domestic violence by women: A methodological, theoretical, and sociology of science analysis. In X. B. Arriaga & S. Oskamp (Eds.), *Violence in intimate relationships* (pp. 17-44). Thousand Oaks, CA: Sage.

Straus, M. A. (2000). *Beating the Devil out of Them: Corporal Punishment in American Families and Its Effects on Children* (2nd ed.) New Brunswick, NJ: Transaction Publishers.

Straus, M. A., & Gelles, R. J. (1990). How violent are American families? In M. A. Straus & R. J. Gelles (Eds.), *Physical violence in American Families: Risk factors and adaptations to violence in 8,145 families* (pp. 95-112). New Brunswick, NJ: Transaction Publishers.

Straus, M. A., Gelles, R. J., & Steinmetz, S. K. (1980). *Behind closed doors: Violence in the American family.* Garden City, NJ: Anchor/Doubleday.

Straus, M. A., & Paschall, M. A. (1999). *Corporal punishment by mothers and children's cognitive development: A longitudinal study of two age cohorts.* Paper presented at the 6th International Family Violence Research Conference. Durham, NH.

Straus, M. A., & Smith, C. (1990). Family patterns and child abuse. In M. A. Straus & R. J. Gelles (Eds.), *Physical violence in American Families: Risk factors and adaptations to violence in 8,145 families* (pp. 245-261). New Brunswick, NJ: Transaction Publishers.

Straus, M. A., & Sweet, S. (1992). Verbal/symbolic aggression in couples: Incidence rates and relationships to personal characteristics. *Journal of Marriage and the Family, 54*, 346-357.

Tjaden, P., & Thoennes, N. (2000). Prevalence and consequences of male-to-female and female-to-male intimate partner violence as measured by the National Violence Against Women Survey. *Violence Against Women, 6*(2), 142-161.

Tuel, B. D., & Russell, R. K. (1998). Self esteem and depression in battered women. *Violence Against Women, 4*(3), 344-362.

Vivian, D., & Langhinrichsen-Rohling, J. (1994). Are bi-directionally violent couples mutually victimized. *Violence and Victims, 9*(2), 107-124.

Waldner-Haugrud, L. K., Gratch, L. V., & Magruder, B. (1997). Victimization and perpetration rates of violence in gay and lesbian relationships: Gender issues explored. *Violence and Victims, 12*(2), 173-184.

Waltz, J. (2002). Dialectical behavior therapy in the treatment of abusive behavior. *Journal of Aggression, Maltreatment, & Trauma, 7*(1/2), 75-103.

Weathers, F. W., Huska, J. A., & Keane, T. M., (1991). *The PTSD Checklist-Civilian Version (PCL-C).* (Available from F.W. Weathers, National Center for PTSD, Boston Veterans Affairs, Medical Center, 150 S. Huntington Avenue, Boston, MA 02130).

Yllo, K. (1993). Through a feminist lens: Gender, power, and violence. In R. Gelles, & D. Loeske (Eds), *Controversies in Family Violence* (pp. 47-62.). Newbury Park, CA: Sage Publications.

SPECIAL ISSUES IN THE TREATMENT OF INTIMATE VIOLENCE PERPETRATORS

Legal and Ethical Issues in the Court-Mandated Treatment of Batterers

Alan Rosenbaum
William J. Warnken
Albert J. Grudzinskas, Jr.

SUMMARY. In the following article, we will explore the nature of the therapeutic relationship as it relates to batterers' treatment programs. We

Address correspondence to: Alan Rosenbaum, PhD, Department of Psychology, Northern Illinois University, DeKalb, IL 60115 (E-mail: arosenb@niu.edu).

The authors gratefully acknowledge the contributions of Paul Appelbaum, MD, and Penny Leisring, PhD, who provided editorial comments and suggestions on earlier drafts of this manuscript. All responsibility for the content and opinions expressed herein, however, resides with the authors.

[Haworth co-indexing entry note]: "Legal and Ethical Issues in the Court-Mandated Treatment of Batterers." Rosenbaum, Alan, William J. Warnken, and Albert J. Grudzinskas, Jr. Co-published simultaneously in *Journal of Aggression, Maltreatment & Trauma* (The Haworth Maltreatment & Trauma Press, an imprint of The Haworth Press, Inc.) Vol. 7, No. 1/2 (#13/14), 2003, pp. 279-303; and: *Intimate Violence: Contemporary Treatment Innovations* (ed: Donald Dutton, and Daniel J. Sonkin) The Haworth Maltreatment & Trauma Press, an imprint of The Haworth Press, Inc., 2003, pp. 279-303. Single or multiple copies of this article are available for a fee from The Haworth Document Delivery Service [1-800-HAWORTH, 9:00 a.m. - 5:00 p.m. (EST). E-mail address: docdelivery@haworthpress.com].

http://www.haworthpress.com/store/product.asp?sku=J146
© 2003 by The Haworth Press, Inc. All rights reserved.
10.1300J146v07n01_12

will consider the impact of obligations created by forces outside the relationship, such as those imposed by legal proceedings. We will discuss the concepts of confidentiality, privilege, and agency and their impact on the therapeutic relationship and the extent to which the therapists' understanding of the role these concepts play may be altered by court orders that impose treatment on a client/patient. Finally, we examine the issues and choices a therapist must make when engaging in court-ordered treatment of batterers, and the implications of those choices for both therapist and client; we will also suggest guidelines to help therapists sort through the often conflicting goals of therapy and the legal process. *[Article copies available for a fee from The Haworth Document Delivery Service: 1-800-HAWORTH. E-mail address: <docdelivery@haworthpress.com> Website: <http://www.HaworthPress.com> © 2003 by The Haworth Press, Inc. All rights reserved.]*

KEYWORDS. Domestic violence, therapeutically based interventions, confidentiality, privilege, agency, court-ordered treatment for batterers, batterers

INTRODUCTION

The relationship between therapist and client/patient is fiduciary. The therapist by virtue of entering the therapeutic relationship undertakes a duty to act primarily for the benefit of the client in matters connected to the therapy. In its usual manifestation, the role of the therapist is well-defined and involves helping and supporting the patient's efforts to make positive changes in his/her life and acting in the client/patient's best interests. The introduction of legal proceedings into a therapeutic relationship can disrupt the therapeutic process and complicate the therapist's perceptions regarding the client's best interests. For example, Dubey (1974) notes: ". . . what may be in a person's best legal interests, i.e., maintenance of dramatic symptoms in order to present a sound case for disability or liability, may be directly contrary to his therapeutic interests, i.e., relinquishing of symptoms" (p. 1093).

The enactment of domestic violence legislation in many states has led to a dramatic increase in the numbers of individuals court ordered to undergo some form of intervention. When individuals are court-ordered into treatment (hereafter "court-mandated"), the therapist is required to balance the often competing interests of the batterer and the legal system. Dealing with court-mandated clients is sufficiently rare and generally restricted to the battering context. Therapists, therefore, may not have received much training regarding the legal and ethical issues encountered when working with this population. Is the therapist an agent of the courts or an advocate for his/her client? Many states now have legislation in place that permits judges to mandate batterers into treatment or intervention programs. In some cases (e.g., Phoenix, Arizona) the batterers' treatment program is offered to domestic offenders as a diversionary program. Batterers are assigned a future court date, by which they must have completed a batterers' treatment program or face prosecution for their offense. In other jurisdictions (e.g., Massachusetts), the treatment mandate is specified as a term of probation, following either a plea or a guilty verdict. From a legal perspective, these alternatives have very different attributes and consequences which are beyond the scope of this article.

In either case, however, mandated treatment presents complicated practical, ethical, and legal considerations for the treater. Most states that allow for court ordering of batterer treatment also have standards in place, or are in the process of developing standards, for the certification of programs. These standards, which vary from state to state, may specify program length and/or content, format (e.g., group vs. individual, gender specific vs. couples), minimum credentials or training for treaters and/or program sponsoring organizations, reporting requirements (e.g., to the victim, probation department, or courts), and the circumstances under which confidentiality is limited. For a complete discussion of batterer program standards, see Geffner and Rosenbaum (2001).

Despite wide use of the term "batterers' treatment" as a generic description of the endeavor, there is substantial support for the idea that this is not treatment in the psychotherapeutic sense of the word, but rather an intervention. In fact, many states (e.g., Massachusetts) have adopted the term "batterer intervention" to describe the treatment option available to the courts. In part, this stems from the fear that partner abuse will be viewed, not as criminal behavior, but as a psychological problem, with a consequent softening of the penalties. It might also be intended to remove batterers' treatment from the realm of mental health professionals, where ethical considerations regarding confidentiality could conflict with the reporting requirements of the statutes in many states. Next is the concern that classifying partner aggression as a psychological problem would permit attorneys to make diminished capacity defenses and allow batterers to divert some responsibility for their behavior to their "mental problems." Finally, the orientation of many well known programs (e.g., Emerge) emphasizes protection of the victim by monitoring the behavior of batterers, a function that would be seen as antithetical to the development of a therapeutic alliance. For purposes of clarity and convenience, the terms treatment and intervention will be used interchangeably in this article. In those instances where a distinction between the two is being made, the exception to this usage will be clear from the text.

The term "batterers' treatment" is of little heuristic value given the broad range of interventions it subsumes. Programs vary in length, orientation, content/curriculum, format, leadership, and philosophy. Some more closely resemble educational driving programs for driving under the influence (DUI) offenders while others are indistinguishable from psychotherapy groups. The credentials required for group leadership are also disparate. Many states (e.g., Massachusetts) fail to specify any minimum professional credential, instead requiring a minimum period of training (which may be as brief as one day) from a recognized program (e.g., Duluth or Emerge). Some, but not all, jurisdictions prohibit ex-batterers from serving as treaters. The legal and ethical considerations discussed in this article pertain primarily to individuals in the mental health professions who are engaged in batterers' treatment with court-mandated participants. Even among the various counseling professions, ethical obligations and statutory and case law requirements vary; thus, social workers observe an ethical code and laws that are different from those of psychologists or psychiatrists.

Court-mandated batterer treatment is a relatively new enterprise, with most of the legislation permitting such mandates having been enacted only within the last decade. As a result, relatively little case law has evolved in this field. This chapter will synthesize existing case law relevant to court-mandated batterers' treatment, case law addressing more general court-ordered treatment, interpretations of the various codes of ethics governing the mental health professions, and the opinions of experts responding to queries regarding hypothetical circumstances. It will be written for mental health professionals, not lawyers, so we will make few assumptions regarding the legal knowledge of the intended readership.

STATUTORY LAW AND CASE LAW

In the spirit of avoiding overly legal descriptions, we begin with a definition for the term "case law." Many people are surprised to learn that much of what we term "the law" is not always written by legislatures after debate and public hearing. Clearly defined rules generated by a legislative body, such as those governing speeding, are known as statutes, and the totality of these are collectively referred to as "statutory law." Statutory rape, for example, is a violation of a very specific written rule prohibiting a legally defined adult from having sexual intercourse with a legally defined child. Testimonial privilege (which allows a patient to refuse to allow testimony in court regarding their psychotherapy), in those jurisdictions that have it, may be statutory or by case law.

Case law, according to Black's Law Dictionary (Black, Nolan, & Nolan-Haley, 1990), is "The aggregate of reported cases as forming a body of jurisprudence, or the law of a particular subject as evidenced or formed by the adjudged cases, in distinction to statutes and other sources of law." More simply stated, case law is an interpretation of prior statutes or rulings previously made by a court, in response to a particular case now before the court. The collection of all these rulings becomes the "case law" of a jurisdiction. Although states generally refer to their own case law, federal case law and case law from other states can be used by a court in making a determination about a specific topic. Case law is often used to help shape state regulations and standards of practice. Much of the law regarding the behavior and liabilities of mental health professionals is drawn from case law. The irony of case law, of course, is that the interpretation comes after the fact. Conduct previously deemed acceptable may, because of a new interpretation, become the basis for liability. Consequently, even the most well meaning, ethically aware therapist can become exposed to a law suit. It also means that until specific cases are actually brought, all one can do is speculate about how to deal with situations that fall outside the dictates of existing law, such as those that form the subject matter of this article.

Although states often refer to case law determinations from other states as a basis for rendering decisions, one state court is not mandated or even obliged to rule in the same manner as a court in another state, even though the issue at hand may be very similar or the same. An interesting example of this is a review of the case law that followed the landmark case of *Tarasoff v. Regents of the University of California* (1974).

In July of 1969, Prosenjit Poddar, a graduate student at the University of California, attended therapy at the Student Health Center of this university. During a session, he informed his therapist, Dr. Lawrence Moore, that he intended to kill an unnamed young woman with whom he was infatuated. The psychologist alerted the campus police and his supervisor to this threat. The campus police found Poddar and, after convincing the police that he was not dangerous, he was released from their custody. Two months later, Mr. Poddar stabbed Tatiana Tarasoff to death. Ms. Tarasoff's family then sued Dr. Moore and the State of California for malpractice, asserting that there were actions that Dr. Moore could have taken that would have prevented the victim's death. The trial court found that no cause of action was created by the facts of the case. In 1974, after determining that Dr. Moore had a special (i.e., doctor-patient) relationship with Poddar, the Supreme Court of California determined that the relationship gave rise to a duty to warn innocent third parties of dangers "emanating from the patient's illness" (*Tarasoff* at p. 559). The Court found that the facts presented could support a claim that the psychologist was negligent in his duty by failing to inform Ms. Tarasoff or her parents of the danger the patient presented. In rendering its decision, the court interpreted the law as imposing upon psychologists in California the duty to warn third parties of serious threats made against them. This ruling allowed the plaintiffs to amend their complaints to comply with the new interpretation. Following a subsequent appeal after the trial court dismissed the amended complaints in what is commonly referred to as *Tarasoff II (Tarasoff v. University of California Regents*, 1976), the court expanded the duty of psychologists in California from duty to warn to duty to protect. As Douglas and Webster (1999) noted, "Tarasoff entrenched in case law the idea that mental health workers ought to have the capacity to isolate and act on information that may have a bearing on future violent conduct" (p. 6).

Although *Tarasoff* set the stage for courts in other states to impose upon clinicians a duty to protect third parties, case law in other states have supported, expanded upon, and, in some cases, rejected the duty established by *Tarasoff*. Since *Tarasoff*, there have been a series of legal determinations in California and other states that have attempted to define what type of duty clinicians owe to society in regard to protecting third parties. In *Jablonski v. United States* (1983), a California case post-dating *Tarasoff*, the court determined negligence when the victim was identified only as a person who was close to the perpetrator of the violent act. In *Peck v. Counseling Services of Addison County* (1985), a

Vermont case, this duty was expanded to the protection of a third party's property. A more concerning ruling occurred in 1980. The finding in *Lipari v. Sears, Roebuck & Company* (1980), a Nebraska case, extended the duty of mental health professionals to protect society at large (i.e., no specific individual had been threatened). It should also be noted that some state courts have rejected the duty of clinicians to protect third parties (e.g., *Boynton v. Burglass*, 1991, a Florida case).

The variability in these findings illustrates how courts in different states differ with regard to how they define the responsibilities of clinicians to protect society. In spite of these various post-*Tarasoff* court decisions, Anfang and Appelbaum (1996) note that, although there are some exceptions, "courts have found a duty to protect only clearly foreseeable victims from clearly foreseeable violent threats" (p. 70). Because of the inter-state variability, clinicians must be aware of the relevant case law in the states in which they practice.

As described above, case law can be used as a foundation in the establishment of state regulations that are germane to mental health professionals. As a result of *Tarasoff*, even states that did not have state specific case law adopted state regulations identifying these duties in anticipation of such cases. In many cases, the language of these state regulations is very specific and clearly defined. Clinicians who practice in states that have certification standards for batterer treatment must be aware that there are instances when these standards deviate from the duties that state regulations impose on mental health professionals (usually licensed mental health professionals). To illustrate this point, let us continue to use the issue of a clinician's duty to warn or protect a third party in Massachusetts (a state where *Tarasoff* responsibilities are established by statute, not case law). The batterer intervention certification standards in Massachusetts (see Commonwealth of Massachusetts Executive Office of Health and Human Services, Department of Public Health, 1995) require programs to evaluate the perpetrator's lethality, and to warn victims and current partners deemed to be at high risk. Further, programs must warn all victims and current partners that any violence could be lethal and that lethality or continued violence cannot be reliably predicted. There are additional requirements to inform in writing, both the Chief Probation Officer in Charge and the referring court and to document all attempts to warn victims and current partners.

By reading this section of the certification standards, clinicians could presume that in Massachusetts they only have a duty to warn a third party if that person is identified to be "at high risk" of being harmed. This assumption would be inaccurate. Psychologists in Massachusetts have a very clearly defined duty to protect a third party of "a clear and present danger" of injury (see Massachusetts General Laws, c. 123, s. 36B). This statute also articulates the precautions that a clinician should use to mitigate the likelihood that the third party would be injured. These precautions include contacting the victim, notifying the police (not the probation department) of the threat, arranging for voluntary or involuntary hospitalization of the client making the threats (if appropriate) or all of the above. A psychologist who responds to a threat of injury to a third party in the manner outlined in the certification standards could be accused of failing to fulfill the statutory requirements. Although they may have warned the intended victim and notified probation, for example, they did not directly contact the police or seek involuntary hospitalization of the batterer. It is important for those who work with court ordered offenders to be aware of the inconsistencies that may exist between certification standards, state regulations, and case law that pertain to the treatment of their clients.

CONFIDENTIALITY AND PRIVILEGE

One example of the disruptive nature of imposing legal concerns on therapeutic practice revolves around the ability of the therapist to protect the privacy of material divulged in the context of the therapist-client relationship. Confidentiality "refers to the right of an individual not to have communications that were imparted in confidence revealed to third parties" (Appelbaum & Gutheil, 1991, p. 4). Privilege, or "testimonial privilege" as it is often referred to, applies only in legal contexts. It is the right of an individual, under certain circumstances, to prevent another person from providing testimony during a legal proceeding about that person based on information that was provided in confidence (Appelbaum & Gutheil, 1991). According to Beck (1990), 49 states now have laws addressing when patient communications are privileged. The language of these laws and the circumstances under which they may be enforced varies from state to state. It is noteworthy, however, that in Federal courts, where Federal Rules of Evidence apply, there is no explicit statutorily-based right to clinician-patient privilege. Instead, as we will soon see, the court has "the power to create privilege on a case-by-case basis" (Appelbaum & Gutheil, 1991).

The therapeutic process requires an alliance between the treater and the patient, and the belief by the patient that the therapist has his best interests at heart. It is for these reasons that confidentiality is the cornerstone of the psychotherapeutic relationship, and that information acquired in a therapist-client relationship is legally protected as privileged communication.

In Jaffee v. Redmond (1996), a case that established a patient's right to prevent a therapist from disclosing clinical information regarding the client, the Supreme Court noted:

> Effective psychotherapy . . . depends upon an atmosphere of confidence and trust in which the patient is willing to make a frank and complete disclosure of facts, emotions, memories, and fears. Because of the sensitive nature of the problems for which individuals consult psychotherapists, disclosure of confidential communications made during counseling sessions may cause embarrassment or disgrace. For these reasons, the mere possibility of disclosure may impede development of the confidential relationship necessary for successful treatment. (p. 10)

Yet despite its importance to the therapeutic process, confidentiality is often poorly protected. A substantial body of case law exists in which mental health professionals have been compelled to divulge information obtained under the expectation that it would be confidential and protected from disclosure by privilege. In situations where the client is court-mandated to treatment, breaches of confidentiality may be more than embarrassing or inconvenient. They may result in serious legal consequences, such as revocation of parole, probation, or an imposition of a prison or jail sentence.

Anytime information in a therapeutic relationship is disclosed to outside parties, particularly if it is released to more than one party, issues of confidentiality and privilege can arise. The batterer may rightfully believe that disclosing angry feelings, alcohol use, or aggressive behavior might cause his probation to be revoked and lead to imprisonment. Such a belief may impair his ability to openly participate in treatment. Is it illegal or even unethical for psychologists to unilaterally share such information with the courts and victims? Are they at any increased risk of litigation from this practice? The following analysis should help provide a framework for resolving such issues in the reader's own jurisdiction.

The concept of confidentiality has evolved over centuries. During the past 30 years, legal scholars have interpreted the U.S. Constitution to imply a "right to privacy." Although the word "privacy" is never actually used in the Constitution, "the Supreme Court has reasoned that the term 'liberty' in the Fourteenth Amendment implies certain privacy rights" (Behnke & Hillard, 1998, p. 26). In addition to these legal reasons, psychologists, as we have already discussed, have been trained to believe that it is necessary for effective treatment that communications between therapist and clients be private and confidential. Although the research on this topic is equivocal (Appelbaum, 1985), it is presumed that without such protection clients will not honestly share their real thoughts and problems in treatment. In doing so, clients would be compromising the therapist's ability to assist them in making the types of changes that they wish to have occur. Considered to be so central to the therapeutic relationship, the Ethical Principles of Psychologists and Code of Conduct (American Psychological Association [APA], 1992) have established guidelines regarding ethical conduct related to preserving confidentiality in the therapeutic relationship.

It should be noted that psychologists and other licensed professionals can undergo disciplinary action by a sanctioning agency (i.e., the American Psychological/Psychiatric Association or National Association of Social Workers) and/or, depending on case law or state statutes, can be sued in civil court over a breach of confidentiality. However, it is not uncommon for state statutes defining who has confidentiality requirements to have no specific provisions for those individuals who provide batterers' interventions or treatment. Massachusetts General Law (c. 233, s. 20K), for instance, explicitly identifies a number of counseling disciplines, including domestic violence victims' counselors, as professionals having confidentiality requirements, but makes no similar provisions for the professionals who treat male batterers. Although some individuals who provide batterer treatment or intervention in Massachusetts may have licensure that mandate confidentiality and privilege via state regulations, others may have no provision under state law or regulations requiring confidentiality.

For those professionals who have confidentiality requirements, the promise of confidentiality is not an absolute principle. In fact, there have always been exceptions to confidentiality, mandated either by state law or regulations. Although states vary with regard to the circumstances under which confidentiality can be breached, clinicians can usually "break" confidentiality for several reasons. These include mandated reporting of instances of child or elder abuse and the threat of injury towards others or toward the client himself or herself. Because of these noteworthy exceptions to confidentiality, APA ethics (APA, 1992), the "aspirational" Specialty Guidelines for Forensic Psychologists (Committee on Ethical Guidelines for Forensic Psychologists, 1991), and state regulations in many jurisdictions require licensed clinicians at the onset of the professional relationship to inform their clients of the circumstances under which they will provide information to others. This warning is usually labeled as the Limits of Confidentiality (see for example, APA, 1992; Massachusetts General Laws, c. 117, s. 129A).

IDENTIFICATION OF AGENCY

In rendering its decision in *Jaffee v. Redmond* (1996), the court was asked to rule on a case where there was a clearly defined client-therapist relationship. Although clinician-client confidentiality is, in many states, protected by statute and has been repeatedly endorsed by case law across states, the interface between the judicial system and the therapist that is created when therapy is court-mandated presents challenges as to when and how information is shared with others. This problem emerges when programs who treat batterers define the client of their services as individuals or institutions other than the batterer himself.

Perhaps the largest philosophical difference between programs that work with domestically violent men is the identification of "agency." Agency, according to Gutheil and Appelbaum (2000), refers to how a clinician (or organization) defines who is the client of their services. Programs that work with domestically aggressive men often differ in whom they define as the "clients" of their services. Some programs view the court as their "client" and report all information discussed in treatment/intervention sessions to probation or other officials of the court. The identification of the court as the client of these programs' services appears to be a logical one, given that the court is the impetus for treatment and the completion of treatment a term of probation. Many programs, as well as some courts, tend to view the programs as extensions of the court or its probation department.

In contrast, other programs identify the batterer as the client of the program. This should not be taken to imply that victim safety is less important to these programs than to others; rather, it identifies the batterer and his aggressive behaviors as the focus of therapeutic intervention. Programs that identify the court as the client of their services tend to employ a social control framework as the focus of their intervention, and focus on providing internal change as catalyst for the cessation of violent behavior. The "batterer as client" model assumes a more traditional treatment approach, including concerns about how sharing information with outside parties impacts the batterer's ability to truthfully share information in treatment. Clinicians who treat batterers from this more traditional framework have greater concerns about how information is disseminated to the court than those programs who identify the court as the client of their services.

However, most programs that work with batterers have, either explicitly or implicitly, what Appelbaum and Gutheil (1991) describe as "split agency." Split agency refers to having more than one identified person or party as clients. In the treatment of batterers, split agency could mean that a program has some allegiance to the court, victim, and/or the batterer. According to Appelbaum and Gutheil, "Split agency is not necessarily a problem; ethically, however, candor is required to delineate the nature of the agency before material is explored in any situation where agency is not limited only to the patient" (p. 21). In other words, prior to entering into any type of intervention or treatment, the individual working with the batterer must inform him of how the information that is discussed in treatment sessions will be used and who will have access to the information.

For psychologists or other licensed professionals who, either by ethical standards, case law, or state statute, have confidentiality and privilege requirements, the clarification of agency is of particular importance. Depending on the treatment program's identification of its role, there may be other information that clinicians should alert batterers to prior to their entering a program. For example, if a batterer's intervention program identifies itself as an agent of the court, it is important for that program to inform the batterer what information will be provided to the court or other parties at the onset of the intervention or treatment relationship. The clearer the program is in identifying agency, the clearer it will be when informing the batterer about who will receive information related to his or her intervention/treatment and the reasons for this disclosure. Licensed professionals (or at least the ones identified by state regulations) could be sanctioned, lose their licenses, and/or be sued, if they reveal information to outside parties without the permission of the batterer. As Behnke and Hillard (1998) assert, "The four words you never want a client to begin a sentence with are: 'You didn't tell me . . .' " (p. 32).

Certification standards that establish the minimum criteria a program must meet before it is eligible to receive court-mandated referrals also require contact with the victim of the abuse and/or current partner of the batterer in many instances. It is no less important that these individuals be notified about how the information they share with the treater will be used. If the program openly reports all information to probation, the victim should be informed of this. It is important to keep in mind that the victim has no obligation to speak with any clinician, and may have legitimate reasons for not doing so. If a victim chooses to share information, s/he should be advised prior to his/her revealing the information of the use that will be made of the statement and the degree of confidentiality (if any) to expect. By failing to inform the victim of the limits of confidentiality, the clinician may be placing him/her at greater risk of injury. If the victim for example, were to report to the treater that the batterer has remained aggressive, believing that the information would be used for treatment purposes only, and not further disclosed, s/he might then find out that the batterer has been rearrested for violating probation. The victim would be justifiably angry that his/her information has been used in a manner not intended. The victim might then incur retaliation from the batterer for "ratting him/her out," suffer a loss of income formerly provided by the batterer, or suffer some other consequence of having an incarcerated partner.

Cooperation between the various agencies involved in domestic abuse cases is viewed as an important strength by many batterers' treatment programs. Austin and Dankwort (1998) recently published a review of standards for batterer intervention programs and noted that "a coordinated community response in ending domestic violence is stated as being necessary in 97% of the standards . . . " (p. 4). Sixty-one percent of the standards require that new incidences of violence need to be reported to the authorities. One of the more extreme examples of this practice is the Emerge program, which provides the courts with weekly attendance reports, periodic progress reports, and immediate notice of any status change (Emerge, 1998). What, if any, are the limits to cooperation between the treatment program and other agencies? On several occasions, the program conducted by Dr. Rosenbaum at UMass Memorial Health Care has been contacted by a probation officer advising that an arrest warrant had been issued for one of the court-mandated group members and requesting that the program notify probation if the group member attended group so that he could be arrested. Does the therapist have any obligation (legal or ethical) to comply with such a request? In these cases, the program has taken the position that it would inform the batterer that a warrant had been issued and advise him to turn himself in to the police or probation, but would not notify either the police or probation department of his arrival at group. In each of the cases, the batterer failed to attend group once the arrest warrant had been issued, effectively extricating the program from this dilemma.

Situations like the one above arise when there is a confusion of agency by a third party. It is, therefore, important to clarify not only the type of information that will be shared with these parties, but the program's view of its relationship with the third party (i.e., the court). Although some programs who view their role as being an extension of the court may have indeed contacted the court of the batterer's whereabouts, other programs, such as the UMass program, do not feel compelled to respond to this demand. Although it is impossible to foresee every possible boundary problem with another agency, open discussion with the other agency or court about what the program will and will not do should be discussed in advance whenever possible. By doing so, the treating program and the other parties will have a clearer understanding of the boundaries that may exist between them, which then can be articulated to the batterer.

INFORMED CONSENT

Although not generally discussed in the context of batterer treatment, the doctrine of informed consent nevertheless still applies for many clinicians. If the intervention is viewed as treatment, the client has a right (absent a court mandate to the contrary) to refuse the treatment and to be advised of the risks and benefits involved in order to properly assess them in coming to an informed decision to participate. The Ethical Principles of Psychologists and Code of Conduct recommend that "Psychologists obtain appropriate informed consent to therapy or related procedures, using language that is reasonable understandable to participants" (APA, 1992, s. 4.03). But how is this issue directly relevant to the treatment of a batterer? In order to understand the necessity for providing and receiving informed consent for treatment, it will be necessary to review how the doctrine of informed consent was established.

Simply stated, the "doctrine of *violenti non fit iniuria*–no harm is done to one who consents–is the legal maxim that underlies the informed consent doctrine" (Ogloff, 1999, p. 409). One of the first court cases to address the issue of informed consent was heard by the Kansas Supreme Court. Although the case was concerned with a physician who was accused of failing to inform a patient of the risks of radiation treatment for cancer, *Natanson v. Kline* (1960), and later *Canterbury v. Spence* (1972), established the parameters about what information should be provided to individuals who are about to engage in any form of treatment. According to Grisso and Appelbaum (1998), "Patients must be told about the nature and purpose of the proposed treatment or procedure, its potential benefits and risks, and the alternative approaches available, along with their benefits and risks" (p. 7).

To determine whether the requirements of informed consent have been met, there should be an assessment of the level of functioning in three elements domains. Melton, Petrila, Poythress, and Slobogin (1997) wrote "Determining whether informed consent is valid requires consideration of . . . disclosure, competency, and voluntariness" (p. 346). But what do these elements actually mean and how do they relate to the treatment of batterers? The first element, disclosure, refers to whether a clinician has provided adequate information about the type of treatment the batterer would receive (including benefits and potential risks) that would allow him or her to make a reasonable decision about attending treatment. The content of the information that must be provided to meet this requirement varies from state to state, but is typically conceptualized either as "whether a reasonable clinician would disclose particular information under the same circumstances" (Melton et al., 1997, p. 346) or, as Grisso and Appelbaum (1998) note, that in patient-oriented disclosures, clinicians "must disclose the information that a reasonable patient would find material to a decision about the proposed treatment" (p. 8). Some states use the "reasonable clinician rule" while others use the "reasonable patient rule." Although there may not be consensus about what type of information should be shared at the onset of batterers' treatment, enough information about the program should be given to the batterer to allow him to decide whether or not he wishes to participate in that program. Even though batterers are often court-mandated into treatment and failure to attend treatment could result in a violation of probation and subsequent incarceration, theoretically they still have a choice regarding whether they attend treatment or not. An unemployed batterer, for example, after being informed of the fee structure for the program, may decide that he would rather go to jail and complete his sentence than participate in treatment. His logic for this decision may be that he will likely fall behind in his payments, be terminated from a program half-way through, and then be sent to jail anyway.

This type of decision-making leads us to a discussion of the other elements of informed consent: the concepts of voluntariness and competency. Simply because a client is informed of the risks and benefits of a form of treatment does not guarantee that they actually understand or fully appreciate the information presented to them to the extent that they can make an informed decision. As with other types of competency evaluations (e.g., competency to stand trial), assessment of the second element, an individual's competency to consent to treatment, is a functional assessment. That is, does the individual have enough intellectual or cognitive capacity to understand the type of treatment he or she is about to receive and the consequences, positive and negative, of participating in a particular type of treatment? Although it is true that in most court-ordered situations assessment of whether a defendant is competent to make informed decisions about participation in a treatment or intervention program is not often an issue, there are times when a more formal assessment of this issue should be pursued. For example, it is conceivable that a cognitively limited individual could be ordered into treatment. If a cognitively limited batterer does not fully understand what is required of him to complete the program, he may become treatment non-compliant because he did not comprehend the "risks" of missing sessions or not talking in group (both behaviors that could result in termination from a certified program in Massachusetts).

The last important element to informed consent is that the client makes his decision to participate in treatment voluntarily, based on his understanding of the type of treatment he or she is about to receive, and that this decision is not coerced. The issue of what constitutes unacceptable levels of coercion is an interesting one. When a batterer enters treatment because his wife threatens to divorce him or have him arrested the next time he is abusive, is the batterer being coerced into treatment? When the court orders a batterer into treatment or intervention program as a term of his probation and informs him that if he fails to attend the program he will go to jail, does this level of coercion invalidate a batterer's consent to treatment?

In response to the first question, Grisso and Appelbaum (1998) suggest that these types of threats would not invalidate the batterer's consent because "family members and others in patient's lives are entitled to make demands on them as conditions for continuing their relationships . . . clinicians need not refrain from initiating treatment because a patient has consented out of concern for the reaction for the loved one" (p. 6). As regards to the second question, when a defendant is found guilty or accepts a plea bargain to a domestic assault, he will likely be asked if he is willing to attend a treatment program as an alternative to going to jail. More often than not, the batterer under these circumstances will agree, often upon the advice of his attorney, to attend court-mandated treatment as an alternative disposition to incarceration. In doing so, he is making an informed choice to participate in the program and has thus "voluntarily" agreed to enter treatment.

Although courts have the power to mandate treatment as a condition of a plea bargain or probation either by state or federal regulations (see Title 18 U.S.C., s. 3563, [2002]), this does not imply that the court can automatically have access to his or her treatment records without the probationer's permission. Even when therapy is court ordered, the patient retains the right to refuse to participate (see *Washington v. Harper*, 1990, where the United States Supreme Court found that even convicted prisoners retained a substantive due process right to refuse treatment, absent a compelling state interest). Communications therefore remain as privileged as the statutes permit, and consent must be obtained in most cases. The qualifying phrase "in most cases" was used because it is always possible for a court to subpoena a record without the patient's consent, and while the therapist can ask that the confidence be protected, it is ultimately up to the courts to decide whether the privilege will be respected. If the court orders the release of information, the therapist is obligated to comply with the court's request or risk the possibility of legal sanctions being imposed upon him or her.

This point is usually moot, however, since most courts/probation departments will compel a probationer to sign a release under threat of imprisonment and, therefore, a signed release will almost always be in place prior to the start of treatment. If not, it will be soon after the therapist informs the court/probation officer that such a release is required before information can be divulged. What, then, should be a therapist's policy regarding a coerced release? Providing that the therapist is not the one doing the coercing, the circumstances under which the release was signed does not, apparently, concern us. Individuals are always making decisions based on their appraisal of consequences and contingencies. The probationer has the choice of not signing the release, even if that might mean going to jail, just as he has the choice of going to jail in preference to participating in a diversionary program.

Many programs require the batterer to sign a release for probation or victim contacts as a pre-condition of treatment. Referring to the Duluth Model, Pence and Paymar (1993) state that "participants refusing to sign the release are not allowed to participate [in the program] and are referred back to the courts" (p. 24). It is also possible, depending on the circumstances, for a batterer to give consent for release of certain information (e.g., his attendance at the program) while protecting other information (e.g., his progress or lack thereof). Again, there are both legal and therapeutic considerations. Batterers may be compelled to sign releases either by the courts or in order to be admitted into a program that the courts have required. Therapists may be able to accept such releases as valid; however, these limits around confidentiality may affect the batterer's willingness to disclose information that might be important to therapeutic progress.

OTHER ETHICAL AND LEGAL DILEMMAS

Mandated reporting of child abuse. The interface between spousal abuse and child abuse poses additional ethical dilemmas. In many states, it is considered abuse/neglect if the child is allowed to witness interparental aggression; it is not necessary for the child to be otherwise abused. Thus, the treater has an obligation to make a report to the child protective services agency if he/she is aware of interspousal aggression. Several questions arise regarding the reporting obligations. First, if the batterer is no longer living in the house and/or is under a restraining order, would the obligation to file still be in force? Massachusetts, for example, requires that the child be at risk from a caregiver; however, a person barred from the home is no longer considered a caregiver (see Massachusetts General Law c. 119, sec. 51A). Certainly, these measures might reduce the likelihood of further instances of this form of abuse/neglect. It might not, however, diminish any negative consequences for the child of having witnessed the abuse. Whether or not this should be a consideration would depend on whether the objective of child protective services is to prevent future exposure or to remedy the consequences of past events. In many cases, the involvement of child protective services is the impetus for the restraining order. Without such agency influence, the probability of re-establishing a family unit might be increased (assuming sufficient resolution of the battering issues).

Police and/or court involvement raises a second issue. Since the police and the courts are mandated reporters of child abuse/neglect, it is reasonable for the treater to assume that if a report to child protective services was indicated, then the police and/or the courts would have made the report. Further, if this is a reasonable assumption, does it eliminate the obligation of the treater to make the report? Does the fact that the police and courts have not made a report to child protective services indicate that such a report is not warranted? In our opinion, neither of these assumptions is acceptable. Whether or not another treater (or mandated reporter) has complied with their legal and ethical obligation does not necessarily alter the obligation of other mandated reporters. The failure of the court or the police to make a report does not excuse other mandated reporters from making a report. Similarly, the assumption that someone else has already filed a report does not necessarily relieve a mandated reporter of responsibility to report. If the therapist has a reasonable basis for believing that a report has been made (e.g., the information comes from a reliable reporter, such as another therapist, school official, or the court), it may not be necessary to file a report. On the other hand, if a parent reports abuse to a therapist but states that a report has already been filed (by a teacher or physician, for example), the therapist might want to confirm this with child protective services. Unfortunately, the statutes are ambiguous regarding the obligations of multiple reporters. Some agencies designate a reporter who files on behalf of the agency, thus avoiding duplication by different treaters within the same organization. When dealing with courts and multiple agencies, this strategy may not be appropriate.

It is important for therapists/treaters to remember that court-mandated batterers are almost always on probation and face the possibility of incarceration for any violation of the terms of probation. Programs that routinely violate confidentiality for even the suspicion that the batterer might become aggressive should be aware that they are taking actions that could substantially impact the life of the batterer and his family. Reports to child protective services fall into this category. While physical abuse or neglect of the child must be reported under state law, exposure to aggression between parents that has occurred in the past is less definite and may allow for greater discretion by the therapist. Therapists should be aware of the consequences of reporting not only for the batterer but also for the female partner. The report could be viewed by the courts and probation as a subsequent offense and compromise the batterer's probationary status. Even if it does not, it could be taken as additional evidence of his aggressiveness and influence future court involvements (e.g., custody or visitation decisions). Child protective agencies often require the mother to obtain a vacate or restraining order against the batterer as a condition for receiving services, thus forcing the batterer out of the house (when it may not be otherwise warranted), an action that could have negative consequences for her (both physically and financially) and further disrupt family functioning (Emerge, 1998).

A related problem concerns how to handle reports by the batterer that the mother is abusing the children. As a mandated reporter, the therapist would ordinarily be obligated to file a report with child protective services. However, batterers in treatment would be aware of this, having been warned of the exceptions to confidentiality at the initiation of treatment, and could intentionally try to cause trouble for their partners by fabricating stories of abuse by the mother. The therapist would thus be colluding with the batterer to harass his victim. Even more concerning would be the fact that a report by a mental health professional might add weight to the report, increasing the possibility of some action by child protective services. On the other hand, victims of abuse may be more likely to abuse or neglect their children, and the possibility that the batterer's report is accurate cannot be discounted. Straus (1990) reported that "the more violent husbands are toward their wife, the more violent the wife is to her children" and that even battered women who had been subjected to minor violence (i.e., pushes and slaps) "had more than double the rate of frequent severe assaults on their children than did wives whose husbands did not hit them" (p. 421). Protection of the children would dictate that a report to child protective services would have to be made.

Standards of care. To the lay person, any outcome that results in continued abuse or in new injury may be viewed as evidence of malpractice on the part of the treater/therapist. If a patient hurts someone else or themselves, the therapist should have predicted and prevented it. Legally, the term "standard of care" is used to ascertain liability. Standard of care refers to the accepted practice with respect to a specific problem. Thus, the judgment is not based on outcome but rather on whether the therapist provided standard, or sub-standard, treatment. This acknowledges that a therapist could do all the right things but the patient could still harm someone, and that under such circumstances, the therapist would not be held liable. Written standards may be developed by professional organizations, or within agencies (e.g., by a hospital, practice, or clinic); however, they are rarely considered definitive. In the area of batterer treatment, the question arises as to whether state standards (if they exist) define the standard of care and whether failure to comply with those standards creates liability for the therapist. Batterer treatment standards typically have been developed by committees that include battered women, representatives of law enforcement and/or the judicial system, victim advocates, representatives from batterer intervention programs, and in some cases, researchers or other experts. Representatives from specific mental health disciplines are not necessarily excluded and may be included because they satisfy one of the other criteria (e.g., a psychologist who operates a batterer treatment program). In any case, the ethical requirements of any particular mental health discipline should guide the development of the standards. State professional associations should lobby long and hard with legislatures regarding the development of such standards. State standards should not be allowed to define the standard of care for the provision of batterer intervention without the input of the various mental health professions. In general, standard of care is discipline specific; thus, psychologists may be held to a different standard of care than social workers or psychiatrists. In our opinion, then, a psychologist who does not comply with certification standards because they are inconsistent with the ethical practice of psychologists should be held to the standard of care practiced by other psychologists and not those defined by state standards for a field that only considers a portion of the discipline's concerns. An exception might be in states (e.g., Utah) where all providers of batterer treatment are required to comply with the certifications standards.

CONCLUSIONS

Regardless of the nature of the intervention, the batterer is often a reluctant participant and may not view the treatment as being in his best interests. Accordingly, he may view the treater not as an advocate, but as an arm of the legal or judicial system, and therefore be reluctant to disclose personal information that might be relevant to his treatment for fear that such information might be used against him. This concern may or may not be well founded. The batterer's liability stems from several sources. First, many programs regularly exchange information with the courts/probation departments. Adams (1994) noted that "generally, state standards of batterer treatment require that programs . . . inform courts about repeat acts of violence, alcohol or drug abuse, attendance, and overall progress" (p. 9). Such programs share the batterer's view that the program is indeed an arm of the law and, as Adams points out, "batterer treatment programs are able to more closely monitor the perpetrator's abusive behavior than the probation officer alone" (p. 5). The batterer may rightfully believe that disclosing angry feelings, alcohol use, or aggressive behavior might cause his probation to be revoked and lead to imprisonment. It should also be noted that state standards that require that programs inform the courts about repeat acts of violence, alcohol or drug abuse, attendance, and overall progress may be asking mental health professionals to violate confidentiality for reasons other than those specified in either their Tarasoff duties or their ethical code.

A second reason for the batterer's suspicions derives from uncertainty regarding the requirements for treatment completion. He may fear that his probation will be extended and his termination from the program delayed if he discloses any negative feelings or behaviors. Such concerns may prevent the batterer from engaging in the therapeutic process and may diminish any potential gains from program participation.

In summary, batterers' treatment subsumes a diverse set of interventions, administered by practitioners representing a variety of disciplines and philosophical orientations. Programs vary with respect to whether they view their roles as management and control of batterers or psychotherapeutic treatment of batterers; whether they view the batterer, the courts, or the victim, as their client; and whether they view themselves as an agent of the legal system or as a supportive change agent for the batterer. Where a treater stands on these various issues will influence important therapeutic constructs such as the confidentiality of information provided by the batterer, which may in turn influence the nature of the information provided by the batterer and the degree to which he is able to engage in, and benefit from, the intervention. Although there is a dearth of case law specific to batterer treatment, relevant case law bearing on psychotherapy in general suggests some guidelines:

1. Batterer treatment programs should be clear about their views regarding agency and communicate this to the batterer at the start of treatment.
2. Full disclosure of the nature and limits of confidentiality should be explained at the initiation of the contact between the batterer and the program. The types of information that will be disclosed and the parties to whom it will be disclosed should be specified.
3. Treaters opting to disclose information for reasons other than those delineated in the ethical guidelines of their professions should obtain a signed release from the batterer.
4. It is reasonable for programs to refuse to treat batterers who refuse to sign releases allowing exchange of information with the courts, victims, or probation officers. A release obtained, even under the circumstance where treatment is contingent upon signing the release, is valid and is not considered to be coerced.
5. Participation is considered to be voluntary, even if the batterer agrees to attend in order to avoid incarceration.
6. Standard of care is defined within each of the disciplines and is not determined by batterer treatment standards, which may be influenced more by political objectives than by therapeutic concerns.

7. Programmatic decisions regarding agency and limiting confidentiality may impact on the willingness of batterers to engage in (as opposed to attend) treatment as well as impact on the effectiveness of the intervention.
8. Victim contacts, however well intentioned, may place the victim in jeopardy and must be carefully reasoned and implemented. Victims should be informed regarding the intended use of the information they provide.
9. Therapists engaging in the treatment of batterers are advised to familiarize themselves with the laws, legal issues, and regulations of their particular state and jurisdiction as these will take precedence over the guidelines of their discipline. It should be apparent from the foregoing discourse that differences from one jurisdiction to another may be substantial.

A number of other important considerations were discussed, especially those regarding mandated reporting of child maltreatment. Although providers are bound by these regulations, concerns were raised regarding reporting the witnessing of aggression by children and the possibility that the batterer could use the treater to harass his partner by falsely representing her behavior and precipitating a report to the authorities.

We are unaware of any research comparing treatment outcomes between programs that protect confidentiality to the extent dictated by the professional ethics of the various mental health disciplines and those that more readily make reports to victims, probation, and the courts. Without empirical tests, we can only speculate that protection of confidentiality would facilitate participation in treatment and improve outcomes. The answers to many of the questions raised in this article await both future research and future lawsuits.

REFERENCES

Adams, D. (1994). Treatment standards for abuser programs. *Violence Update, 5*(1), 5-9.

American Psychological Association. (1992). *Ethical principles of psychologists and code of conduct.* Washington, D.C.: Author.

Anfang, S. A., & Appelbaum, P. S. (1996). Twenty years after Tarasoff: Reviewing the duty to protect. *Harvard Law Review, 4,* 67-76.

Appelbaum, P. S. (1985). Confidentiality in the forensic evaluation. *International Journal of Law and Psychiatry, 7,* 285-300.

Appelbaum, P. S., & Gutheil, T. (1991). *Clinical handbook of psychiatry and the law* (2nd Ed.). Baltimore: Williams and Wilkins.

Austin, J., & Dankwort, J. (1998). *A review of standards for batterer intervention programs*, VAWnet (Violence Against Women Online Resources).

Beck, J. C. (1990). *Confidentiality versus the duty to protect: Foreseeable harm in the practice of psychiatry*. Washington, D.C.: American Psychiatric Press.

Behnke, S. H., & Hillard, J. T. (1998). *The essentials of Massachusetts mental health law: A straightforward guide for clinicians of all disciplines*. New York: W.W. Norton and Company.

Black, H. C., Nolan, J. R., & Nolan-Haley, J. M. (1990). *Black's law dictionary* (6th Ed.). St. Paul, MN: West Publishing Company.

Boynton v. Burglass, 590 So.2d 446 (Fla. App. 1991).

Canterbury v. Spence, 464 F.2d. 772 (D.C., 1972).

Committee on Ethical Guidelines for Forensic Psychologists. (1991). Specialty guidelines for forensic psychologists. *Law & Human Behavior, 15*(6), 655-666.

Commonwealth of Massachusetts Executive Office of Health and Human Services, Department of Public Health. (1995). *Massachusetts guidelines and standards for the certification of batterer intervention programs*. Boston, MA.

Douglas, K. S., & Webster, C. D. (1999). Predicting violence in mentally and personality disordered individuals. In R. Roesch, S. Hart, & J. R. P. Ogloff (Eds.), *Psychology and law: The state of the discipline* (pp. 175-239). New York: Kluwer Academic/Plenum Publishers.

Dubey, J. (1974). Confidentiality as a requirement of the therapist: Technical necessities for absolute privilege in psychotherapy. *American Journal of Psychiatry, 131*(10), 1093-1096.

Emerge. (1998). *Emerge program manual: First stage groups for men who batter*. Cambridge, MA: Author.

Geffner, R. A., & Rosenbaum, A. (2001). Domestic violence offenders: Current interventions, research, and implications for policies and standards [Special Issue]. *Journal of Aggression, Maltreatment, & Trauma, 5*(2).

Grisso, T., & Appelbaum, P. S. (1998). *Assessing competency to consent to treatment: A guide for physicians and other health professionals*. New York: Oxford University Press.

Gutheil, T. G., & Appelbaum, P. S. (2000). *Clinical handbook of psychiatry and the law* (3rd Ed.). Philadelphia: Lippincott Williams & Wilkins.

Jablonski v. United States, 712 F.2d 391 (9th Cir. [Cal.] 1983).

Jaffee v. Redmond, 518 U.S. 1, 116 S.Ct. 1923 (Ill., 1996).

Lipari v. Sears, Roebuck & Company, 497 F.Supp. 185 (Neb., 1980).

Massachusetts General Law, c. 117, s. 129A.

Massachusetts General Law, c. 119, s. 51A.

Massachusetts General Law, c. 123, s. 36B.

Massachusetts General Law, c. 233, s. 20K.

Melton, G., Petrila, J., Poythress, N. G., & Slobogin, C. (1997). *Psychological evaluations for the courts: A handbook for mental health professionals and lawyers* (2nd Ed.). New York: The Guilford Press.

Natanson v. Kline, 350 P.2d 1093 (Kan., 1960).

Ogloff, J. R. P. (1999). Ethical and legal contours of forensic psychology. In R. Roesch, S. Hart, & J. R. P. Ogloff (Eds.), *Psychology and law: The state of the discipline* (pp. 403-422). New York: Kluwer Academic/Plenum Publishers.

Peck v. Counseling Service of Addison County, 499 A.2d 422 (Vt., 1985).

Pence, P., & Paymar, M. (1993). *Education groups for men who batter: The Duluth model*. New York: Springer Publishing Company, Inc.

Straus, M. A. (1990). Ordinary violence, child abuse, and wife beating: What do they have in common? In M. A. Straus & R. J. Gelles (Eds.), *Physical violence in American families* (pp. 403-424). New Brunswick, NJ: Transaction Publishers.

Tarasoff v. Regents of the University of California, 529 P.2d 553 (Cal., 1974).

Tarasoff v. Regents of the University of California, 551 P.2d 334 (Cal., 1976).

Title 18 United States Code, Crimes and Criminal Procedure Part II Criminal Procedure Chapter 227. Sentences Subchapter B. Probation, sec. 3563 Conditions of Probation (2002).

Washington v. Harper, 494 U.S. 210, 110 S. Ct. 1028 (Wash., 1990).

Voices from the Group: Domestic Violence Offenders' Experience of Intervention

Mindy S. Rosenberg

SUMMARY. This article presents experiential reactions of male and female domestic violence perpetrators one year after completing a 52-week court-mandated intervention program. Data were derived from in-depth interviews as part of a larger research study looking at recidivism and other outcomes in a probation department with a domestic violence court and a coordinated legal, programmatic and community response. Overall, elements that were most helpful in domestic violence intervention were primarily relational ones, such as group support and therapist/facilitator alliances, and secondarily, specific strategies of handling anger and other emotions, and interpersonal communication. The discussion focuses on the implications of these findings for therapists and facilitators involved in providing services for this population. *[Article copies available for a fee from The Haworth Document Delivery Service: 1-800-HAWORTH. E-mail address: <docdelivery@haworthpress.com> Website: <http://www.HaworthPress.com> © 2003 by The Haworth Press, Inc. All rights reserved.]*

Address correspondence to: Mindy S. Rosenberg, 1505 Bridgeway, Suite 105, Sausalito, CA 94903 (E-mail: mindyrosenberg@yahoo.com).

[Haworth co-indexing entry note]: "Voices from the Group: Domestic Violence Offenders' Experience of Intervention." Rosenberg, Mindy S. Co-published simultaneously in *Journal of Aggression, Maltreatment & Trauma* (The Haworth Maltreatment & Trauma Press, an imprint of The Haworth Press, Inc.) Vol. 7, No. 1/2 (#13/14), 2003, pp. 305-317; and: *Intimate Violence: Contemporary Treatment Innovations* (ed: Donald Dutton, and Daniel J. Sonkin) The Haworth Maltreatment & Trauma Press, an imprint of The Haworth Press, Inc., 2003, pp. 305-317. Single or multiple copies of this article are available for a fee from The Haworth Document Delivery Service [1-800-HAWORTH, 9:00 a.m. - 5:00 p.m. (EST). E-mail address: docdelivery@haworthpress.com].

http://www.haworthpress.com/store/product.asp?sku=J146
© 2003 by The Haworth Press, Inc. All rights reserved.

10.1300J146v07n01_13

KEYWORDS. Domestic violence, batterer intervention, evaluation

Partly as a result of a terrible domestic violence tragedy, and partly in reaction to a growing concern over the way domestic violence cases had been handled, a Northern California county created a coordinated criminal justice and community response in the mid-1990s to the problem of domestic violence. This coordinated approach includes a specifically designated court (judge, defense, and prosecution team) to oversee misdemeanor cases, a domestic violence unit within the probation department, and community programs that provide mandated group intervention for men and women convicted of domestic violence. Conviction of domestic violence results, at a minimum, in a three-year probation term, a $200 fine, community service, and one year of weekly two-hour group intervention sessions. In January 1999, the county probation department hired the author to conduct a general outcome study on probationers who had attended its domestic violence intervention programs (Rosenberg, 2001). While most outcome studies on domestic violence treatment focus on re-offenses (Dutton, Bodnarchuk, Kropp, Hart, & Ogloff, 1997; Gondolf, 2000; Hanson & Wallace-Capretta, 2000), there is no qualitative information in the literature on the experiences of offenders who are required to attend treatment. To address this gap in knowledge, the author conducted in-depth interviews with a group of probationers and their victims. This article discusses the findings from those interviews, focusing on the probationers' perceptions of their intervention programs and their victims' perceptions of safety. For a full discussion of the methodology and results of the outcome study, the interested reader is referred to Rosenberg (2001).

METHODOLOGY

The interview data from domestically violent men, women, and their victims were collected as part of a larger study of the recidivism outcomes of court mandated domestic violence offenders (Rosenberg, 2001). A brief overview of the larger research study will first be presented, followed by a more detailed review of the interview data gathered from a subset of the larger sample.

Between 1999 and 2000, the author and another researcher reviewed the probation files of men and women who were convicted of domestic

violence in 1997. We chose 1997 as the starting date for probation because it enabled us to document probationers' experiences over time
and to include data on both program completion and recidivism one-
year post-program completion. Since some probationers took longer
than 52 weeks to complete their intervention program due to a variety of
problems along the way (e.g., probation violations, being terminated
from one program and ordered to restart the same or a new program,
etc.), the 1997 probation start date provided a long enough follow-up
period to describe the different experiences of domestic violence offenders during their three-year probation period.

The first consecutive 224 probationer files that could be located were
included in the total sample. Variables relevant to the hypotheses under
consideration for the larger study were extracted from the files (e.g.,
prior criminal history, alcohol and substance use history, etc.). The total
sample of probationers and their victims was then contacted by telephone and asked to participate in a confidential interview, either in person or over the telephone. While the probationer interview covered a
range of topics, including trauma history, quality of life since arrest, and
physical and psychological violence since program completion, this
chapter will focus on probationers' perceptions of their treatment programs. Victims were also interviewed about variety of topics related to
domestic violence; we will report here on their perceived level of safety
following their partners' completion of treatment.

Each probationer and victim was contacted by one of two researchers, who explained the purpose of the interview, assured confidentiality
of any information provided, and gained informed consent from the participant. In all, 70 probationer interviews were completed (31% of the
sample), given the time constraints of the project. Eighty-one percent of
the perpetrator sample was male ($n = 57$) and 19% ($n = 13$) was female.
Each probationer had been assigned to one of six certified domestic
violence intervention programs operating in the county. The intervention programs included process-oriented clinical approaches, cognitive-behavioral approaches (see Dutton, 2002), and educational
approaches. Although programs differ in theoretical approaches, much
of the content is dictated by state law, resulting in reasonable consistency in the most common interventions used to bring about the cessation of violent behavior (e.g., time outs, recognizing triggers to anger
and patterns of escalation, emotion regulation, communication skills,
etc.).

A total of 180 victims were identified by name, although not all
victims had additional contact information such as addresses and

telephone numbers. In all, 62 victim interviews were completed (approximately 28% of the sample). Statistical analyses to determine whether the interviewed group of probationers differed significantly from the non-interviewed probationer group on specific variables of interest revealed essentially no differences. The groups did not differ on general level of functioning or on historical variables such as prior domestic violence, prior violent crimes, or prior alcohol and drug abuse. The only variable that differentiated the groups was their number of prior non-violent crimes, in that those interviewed tended to have committed fewer non-violent crimes than those not interviewed.

When reoffense rates were examined, however, an interesting finding emerged. Those in the interviewed group were significantly more likely to have committed some form of domestic violence *post-arrest* than those who were not interviewed. The time period examined began at arrest and continued through program completion. Forty-seven (65%) of those interviewed had perpetrated domestic violence post-arrest, compared to 25 (35%) of those not interviewed. When *post-program completion* reoffense rates were analyzed, however, no significant differences emerged. In summary, the group of probationers interviewed had committed slightly fewer non-violent crimes but more domestic violence reoffenses post-arrest than the non-interviewed group. Other critical variables did not differentiate the two groups. The concern of whether the interviewed group was a more compliant, "goody-goody" group than those not interviewed was not supported by the data.

RESULTS

Reactions to the Domestic Violence Intervention Program

Qualitative data were collected from probationers' responses to several questions: what were the most helpful parts of the program they attended; whether they had learned anything from the program that they still used today; how they felt about the length of the program; and whether there were any drawbacks to the program. After asking these open-ended questions, the interviewer probed for feedback on various program elements that might have been significant to the probationer's experience, such as gaining group members' support, talking about one's personal situation, learning new coping tools, and gaining information about the legal system and other resources.

Most helpful parts of the program. Table 1 lists the program elements that probationers felt had been most helpful in addressing their violence. Respondents frequently listed more than one aspect. The most frequently mentioned helpful aspects appear to fall into two categories. The first is group support, which includes relationship development between group members and group leaders, personal expression of concerns in the group, participants' support, feedback from others, listening to others' stories, making a connection with the group leader, viewing the group leader as a role model, and sharing feelings and expressing oneself to others.

The development of group cohesion, or a strong sense of rapport between group members, and the ability of the group leader to facilitate individual and group expression each played a significant role in change for many men and women (see Dutton, 2002). Some group leaders encouraged a "buddy" system and passed around members' telephone numbers in case people needed help (e.g., rides, employment information, or extra support). Many probationers commented that the weekly contact and personal sharing with other people decreased their isolation and made them feel the group was "like a family." Several respondents said that they stayed in touch with other group members after the program ended and now considered them close friends. There were three people (two men and one woman) who felt that the groups were "too mixed in terms of level of violence" or participants had such "different experiences" that they felt out of place and had difficulty relating to the other members.

The second category of helpful treatment aspects included the specific skills and information learned in the group. Respondents described tools they learned to change their violent and other potentially dangerous behavior (e.g., coping tools to deal with anger, including time-outs, and information on different forms of violence and abuse, such as psychological abuse).

Skills still used today. Table 2 lists probationers' responses to the question of whether they continued to use any skills after their program had ended. The most consistent skill learned (and remembered) by participants was the "time-out" (Sonkin & Durphy, 1997), followed by a variety of other methods to manage anger and intense emotions. Many said they used time-outs in stressful work situations as well as in personal situations at home. Several probationers described how their group experience led them to change their behavior at work. For example, some respondents said they now handled angry customers or bosses differently, by not engaging with them or becoming defensive. Both

TABLE 1. Percentage of Respondents Reporting That Specific Program Elements Were Helpful ($N = 70$)

Probationer response	Percent reporting
Group support/feedback/others' stories	96%
Connection with the group leader/role model	86%
Learning new coping tools for anger, e.g., time-outs	81%
Learning about different forms of abuse, e.g., power & control	61%
Sharing feelings/expressing oneself	41%
Learning to recognize minimization and denial	33%
Taking responsibility for one's behavior	23%
Identifying triggers for anger/anger signals	20%
Attention to childhood trauma	19%
Increased awareness of self (needs, etc.) and others	19%
Remaining clean and sober/learning about effects of alcohol	14%
Learning different perspectives on relationships/women	13%
Thinking about consequences of actions/keeping safe	13%
Communication skills	10%
Videos, handouts	6%
Stopping before escalating arguments	6%
Using adjunct resources (therapy, medication)	6%
Recognizing one can control one's own reactions but not others'	4%
Relaxation exercise at beginning of group	1%
Homework assignments	1%
Slowing down to evaluate one's life	1%
Redefining what is means to be a man	1%
Connecting relapse prevention and domestic violence	1%
Discipline of needing to be on time for group	1%
Pledge said at the end of group	1%

men and women reported that they could now remove themselves from an argument before it escalated. They took time-outs to gain perspective and calm down before returning to a discussion. Before attending the group, they had been unable to do this.

Group participants also mentioned that they continued to use communication skills to express thoughts and feelings before their anger es-

TABLE 2. Percentage of Respondents Reporting That They Utilized Skills Learned in Program (*N* = 70)

Probationer response	Percent reporting
Coping skills to manage anger (e.g., time-outs)	84%
Communication skills	30%
Calm down, stop, think/consider consequences	14%
Recognize triggers to anger/anger signals	14%
Set boundaries/separate from situation	14%
Take responsibility/recog. one's role in arguments	13%
Don't escalate/diffuse arguments	9%
Think of class/review program material	9%
Make sure to be in safe situations	9%
Stay clean and sober	9%
Recognize power and control issues	9%
Find time for oneself/self discovery	9%
Control one's reactions/behavior	6%
Increase flexibility/patience	6%
Recognize other viewpoints	6%
Remain in touch with/acknowledge feelings	4%
Develop new ideas (re: women and relationships)	1%
Remember jail as a consequence	1%
Using adjunct services (couples therapy)	1%
Practice relaxation	1%

calated. Both men and women commented on their improved ability to talk with their partners and other people in their lives (e.g., employer, employees, etc.), rather than storing up or "stuffing" (Sonkin & Durphy, 1997) their thoughts and feelings.

Program length. The appropriate length of domestic violence intervention has been a hotly debated issue across the country. Program length has varied from 12 to 52 weeks, with an average of approximately 32 weeks. Currently, state mandates dictate program length, but the rationale directing one state to choose 16 weeks and another to choose 36 weeks is often arbitrary. The research on program effectiveness and treatment length suggests there are diminishing returns after 30-36 weeks of intervention (e.g., Dutton et al., 1997). However, most of these outcome studies focus on rates of physical violence and neglect other important outcomes, such as victims' perceptions of safety.

In California, the mandated program length is a minimum of 52 weeks. Among our sample of men and women, most (60%) strongly supported having 52-week programs. Several people said that they wished their program had been even longer. Only four people (6%) felt the program was too long. When those who endorsed having 52 weeks of treatment were asked to explain their support, they most often described a gradual process in which they loosened their defenses, developed trust, accepted responsibility, and eventually were able to take advantage of what the program had to offer (see Wallace & Nosko, 2002). Generally, the men mentioned that it took them between three and six months for this process to unfold. Probationers described an initial stage of treatment in which they felt angry at probation, their victim, or some other person whom they held responsible for their arrest. Some initially felt that their situation was different from that of other group members (e.g., they were not as violent as others, they did not have a problem with alcohol or drugs like others, etc.), which they interpreted as meaning that they did not need the group. Some men reported that, during this initial phase, the group "felt like a burden," they "were scared to speak in front of other men," or the group felt "forced on them by the system because [the violent incident] wasn't [their] fault." After approximately 6 months (or less for some participants), the majority of participants reported that the "time flew by," they "looked forward to going," they were able to "find personal meaning in attending the group," and "it was hard to leave." Some participants voiced the idea that fewer than 52 weeks would have left them still feeling defensive and unable to absorb the material in a deep and meaningful way.

Unlike men, women did not mention time as a factor in their capacity to "connect" with the group. Although the women also described a process of developing trust in others and gradually loosening their protective defenses, they appeared to have an easier time initially with sharing personal information and their emotions than did the men. In fact, several men stated articulately that men, in general, need more time than women to become comfortable sharing personal information with one another. For the majority of men, the group was the first time they had ever shared their private feelings and thoughts with others.

Program drawbacks. Table 3 represents probationers' views on the negative aspects of their mandated programs. About one-third of respondents said there were no specific drawbacks to the program they attended. Several mentioned the cost of the group as a drawback (all

TABLE 3. Percentage of Respondents Reporting on the Negative Aspects of Program (*N* = 70)

Probationer response	Percent reporting
No drawbacks to program	49%
Money related (too expensive)	27%
Wanted partner involvement	16%
Wanted more content (e.g., solutions, applications to life)	13%
Time related (sessions too long, 52 weeks too long)	10%
Job related	9%
Needed more time (for check-in, to work on problems)	6%
Program structure (more structure, check-in too long)	6%
Wanted more feedback (re: homework, life issues)	4%
Not enough confrontation by group leader	4%
Group room not comfortable enough (furniture, etc.)	4%
Mix of group inappropriate/men too violent	1%
Boring listening to other people's stories	1%
Re-enacted incident too frequently	1%
Worried about group information getting back to probation	1%
Too strict (no breaks, punctuality, payment)	1%
Needed individual therapy/felt out of place	1%
Too much time bringing new people up to date	1%
Repetitive	1%
Facilitators inconsistent/didn't like rotation of leaders	1%

groups used a sliding scale to set weekly fees), but most probationers seemed to think that the program cost was fair and manageable. One of our hypotheses for the larger outcome study was that probationers would be more likely to increase their income between arrest and follow-up than to lose or not change in income. This hypothesis was confirmed (Rosenberg, 2001).

A small number of participants mentioned that they wanted their partners involved in the treatment at some point, particularly if the couple was planning to stay together. These participants explained that while they had learned new ways of handling their anger, their partners had not, and this limited the progress they could make as a couple in improving their communication and problem-solving skills.

Victims' Perception of Safety

We interviewed 62 victims of probationers' violence, approximately two years after probationers had completed treatment. When victims were asked about their current perceptions of safety regarding the probationer, approximately three-quarters of the victims felt either "extremely" or "very safe" with the probationer ($n = 48$). A small percentage, 8% ($n = 5$), felt "not at all safe" or "marginally" safe with the probationer, while 5% ($n = 3$) felt "somewhat safe." Six (9%) victims felt the question was not relevant because they no longer had contact with the probationer.

DISCUSSION: BEYOND SKILLS AND INFORMATION

One important finding from this study is that most perpetrators reported that relationships–both with fellow participants and with group leaders–played a critical role in addressing the violence in their lives. Although teaching new techniques, such as anger management, may help to reduce domestic violence, this study suggests that there is more to changing violent behavior than imparting information. Therapy and intervention occur within the context of a relationship. As years of outcome research have already suggested, the therapeutic relationship is critical to positive therapy outcome (Horvath & Luborsky, 1993). Likewise, the cohesiveness of a group (built on relationships between group members) is associated with the success of group psychotherapy (Yalom, 1994).

Research suggests that witnessing and being a victim of trauma in childhood may contribute to the development of an abusive personality (Dutton, 1998, 2000). The wounds, disappointments, and emotional pain that give rise to violence are those that develop within the context of close relationships. Therefore, it makes sense that if healing is to occur, it will occur within the context of a relationship (e.g., between group members and between group members and group leaders). Unfortunately, the role of the therapeutic relationship in treatment outcome has been missing from the domestic violence literature to date. This study suggests that, according to participants themselves, the creation of supportive relationships is critical to effective domestic violence treatment. Focusing more on the development of such relationships may help improve the outcomes of batterer intervention programs.

However, many probationers felt that it took time to build these new relationships in which they felt comfortable discussing their problems and feelings. Providers of batterer treatment around the country whose programs are shorter than California's may wonder why 52 weeks of treatment are deemed necessary. Indeed, if a program is only teaching anger management skills or power and control issues, less time might be adequate. However, one unintended outcome of California's longer treatment programs may be that probationers have the opportunity to experience ongoing and relatively long-term relationships with fellow group participants and their group leader. This experience may ultimately contribute most to changes in behavior, perhaps beyond even the skills or knowledge that probationers gain.

To give anger management skills their due, we must highlight one finding that we anticipated but think merits reiteration. The vast majority of the probationers interviewed reported that anger management skills such as time-outs were the most helpful techniques they had learned in their group. They mentioned these tools far more frequently than they mentioned acquiring knowledge about patriarchal beliefs or new gender attitudes. Researchers and advocates have long debated the roles that patriarchal attitudes and emotion dysregulation play in domestic violence (Dutton, 1994; Schore, 1994). This study suggests that, in the eyes of program participants themselves, improving emotion regulation is critical to effective domestic violence treatment.

STUDY LIMITATIONS AND CONCLUSION

There are limitations to the current study. First, and most notably, only a sub-sample of perpetrators and victims were interviewed in-depth, given the time limitations of the grant that funded the research and the difficulty tracking down transient participants. The data that is missing are from probationers who were terminated from programs at various points along intervention process and eventually sent to jail to complete their sentence. Probationers who were terminated and then re-started a program or were transferred to another program were included in the interview sub-sample. However, those who were sent straight to jail without program intervention or those who began a program, violated probation multiple times or committed a severe enough offense to have their probation terminated were difficult to find and therefore, were not interviewed. Certainly, we could learn a great deal from these "hard to treat" probationers. For example, being able to identify program ele-

ments that maximize the chances of a good "match" between probationer and intervention mode, or similarly, that exacerbate negative
outcomes would have been important to understand from this under-
studied group of probationers.

Similarly, the victims were even more difficult to track down. On the
one hand, they may have had more incentive to "hide" due to ongoing
danger from their partners, as well as a desire to start a new life away
from their past partners. Second, although probation attempts to keep in
regular contact with victims to gather ongoing information about victim
safety, there is no legal reason why victims need to keep in touch with
probation. Again, information from the victims who choose to stay with
their partners who did not complete a program or who were sent straight
to jail would have been crucial to explore further.

Personal feedback about program intervention, although somewhat
biased in terms of sample selection, can still offer the program providers
useful information regarding the expected and unexpected elements
that contribute to positive treatment outcomes. We know that the time
honored anger management strategies are very effective in giving probationers specific tools in stopping interpersonal violence. However,
what is frequently overlooked and appears to be very significant from
the clients' point of view is the interpersonal aspects of the treatment
experience–relationship with fellow group members and with the treatment provider.

REFERENCES

Dutton, D. G. (1994). Patriarchy and wife assault: The ecological fallacy. *Violence &
Victims, 9*(2), 125-140.

Dutton, D. G. (1998). *The abusive personality: Violence and control in intimate relationships*. Guilford Press: New York.

Dutton, D. G. (2000). Witnessing parental violence as a traumatic experience shaping
the abusive personality. *Journal of Aggression, Maltreatment & Trauma, 3*(1),
59-67.

Dutton, D. G. (2002). Treatment of assaultiveness. *Journal of Aggression, Maltreatment, & Trauma, 7*(1/2), 7-28.

Dutton, D. G., Bodnarchuk, M., Kropp, R., Hart, S., & Ogloff, J. (1997). Wife assault
treatment and criminal recidivism: An eleven-year follow-up. *International Journal of Offender Therapy and Comparative Criminology, 41*(1), 9-23.

Gondolf, E. W. (2000). A 30-month follow-up of court-referred batterers in four cities.
International Journal of Offender Therapy and Comparative Criminology, 44(1),
111-128.

Hanson, R. K., & Wallace-Capretta, S. (2000). *A multi-site study of treatment for abusive men. User Report 2000-05.* Ottawa: Department of the Solicitor General of Canada.

Horvath, A. O., & Luborsky, L. (1993). The role of the therapeutic alliance in psychotherapy. *Journal of Consulting and Clinical Psychology, 61,* 561-573.

Rosenberg, M. S. (2001). *Domestic violence in Sonoma County.* Report prepared for Sonoma County Adult Probation, Santa Rosa, CA.

Schore, A. N. (1994). *Affect regulation and the origin of the self: The neurobiology of emotional development.* Mahwah, NJ: Erlbaum.

Sonkin, D. J., & Durphy, M. (1997). *Learning to live without violence: A handbook for men.* San Francisco: Volcano Press.

Wallace, R., & Nosko, A. (2002). Shame in male spouse abusers and its treatment in group therapy. *Journal of Aggression, Maltreatment, and Trauma, 7*(1/2), 47-74.

Yalom, I. (1994). *The theory and practice of group psychotherapy.* Basic Books: New York.

Index

Abandonment, 109-110. *See also*
   Attachment theory
   threats of, 35-36,53
Aboriginal men, 237-256
   Change of Seasons model, 238,
      248-252
   community and program
      development, 252-254
   cultural awareness and therapy,
      240-241
   culturally appropriate initiatives,
      253
   group facilitator, 247-248
   history of oppression, 238-240
   models of treatment, 241-248
   ritual and ceremony in therapy,
      245-247
   systems thinking and Native
      American worldview,
      241-242
   Wilber's transpersonal psychology,
      243-245
Abuse
   child. *See* Abuse history; Child
      abuse; Child witnesses
   forms of, 11
Abuse cycles, 16. *See also* Borderline
      personality disorder
Abuse history, 5-6,15,93,177
   attachment and, 118-119,123
   in borderline personality disorder,
      83
   of female-to-male batterers, 262
   significance vs. shaming, 52-53
Abusers, research literature, 51-54
Abusiveness. *See also* Violence
   as addiction, 20,180
Abusive personality, 109

Adaptive behaviors, 87. *See also* Skills
      development
Addiction, abusiveness as, 20,180
Adult Attachment interview, 124-126
Adult attachment style, as resembling
      infant, 108
Affect
   after psychoanalytic psychotherapy,
      42
   contagiousness of, 49
Affect theory, attachment theory and,
      47-74. *See also* Social group
      work
Agency, split, 290
Agency issues, 289-292
Aggression
   definition of, 140-141
   vs. assertion, 150
American Psychological/Psychiatric
      Association. *See* APA *entries*
Anger
   cognitive-behavioral model of, 149
   as defensive script, 50-51
   levels of, 149
   shame and, 50-51
Anger control, 149
Anger diary, 12-14
Anger/emotion dysregulation, in
      borderline personality
      disorder, 78,81-84
Anger escalation/de-escalation, 267
Anger signs, 265
Anger suitcase, 266
Antisocial personality disorder, 21
   Linehan's biosocial theory and, 84
Anxiety, about psychotherapy, 113,
      121-122
Anxious attachment style, 273

© 2003 by The Haworth Press, Inc. All rights reserved.

SPECIAL 25%-OFF DISCOUNT!

Order a copy of this book with this form or online at:
http://www.haworthpress.com/store/product.asp?sku=4954
Use Sale Code BOF25 in the online bookshop to receive 25% off!

Intimate Violence

Contemporary Treatment Innovations

____ in softbound at $26.21 (regularly $34.95) (ISBN: 0-7890-2019-X)
____ in hardbound at $44.96 (regularly $59.95) (ISBN: 0-7890-2018-1)

COST OF BOOKS _____

Outside USA/ Canada/
Mexico: Add 20% _____

POSTAGE & HANDLING _____

(US: $4.00 for first book & $1.50
for each additional book)
Outside US: $5.00 for first book
& $2.00 for each additional book)

SUBTOTAL _____

in Canada: add 7% GST _____

STATE TAX _____

(NY, OH, & MIN residents please
add appropriate local sales tax

FINAL TOTAL _____

(if paying in Canadian funds, convert
using the current exchange rate,
UNESCO coupons welcome)

❏ **BILL ME LATER:** ($5 service charge will be added)
(Bill-me option is good on US/Canada/
Mexico orders only; not good to jobbers,
wholesalers, or subscription agencies.)

❏ **Signature** _____

❏ **Payment Enclosed: $** _____

❏ **PLEASE CHARGE TO MY CREDIT CARD:**

❏ Visa ❏ MasterCard ❏ AmEx ❏ Discover
❏ Diner's Club ❏ Eurocard ❏ JCB

Account # _____

Exp Date _____

Signature _____

*(Prices in US dollars and subject to
change without notice.)*

PLEASE PRINT ALL INFORMATION OR ATTACH YOUR BUSINESS CARD
Name
Address
City   State/Province   Zip/Postal Code
Country
Tel   Fax
E-Mail

May we use your e-mail address for confirmations and other types of information? ❏Yes ❏No
We appreciate receiving your e-mail address and fax number. Haworth would like to e-mail or
fax special discount offers to you, as a preferred customer. **We will never share, rent, or
exhange your e-mail address or fax number.** We regard such actions as an invasion of
your privacy.

Order From Your Local Bookstore or Directly From
The Haworth Press, Inc.
10 Alice Street, Binghamton, New York 13904-1580 • USA
Call Our toll-free number (1-800-429-6784) / Outside US/Canada: (607) 722-5857
Fax: 1-800-895-0582 / Outside US/Canada: (607) 771-0012
E-Mail your order to us: Orders@haworthpress.com

Please Photocopy this form for your personal use.
www.HaworthPress.com

BOF03